HET's Manual of
Pelvic Floor Rehabilitation

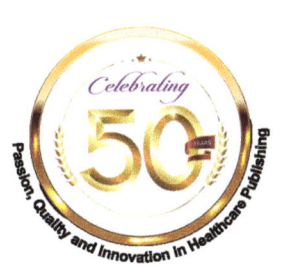

HET's Manual of
Pelvic Floor Rehabilitation

Het Desai MPT
Loma Linda University, California, USA
Chairman and Founder of
International Institute of Pelvic Floor Research
Rehab and Education (IIPRE), WOW Group of Businesses
WOW Experience Research and Development
World Pelvic-Floor Organisation (WPO)

Forewords
Dr Vineet Mishra
Dr Alpesh Gandhi
Dr Haresh U Doshi
Dr Mrugesh Vaishnav
Dr Mona P Desai
Dr Jagdish Gandhi
Dr Sunita Patel (PT PGDip HSC)
Dr Dhara Shah (MPT)
Dr Jigar Shah (MPT)
Dr Jayadeep Singh Rathod (MPT)

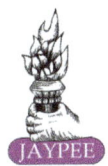

JAYPEE BROTHERS MEDICAL PUBLISHERS
The Health Sciences Publisher
New Delhi | London

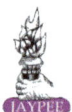 **Jaypee Brothers Medical Publishers (P) Ltd**

Headquarters

Jaypee Brothers Medical Publishers (P) Ltd
4838/24, Ansari Road, Daryaganj
New Delhi 110 002, india
Phone: +91-11-43574357
Fax: +91-11-43574314
Email: jaypee@jaypeebrothers.com

Overseas Office

J.P. Medical Ltd
83 Victoria Street, London
SW1H 0HW (UK)
Phone: +44 20 3170 8910
Fax: +44 (0)20 3008 6180
Email: info@jpmedpub.com

Website: www.jaypeebrothers.com
Website: www.jaypeedigital.com

© 2020, Jaypee Brothers Medical Publishers

The views and opinions expressed in this book are solely those of the original contributor(s)/author(s) and do not necessarily represent those of editor(s) of the book.

All rights reserved. No part of this publication may be reproduced, stored or transmitted in any form or by any means, electronic, mechanical, photocopying, recording or otherwise, without the prior permission in writing of the publishers.

All brand names and product names used in this book are trade names, service marks, trademarks or registered trademarks of their respective owners. the publisher is not associated with any product or vendor mentioned in this book.

Medical knowledge and practice change constantly. This book is designed to provide accurate, authoritative information about the subject matter in question. However, readers are advised to check the most current information available on procedures included and check information from the manufacturer of each product to be administered, to verify the recommended dose, formula, method and duration of administration, adverse effects and contraindications. It is the responsibility of the practitioner to take all appropriate safety precautions. Neither the publisher nor the author(s)/editor(s) assume any liability for any injury and/or damage to persons or property arising from or related to use of material in this book.

This book is sold on the understanding that the publisher is not engaged in providing professional medical services. If such advice or services are required, the services of a competent medical professional should be sought.

Every effort has been made where necessary to contact holders of copyright to obtain permission to reproduce copyright material. If any have been inadvertently overlooked, the publisher will be pleased to make the necessary arrangements at the first opportunity. The **CD/DVD-ROM** (if any) provided in the sealed envelope with this book is complimentary and free of cost. **Not meant for sale.**

Inquiries for bulk sales may be solicited at: jaypee@jaypeebrothers.com

HET's Manual of Pelvic Floor Rehabilitation

First Edition: **2020**
ISBN: 978-93-88958-62-2

Dedicated to

Millions of Silent Sufferers

Author's Profile

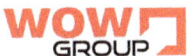

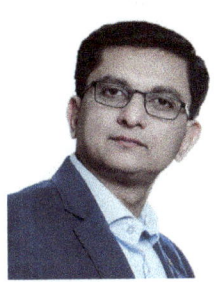

Dr Het Desai MPT-USA
Entrepreneur, Innovator, Author
Life Mission: Step outside the box to improve lives.
Special Interest: Fitness-Boxing, Reading, Listening, Innovation and Entrepreneurship—To make a Visionary Impact."

Chairman and Founder:

- WOW IIPRE (International Institute of Pelvic Floor Research, Rehab and Education)—Recognized by Central Government of India which provides exclusive training to medical and paramedical professionals for pelvic floor rehabilitation. (With pot. of 100 crore Indian Rupees/year).
- WOW Experience Research and Development—Received the Certificate of Recognition by Central Government of India for developing (under patent)—innovative technologies.
- WOW Group of Businesses.
- WPO—World Pelvic-Floor Organisation

Work Experience:

More than 12 years of experience as an entrepreneur and devoted professional for Pelvic Floor Rehab. Worked in different private settings in America.

Innovations-Intellectual Property (IP):

- "WOW PF 360" pelvic floor muscles exerciser/rehab technologies for doctors, urogynec surgeons, other medical practitioners, therapists and pelvic rehab specialists.
- "WOW Woman" 3 minutes pelvic floor muscles exerciser for toning and tightening of pelvic floor (-vaginal) muscles in women.
- "WOW Man" pelvic floor muscles exerciser for men to help with ED, PME, urinary incontinence, etc.
- Above mentioned are the revolutionary, noninvasive and under patent pelvic floor rehab technologies which are recognized by "Department of promotion of industry and internal trade, Ministry of Commerce & Industry Government of India".
- WOW Vagina-Fit (PFME)—a unique transvaginal objective testing and training (proprioceptive and resistive) gadget for female patients (for Vaginal laxity).
- WOW Vagina-Dilate (PFMRE)—all in one dilator which can be used for objective testing and training in beginner, intermediate and advanced cases of hypertonus pelvic floor muscles in conditions like endometriosis, interstitial cystitis, vaginismus, dyspareunia, chronic pelvic pain, etc.
- WOW Group App—a mobile application for pelvic floor muscle exercises with visual & auditory cues which can also provide progress report to customise efficient home exercise program for patients.

Academic Contribution-Intellectual Property (IP):

- Het's MMT (Manual Muscle Testing Scale): Het's MMT is a unique transvaginal/transrectal manual muscle testing scale which can help doctors to evaluate strength and relaxation component of pelvic floor muscles, it can be used for hypotonus or hypertonus pelvic floor dysfunctions.
- Het's FMT (Functional Muscle Testing and Training): An innovative and objective way to measure the functionality of pelvic floor muscles by using WOW Vagina-Fit for hypotonus conditions and WOW Vagina-Dilate for hypertonus conditions.
- Het's SERF assessment scale: Scale to evaluate strength, endurance, repetitions and fast twitch muscle fiber activity of pelvic floor muscles.
- HPPG: Het's Providers Protection Guidelines.
- Het's Ring clock assessment: Pelvic floor assessment technique for urogenital and anorectal triangle in male and female patients and non- invasive ring clock assessment for pediatric patients.
- Het's RR (Reflexive Results) scale: The scale to set up ultimate goal for progression in the treatment of pelvic floor muscle dysfunctions.
- Het's FSF (Female Sexual Function) scale: The scale is designed to score (rate) the female sexual health, it covers the questions directly or indirectly related to hypertonus and hypotonus pelvic floor muscle dysfunctions.
- Het's MSF (Male Sexual Function) scale: The scale is designed to score (rate) the male sexual health.

Author:

- HET's Manual of Pelvic Floor Rehabilitation.

Please visit www.visionwowgroup.com

Author's Vision

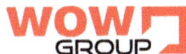

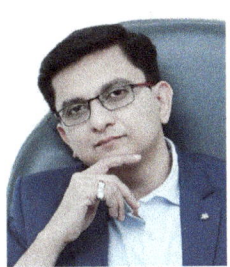

Dr Het Desai MPT-USA

Millions of people, all over the world silently suffer from pelvic floor dysfunctions. It is a cultural taboo even to talk about it.

"My vision is to courageously break the cultural taboo and make pelvic floor rehab accessible to every single woman and man on the globe through innovative technologies and services".

Its extremely fulfilling to devote myself to a vision which is much larger than just me, my life and my time on this earth. This book, innovations, services, technologies and initiation of movement will continue to serve humanity even after my life. This is a revolutionary war against "Silent Sufferings".

I want to invite all of you to join hands to take a solid stand against silent sufferings and help making a positive impact on millions of lives.

Foreword

The pelvic floor provides support for the organs in the pelvis, helps control the bowel and bladder, plays a role in sexual activities, provides stability by its attachment to various ligaments in pelvis and provide postural support to the trunk. Pelvic floor physical therapists have focused on rehabilitation of the weak or tight pelvic floor muscles. With recognition that many urogynecological symptoms arise from presence of short, painful pelvic floor, the role of the medical and surgical as well as physical therapy is expanding. 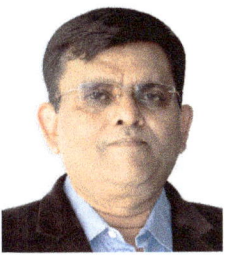 If you are reading this Foreword, then you are reading a book that contains every aspects related to pelvic floor in terms of its anatomy, physiology, functions, dysfunctions and how it can be corrected by rehabilitation or medical and surgical approach. **The author Het Desai is also an innovator of multiple noninvasive, under patent pelvic floor rehabilitation technologies, entrepreneur, and well recognized in the field of urogynecology, physical therapists and pelvic rehabilitation specialists.** He is also the chairman and founder of WOW group of businesses and IIPRE-International Institute of pelvic floor research, rehabilitation and education. Pelvic floor rehabilitation technologies and IIPRE invented by him, are recognized as a start up from Central Government of India. The contents of the book ranges from basic to futuristic vision in the field. In these 5 sections including all chapters, one will envision every minute concepts ranging from basic anatomy up to the most advanced approaches of rehabilitation, in a clear detailed and illustrative manner through the writing as well as photographs. We all have been using Oxford MMT scale for pelvic floor muscle evaluation. We understand the limitations of Oxford MMT scale which helps to assess only contractile portion of pelvic floor muscles. However, Het's MMT scale empowers the clinicians to assess contractile and relaxation part as well which could greatly benefit to treat patients with vaginismus, dyspareunia or any type of conditions which can lead to hypertonicity of pelvic floor muscles. **We are so much proud that Het has invented much more efficient Het's MMT SCALE, Het's SERF assessment technique, Het's ring clock assessment techniques, Het's RR-reflexive results levels and much more.** These academic contributions will help to empower pelvic floor rehabilitation specialists and serve humanity. **Apart from Het Desai, who else do you know in the whole world of pelvic floor rehabilitation experts who has made such valuable contributions!**

A wise mentor once said "You are only as good as tomorrow". That single sentence should inspire each of us as we arise every morning to provide relief to those who suffer. Till that, we must seek methods to relieve suffering, to heal without harming, to cure without substituting one malady for another. Urogynecology empowers each one of us to provide all individuals seeking our cares with a kinder, gentler solution regarding their problem. **I highly recommend medical and paramedical providers like gynecologists, urogynecologists, sexologists, physical therapists to provide complete care to your patients by adding pelvic floor rehabilitation to your practice. HET's manual of pelvic floor rehabilitation will be the ultimate guide you will need to empower your practice and benefit your patients with new level of care.**

My heart felt congratulations to Het Desai who has provided a comprehensive guide of immense value to me, to you and to all of our patients. Read "HET's Manual of Pelvic Floor' Rehabilitation" well, apply its principle earnestly and bless your patients with complete care, more than they expect.

Dr Vineet Mishra MD (Obstetrician and Gynaecology)
Founder President of SAFUG South Asian Federation of Urogyneacology
Founder member of Gynecological Endocrine Society of India
Director and Professor and HOD (Obstetrics and Gynecology) IKDRC-ITS
Ahmedabad, Gujarat, India

Foreword

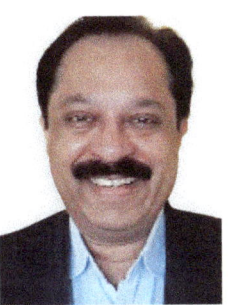

Approximately, 35 million women suffer from urinary incontinence, 54% from some type of female sexual dysfunctions and 9 out of 10 mothers from vaginal laxity. Almost every single woman is likely to suffer from some kind of pelvic floor dysfunction in her lifetime. Medical science has advanced in many areas in recent years including cosmetic gynecology. However, pelvic floor rehabilitation is clearly missing the link. Inner (perineal) health should be blessed by pelvic floor rehab. **"HET's manual of pelvic floor rehabilitation." is absolutely amazing book which offers detailed evaluation and efficient rehabilitation protocols in a most simplified fashion. Oxford scale for pelvic floor muscle testing has been used from ages without realizing a huge limitation. The gap is bridged by Het's MMT scale which also measures relaxation component along with the contractile component.** I also appreciate Het's visionary initiation of WOW IIPRE, International Institute of Pelvic Floor Research, Rehab and Education. If patients do not want to opt for surgery or if she wants to delay surgery or even for postsurgical conditions along with prenatal/postnatal conditions, pelvic floor rehab can help patients with complete care beyond their expectations. **Het Desai has also innovated multiple under patent, noninvasive and highly efficient technologies like PF 360 which also earned a certificate of recognition from Central Govt of India as a startup. I congratulate Het Desai on bringing awesome lights on the untouched and underserved area of pelvic floor rehabilitation through his book and visionary innovations.** I strongly recommend this book to every gynecologists, urogynecologists, sexologists, therapists, medical and para medical professionals to help silent suffering of millions of lives (from, hypertonus-hypotonus pelvic floor dysfunctions to sexual dysfunctions) by offering them pelvic floor rehabilitation care.

Dr Alpesh Gandhi MD (Obstetrician and Gynaecology)
President Elect, FOGSI-2020
Federation of Obstetric and Gynaecological Societies of India

Foreword

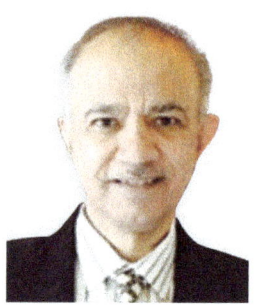

HET's Manual of Pelvic Floor Rehabilitation is a precious as well as enormous collection of scientific material on a subject not much discussed or described due to various reasons. Manual is divided into 5 broad sections and covers every details of pelvic floor dysfunction for male and female, pediatric to old age and from basics like anatomy and physiology to medical and surgical management. **I being a teacher and an author since 35 years realize that huge efforts and in depth knowledge are required for preparing such manual. Recognition of IIPRE by Government of India speaks for its worth.** I congratulate Het for this endeavor and wish him all the best.

Dr Haresh U Doshi MD (Obstetrician and Gynaecology)
Vice President
FOGSI (Federation of Obstetric and Gynaecological Societies of India)

FOREWORD

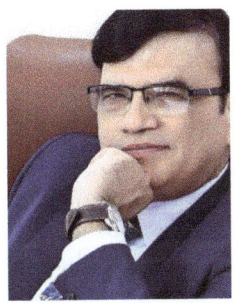

HET's Manual of Pelvic floor rehabilitation is first of its kind book for medical and paramedical professionals including psychiatrists and sexologists. Along with the psychiatric care, this book can greatly help to understand and treat unique dimensions of sexual dysfunctions in male and female patients. Patients with conditions like vaginismus, dyspareunia, hypoactive sexual desire disorders, erectile dysfunction and premature ejaculation can be blessed by the principles of this book. **I highly recommend this book to every single psychiatrist and sexologist and I** would also encourage them and other medical professionals to intensively start working with Certified Pelvic Rehab Practitioners in the best interest of patients with sexual dyfunctions.

Dr Mrugesh Vaishnav MD (Psychiatrist)
National President of Indian Psychiatry Society
Direct Council Member Council of Sex Education and Parenthood

Foreword

As a female doctor, I completely understand and empathise personal health issues that most women go through during some or other stages of their lives. We talk a lot about women empowerment but according to me a "Woman" is really empowered after she is physically and mentally healthy and that includes perineal health as well. There are so many health problems which a woman faces right from laxity of pelvic floor muscles after pregnancy and delivery of a child to spasm or tightness of pelvic floor muscles. Our society is still very orthodox and no one addresses such problems of women which would bring a drastic change if improved or corrected.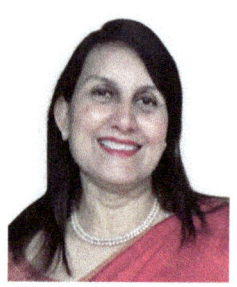

The technologies innovated by Het Desai will not only help perineal sufferings but they will also make a positive difference to overall quality of lives of millions of women.

Het Desai has done Masters from Loma Linda University, California USA. **After years of hard work and experience he has come up with complete revolutionary and unique technologies and visionary formation of WOW IIPRE.**

WOW IIPRE, i.e. International Institute of Pelvic Floor Research, Rehab and Education is an awesome step to empower pelvic floor education amongst medical professionals.

The book "HET's Manual of Pelvic Floor Rehabilitation" has beautifully simplified the subject which will open new doors to opportunities.

I sincerely request medical professionals to read this book which would definitely aid us to start new heights of care for the benefit of the patients in our practice.

Dr Mona P Desai
National President of Indian Medical Association
Woman Doctor's Wing
Indian Medical Association

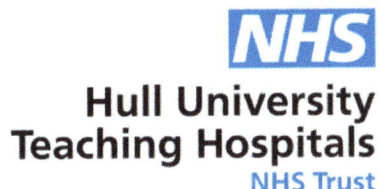

Foreword

The concept of pelvic floor rehabilitation in scientific form is somewhat of a new entity. However, the implication of such noninvasive therapy and excellent outcomes leads to more acceptance and practice of this therapy. After an excellent training and qualification of MPT from Loma Linda University, California, USA, Het has decided to share his experience and interest in innovation and research activities in the form of this manual which is aimed at a wide readership including professionals who work directly or indirectly with pelvic floor muscles like physiotherapists, urogynecologists, sexologists and colorectal surgeons. One striking feature of this book is transferring the concept of rehabilitation therapy in a most clear description. The concise, colorful drawings and pleasure as well as understanding to the principles of anatomical and physiological importance.

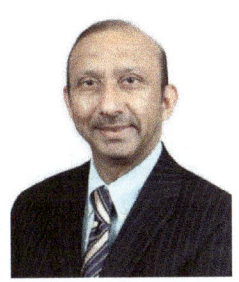

This book is well divided into a number of sections which includes female pelvic floor dysfunction, male pelvic floor dysfunction and pediatric pelvic floor that follows fitness rehabilitation and management strategies. Further layout of the sections in various chapters is done in a logical way of functional anatomy, assessment of pelvic floor and types of various pelvic floor dysfunctions that markes this book easy to read and refer back to. Each of the chapters follows multiple-choice questions to test knowledge acquired as well as a very useful aid for a quick revision.

I have no doubt that this piece of work will be well received by the intended readership. **I congratulate Het Desai for offering this manual to the therapists and clinicians who may be already familiar with the concept of rehabilitation and those who are still new to this mode of management and wish to learn more in a comprehensive manner. This manual will be a treasure for them.**

It is very pleasing to note that Het has been the Founder of IIPRE (International Institute of Pelvic Floor Research, Rehabilitation and Education) and that the IIPRE has received a certificate of recognition from the Central Government of India.

Dr Jagdish Gandhi MD, FRCOG
Lead Consultant Urogynecologist,
Hull University Teaching Hospitals NHS Trust
Anlaby Road, Hull
United Kingdom

Foreword

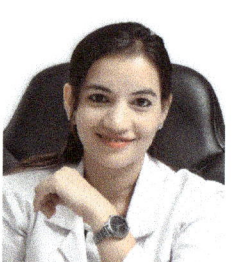

"HET's Manual of Pelvic Floor Rehabilitation" is an absolutely divine book for physical therapists, gynecologists, urologists, sexologists, colorectal surgeons or any other medical professional who is interested in pelvic floor rehabilitation. I do not have words in my vocabulary to praise it enough. There are many books all over the world for different expertise of medical science. However, when it comes to addressing silent sufferings due to pelvic floor dysfunctions, this book has a potential to uplift understanding of professionals, add quality to millions of lives and earn blessings as well. Het Sir has invested years of experience, wisdom and unshakable focus to simplify this book. **This book is not only contents, its years of experience.** There might be some scattered information about pelvic floor rehabilitation in few parts of the world, however, this is first of its kind which will empower readers from basic to advance information about pelvic floor rehabilitation in most simplified way. The book is not only based on theoretical part, it is a complete hands on training system. **This book literally focuses on missing link of special and complete care of urogynec, anorectal and genitourinary well-being.** I strongly believe that medical world has received a very good grading system in the form of Het's MMT, in which Sir has focused not only on the contractile property of the skeletal muscle but also on its relaxation. **I would love to request every medical and paramedical professional, especially pelvic floor rehabilitation professionals to specifically learn about "Het's MMT (transvaginal and transrectal manual muscle testing)" and implement it with every single patient of yours and they will be greatly benefited.** Also, I am privileged to be a beautiful part of the journey of this book.

I consider Het Sir as **"A FATHER OF PELVIC FLOOR REHABILITATION", my guru, my mentor and feel truly grateful for his visionary approach for everything he does. I have been blessed to be trained directly under him. I feel fortunate to be born in his Era and to be around his Aura.** To reach his goal is not an accomplishment for him but in fact, it is a beginning of a new journey that opens up a new world of possibilities and opportunities. **Het Sir has the courage and audacity to see, think, step and work outside the box which will greatly benefit humanity in a long run. His work is a complete blend of logic, intuition and experience. I feel that we are known by our profession but, in nearby time this profession of Physical Therapy will be known by the name of Het Sir.**

I want to personally thank Het Sir for his great contributions like this book under patent pelvic floor rehabilitation smart technologies and many innovations which will do well to millions of people. I strongly recommend this book to anyone and everyone who is passionate about women's health or genitourinary health. You simply cannot afford to miss "HET's Manual of Pelvic Floor Rehabilitation"

Dr Sunita Patel (PT PGDip HSC)
Pelvic Floor rehabilitation Specialist,
CEO, WOW IIPRE
International Institute of Pelvic Floor Research, rehabilitation and Education
Delhi, India

Foreword

Pelvic floor rehabilitation is a wonderful branch of science which has yet not been fully discovered. But the book, **HET's Manual of Pelvic Floor Rehabilitation has simplified the complexity of the pelvic floor rehabilitation. This book is written in such a way that it will be useful for all the faculties of Medical and Paramedical.**

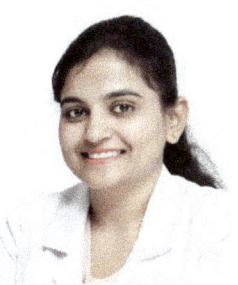

The Author of this book, Dr Het Desai Sir, has a varied experience of treating thousands of patients with pelvic floor dysfunction over the years, and this experience is reflected in book especially in the assessment and treatment chapters. There may be few books available for pelvic floor dysfunction, but this book is the best of all other books. **The assessment techniques like Het's MMT, Het's SERF assessment and ring clock assessment are one of the greatest gift to pelvic floor rehabilitation world from Dr Het Desai Sir. These assessment techniques are really very useful in assessing the complex pelvic floor.**

Moreover, the treatment which is explained in this book is very much up to the mark. **This book is written in very simple and easily understandable manner**. It will be highly useful for not only those who want to build a career in pelvic floor but also for those who just want to gain a decent understanding of pelvic floor rehabilitation. **This book is till now "The To Go Book" for the pelvic floor rehabilitation.** In my opinion, this book should be introduced as a textbook for Medical and Paramedical Courses.

I do not have enough words to write about Het Sir and his qualities but I must say that I am very lucky to be a part of his team. **A team whose Leader is a Visionary person – "Het Sir", is not just an ordinary human being, in fact he is a Leader, Entrepreneur, and an Innovator. He is a pure soul who always believes in spreading positivity. A person who has the strength to change the whole world. He always dreams of a better world and is constantly working to develop a WOW World for every being on this planet. He has the courage to step outside the box for the betterment of others.**

Dr Dhara Shah (MPT)
Pelvic Floor Rehabilitation Specialist
HOD WOW IIPRE
International Institute of Pelvic Floor Research, Rehab and Education
Mumbai, Maharashtra, India.

Foreword

Hello friends I am a proud friend of Het Desai who people know as an innovator, an entrepreneur, a philanthropist, a writer and an amazing orator but I would like to use this opportunity and introduce everyone to a different Het Desai. Let me tell you about Het or as I call him "happy" a friend and a person whom I have known for more than 20 years.

Let's talk about the person Het, I have not met a person in my life around me who has so much self-belief on his thoughts and ideas. Since the time when we were students, he was very determined and persistent towards whatever goals he would set for himself, and would not stop until he has achieved it.

Het the friend is always there, a friend who would not shy away from being completely blunt and direct in informing his closest friend about his mistake but he is also the person who will be standing right next to him in facing the result of the mistake. I have had many fights and arguments with Het as all friends do but he is also the first person I turn to when I am confused about anything because I know his advice might not be the nice thing to hear but it will be the correct one.

I remember the first time Het discussed the idea of pelvic floor rehabilitation with me, at that time I was skeptical but he had complete faith in his thoughts. Over the period of time because he was pursuing the subject, I started noticing things that he had noticed in society. I remember I had talked to him about the social taboos he might have to face when spreading awareness about the problems arising due to chronic weakness of pelvic floor muscles. Apparently, he stuck to his plans and processes and I am happy to see that he is finding success in his goals. I reside and practice in America; here it is a bit easier for women to express complaints like pelvic floor weakness as the social constraints are less in discussing feminine problems. I am privileged to be able to review this book and its content. **I can say that this book is very precise, simple to understand, full of knowledge and opens up new opportunities in the field of rehabilitation. Combination of this book and appropriate hands on training by certified clinicians and use of proper equipment will help any clinicians to step in to the world of pelvic floor rehabilitation. In my 19 years as a physical therapist I have not come across any planned process that treat this problem and I am proud that my friend has taken the initiative to tackle this problem. I wish him best for his book "HET's Manual of Pelvic Floor Rehabilitation" and hope it helps train professionals to help their patients.**

Dr Jigar Shah MPT
Michigan, USA

Foreword

HET's Manual of Pelvic Floor Rehabilitation is a very simplified, amazing book which describes various dysfunctions of pelvic floor in male, female and children. I have read many books, have taught my students from various materials and instruments we get with advantage of advance technology in this modern era but have not come across any simple but very specific book like HET's Manual of Pelvic Floor Rehabilitation.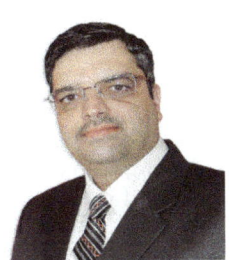

I have been in physical therapy field since last 18 years, have travelled Australia, England and many other countries for quest of my knowledge and passion for physical therapy. Currently I am practicing in USA and still working on the goal of making changes in the world for betterment. **Even after this many years of practicing as therapist and working with many entrepreneurs and senior clinicians I can proudly and confidently say that I have not met any person who is as passionate, focused and dedicated as Het Desai in field of physical therapy.** He has dedicated his better part of his life and professional career behind his goal of innovation, research and education to improve life of every human being around the world.

We have seen so many good educational institutes these days which uses all of the advance technology available in the world to empower their students, but it comes at very high cost, this is where the HET's "Manual of Pelvic Floor Rehabilitation" is different. It provides cutting-edge, very precise knowledge about pelvic floor muscles, various pelvic floor dysfunctions, detailed assessment techniques and very effective treatment techniques without extravagant expenses. Each chapter of the book has been influenced by Het's undaunted focus and vision for the education. I was impressed by the way book was structured like no other with small questionnaire at the end of chapter to not only highlight the important areas of the chapter but help in process of learning it. I cannot emphasize enough to read this book if you are related to any corner of healthcare field. I would recommend this book and to learn all techniques for all gynecologists, surgeons, rehabilitation practitioners and any one who wants to become a pelvic floor rehabilitation practitioner. As a human being age affects all of us and WE CAN definitely do better than what we are doing now in area of pelvic floor rehabilitation. **To improve in life everyone needs a GURU or Mentor who can guide us in right direction which we have now for pelvic floor, HET's *"Manual of Pelvic floor Rehabilitation"*.** As a clinical educator I must say that this book and all the clinical knowledge with appropriate courses can make you a leading clinician in pelvic floor rehabilitation in no time.

Dr Jayadeep Singh Rathod MPT, Clinical manager
Sure Cure LLC
Michigan, USA

Message

Many patients are suffering from upper urinary tract symptoms due to pelvic floor problems. Dr Het Desai is specialized in managing pelvic floor rehabilitation. I find this book very informative and useful.

I congratulate Dr Het Desai for specializing and following a very important aspect of pelvic floor problem. **This will go long way in helping doctors as well as patients.**

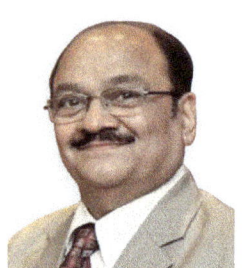

Dr Mahesh Desai
MS, FRCS, FACS Consultant Urologist
Gujarat, India

I want to congratulate my brother, Dr Het Desai for contributing one of the most revolutionary books "Het's Manual of Pelvic Floor Rehabilitation" on such an important and yet worldwide ignored, under served and highly needed subject of medical science. I found this book extremely informative and greatly beneficial. **Implementation of the principles and technologies of this book can add great value to the patients of pelvic floor rehab specialists, therapists, gynecologists, urogyncologists, psychiatrists, sexologists, urologists, oncologists, gastroenterologists and many more medical specialties.** I wish him best.

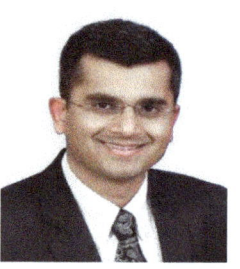

Dr Harit Desai
Temecula, California, USA

"I found this book to be engaging and show how to manage the pelvic floor so it brings out the best overall health for improved quality of life."

Dr Chad Glover MS RCEP-EIM3
American College of Sports Medicine
Registered Clinical Exercise Physiologist
California, USA

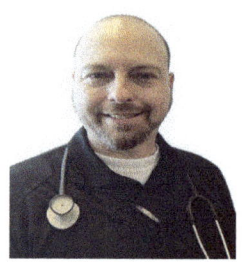

Preface

HET's Manual of Pelvic floor Rehabilitation provides a complete overview of the clinical assessment, diagnosis and rehabilitation of pelvic floor dysfunctions.

Millions of women, men and children all over the world silently suffer from different types of pelvic floor dysfunctions. There is huge demand for pelvic floor rehabilitation specialists all over the world. Pelvic floor rehabilitation is unfocused, unattended, unrecognized, unidentified area of medical practice which addresses global problems, it is a demand of the day and has huge potential. Majority of rehabilitation specialists are just busy practicing basic physical therapy like ortho, neuro, pediatric, cardiac and women's health rehabilitation. Unfortunately most of the practitioners who practice women's health are also limited to external exercises and rehabilitation techniques. Transvaginal and transrectal evaluation and rehabilitation are extremely result oriented. Most of the rehabilitation specialists are completely unaware of their own potential to get superspecialization in the world of rehabilitation. This book is just a small effort towards a higher purpose. It is a beginning to bridge the gap between tremendous demand and limited supply which will create win-win approach for patients, medical professionals and rehabilitation specialists. This book will empower the readers to be "Game Changers" in the world of rehabilitation by mastering perineal/pelvic floor rehabilitation beyond basics (urogential, urogyne and anorectal rehabilitation).

This book will help physical therapist students, practicing physical therapists or medical professionals to reinvent the world of pelvic floor rehabilitation with needful details about the anatomy, physiology, causes of pelvic floor dysfunctions, associated pathologies, types of pelvic floor muscle dysfunctions (hypertonus, hypotonus, incoordination types of pelvic floor dysfunctions) and sexual dysfunctions in female and male along with different pelvic floor dysfunctions in female, male and pediatric population.

This book also mentions different efficient techniques of pelvic floor evaluation, methodologies and treatment options for common pelvic floor muscles condition like stress urinary incontinence, urge urinary incontinence, vaginal laxity, pelvic organ prolapse, sexual dysfunctions, pelvic pain, muscles spasms in female; conditions like erectile dysfunction, premature ejaculations, postvoidal dribbling, prostatitis, postprostatectomy rehabilitation and pelvic pain in male, along with enuresis and encopresis like conditions in children. Also helps to get details about multiple types of biofeedback techniques and other treatment options along with different types of rehabilitation devices or pelvic floor muscle exercises. They could be used in clinical practice for pelvic floor rehabilitation. This book is designed to simplify the complexity of pelvic floor muscles which will provide interested readers with scientific and clinical fundamentals of pelvic floor rehabilitation and it will ultimately add quality of life, health and happiness to millions.

Het Desai

Acknowledgments

First and foremost, I would love to thank my daughter Aishi, who helped me realize that every woman is a darling of her daddy. Its a great satisfaction if I can use myself to contribute well-being towards silent sufferings of millions of lives.

I would love to thank my beloved parents, my father, my guru, Dr Vidyut Desai and my mother Dr Anupa Desai, my wife Jalpa Desai, my brother Dr Harit Desai, grandparents, whole family and friends.

I would also like to specially thank Dr Sunita, CEO of International Institute of Pelvic Floor Research, Rehabilitation and Education (IIPRE), who has stood by the whole journey of book and passionately contributed to simplify the complexity of pelvic floor muscles.

I would also like to thank all colleagues and the team of WOW group for supporting and inspiring me. I also want to thank Dr Akshay Shah for contributing chapter of medical management. I am also grateful to Dr Alpesh Gandhi, Dr Mona P Desai and Dr Mrugesh Vaishnav, Dr Dilip Gadhavi, Dr Haresh U Doshi, Dr Vineet Mishra, Director, Institute of Kidney Diseases and Research Centrer, Dr Jagdish Gandhi,Lead Consultant Urogynaecologist Hull University Teaching Hospital, NHS Trust, Hull, United Kingdom, Dr Jayadeep Singh Rathod, Dr Jigar Shah, Dr Dr Mahesh Desai and Dr Chad Glover, (MS) Dr Nita Agrawal, Dr Digant Patel, Dr Ankur Patel for their great support.

I would also like to thank Dr Hiralal Konar and Mrs Madhusari Konar for their valuable contribution in terms of figures from their book Dr DC Dutta's "Textbook of Gynecology" 7th Edition.

I would also like to thank Dr Dhara Shah for her devotional help in setting up the MCQ's and to edit this book.

I sincerely thank my team who helped me to design revolutionary pelvic floor exercise products like WOW PF 360 and many more. IT team Dharamdeep Singh and team, graphic designer team Mayur, product designer Harsh Mevada, team of die creators Ritesh and Ashok, team of motor generators Hemal, Dharmendra Singh, Mr Kanjia and team of engineers, team of patent attorneys Mr Brahmbhatt and Harpreet singh, team of criminal advocate of Gujarat High Court, Mr Rajesh Goswami, team of civil attorney Mehul and Hitesh, team of CA, PM Patel group Rahul and Premji Uncle, Hardik bhai for pictures and editing work. The work of book and products were designed simultaneously as both intellectually feeded each other. Also appreciate blessings and learnings from my family in USA Dr Ratilal Gajera, Kishore uncle, Dr Hemanginiben, Dr Kamlesh bhai and family.

My special thanks to Shri Jitendar P Vij (Group Chairman), Mr Ankit Vij (Managing Director), Mr MS Mani (Group President), Dr Madhu Choudhary (Publishing Head-Education), Ms Pooja Bhandari (Production Head), Ms Sunita Katla (Executive Assistant to Group Chairman and Publishing Manager), Dr Astha Sawhney (Development Editor), Ms Seema Dogra (Cover Visualizer), Mr Sharad Patel (Commissioning Editor), Mr Rajesh Sharma (Production Coordinator), Mr Kulwant Singh (Typesetter), Mrs Ritika Ahuja (Proofreader) and Mr Rajesh Ghurkundi (Graphic Designer) the whole team of M/s Jaypee Brothers Medical Publishers (P) Ltd, New Delhi, India.

At last but not least, I would like to thank everyone who has directly or indirectly helped me to complete this book.

Contents

Section 1: Female: Pelvic Floor Dysfunction

Chapter 1. Quick Reminder: Functional Anatomy — 3
- Urinary Tract 3
- Bladder 3
- Urethra 5
- Uterus 7
- Ovaries 8
- Fallopian Tubes 9
- Uterine Ligaments 9
- Rectum 10
- Anus 11
- Overview of Female Reproductive System 11
- Vulva 11

Chapter 2. Pelvic Floor Muscle and Functions — 14
- Pelvic Floor Muscle Layers 14
- Functions of Pelvic Floor Muscles 17

Chapter 3. Pelvic Floor Muscles Dysfunction and Types — 22
- Pelvic Floor Muscles Dysfunction 22

Chapter 4. Assessment of Pelvic Floor Muscles — 27
- Subjective History 27
- Other Keypoints in Pelvic Floor Evaluation 28
- Pelvic Rehab Clinic 31
- General Questions 32
- Bladder Health Sample Assessment 32
- Sample form for Vaginal Laxity and Pelvic organ Prolapse 34
- Het's FSF Scale (Pain-Hypertonus) (Female Sexual Function) 34
- Het's FSF Scale (Laxity-Hypotonus) (Female Sexual Function) 37
- Interpretation of Het's FSF Scale 40
- Objective History 42
- Het's MMT Grade for Pelvic Floor Muscles 43
- Het's—Manual Muscle Testing (MMT) Grading—Pelvic Floor Muscles 43
- Wow Vagina-Fit 45
- Wow Vagina-Dilate 48
- Procedure: During Transvaginal Examination 52
- Vaginal Pelvic Floor Muscle Examination—One or two Fingers? 53
- Het's Ring Clock Assessment 55
- Het's Ultimate Goal: Full Curve (From −3 to 3, from Complete Relaxation to Complete Contraction) 59

- Het's Assessment Level for Pelvic Floor Muscle   60
- Other School of Thoughts   61
- Laycock Quantitative Assessment Scale (Perfect)   61

Chapter 5. Hypertonus Pelvic Floor Dysfunction (Vaginal Spasm and Health Issues) — 64

- Pudendal Neuralgia   64
- Tension Myalgia   64
- Coccydynia   65
- Levator Ani Syndrome   65
- Proctalgia Fugax   65
- Hemorrhoids   65
- Anismus   65
- Pelvic Inflammatory Disease   65
- Endometriosis   66
- Coccygeus-levator Spasm Syndrome   67
- Vulvodynia   67
- Vulvar Vestibulitis   67
- Interstitial Cystitis   68
- Urethral Syndrome   68
- Urgency-frequency Syndrome   68
- Hypertonus Pelvic Floor Muscle   69
- Constipation   69
- Inflammatory Bowel Disease   69
- Irritable Bowel Syndrome   70
- Vicious Cycle: Pelvic Floor Muscle Painful Tightness and Anxiety   70

Chapter 6. Hypotonus Pelvic Floor Dysfunction (Vaginal Laxity and Health Issues) — 72

- Causes of Hypotonus Pelvic Floor Muscle   73
- Pregnancy, Labor, Childbirth, and Vaginal Laxity   74
- Vaginal Laxity   77
- Research and Statistics for Urinary Incontinence   84
- Pelvic Organ Prolapse   86
- Hemorrhoids and Pelvic Floor Muscles   94
- Medical Research: Vaginal Looseness and Bulging of Organs (Pelvic Organ Prolapse)   95

Chapter 7. Female Sexual Dysfunction (Pelvic Floor and Female Sexual Dysfunction) — 99

- Female Sexual Health Disorder   99
- Functional Anatomy   100
- Female Sexual Dysfunction   107
- Female Sexual Function Index   113
- Significance of Pelvic Floor Muscle in Female Sex Health   113
- Vaginal Spasms And Female Sex Health   115
- Oncology And Female Sexual Dysfunction   115

- Menopausal Changes   116
- Radiotherapy, Chemotherapy, and Female Sexual Dysfunction   116
- Vaginal Laxity and Female Sex Health   116
- Urinary Incontinence and Female Sex Health   117
- Postsurgical Sexual Problems   117
- Research Findings about Female Sex Health   118
- Orgasm and Pelvic Floor   121

Section 2: Male: Pelvic Floor Dysfunction

Chapter 8. Quick Reminder: Functional Anatomy — 125
- Bladder and Voiding   125
- Urethra   126
- Prostate   126
- Scrotum   127
- Testicles   128
- Epididymis   128
- Spermatic Cords and Ductus Deferens   128
- Seminal Vesicles   130
- Ejaculatory Duct   130
- Cowper's Glands   130
- Penis   130
- Semen   130
- Nerve Supply   131

Chapter 9. Pelvic Floor Muscles and Functions — 133
- Pelvic Floor Muscle Layers   133
- Functions of Pelvic Floor Muscles   136

Chapter 10. Pelvic Floor Muscles Dysfunction (Types of PFD) — 139
- Pelvic Floor Dysfunction   139
- Types of Pelvic Floor Dysfunction   140
- Other Classifications of Pelvic Floor Dysfunction   141

Chapter 11. Assessment of Pelvic Floor Muscle — 143
- Subjective   144
- Het's MSF Scale Male Sexual Function (MSF)   144
- Interpretation of Het's MSF Scale   148
- Objective   149
- Disclaimer   149
- Self Test   150
- Het's—Manual Muscle Testing (MMT) Grading—Pelvic Floor Muscle   151
- Male Pelvic Floor Hypertonus Dysfunction And Trigger Point Symptoms   153

Chapter 12. Hypertonus Pelvic Floor Dysfunction (Pelvic Pain and Health Issues) — 156
- Pelvic Pain   156

| Chapter 13. | Hypotonus Pelvic Floor Dysfunction (Erectile Dysfunction and Other Health Issues) | 162 |

- Causes   163
- Hypotonus Dysfunction   163

Section 3: Pediatric Pelvic Floor

| Chapter 14. | Normal Continence Development, Enuresis and Encopresis | 175 |

- Enuresis   176
- Het's Assessment Level for Pelvic Floor Muscle   176
- Encopresis   178

Section 4: Pelvic Floor Muscle: Rehabilitation

| Chapter 15. | Different School of Thoughts on Kegel and Pelvic Floor Rehabilitation | 185 |

- Pelvic Floor Muscle Training Protocols   185

| Chapter 16. | Foundation for Pelvic Floor Rehabilitation | 188 |

- Treatment   188
- Pelvic Floor Muscles Versus Accessory Muscles   194
- Modalities   196
- Mobilization or Manual Therapy   199
- Home Exercise Plan   199
- WOW Pelvic Floor 360   199
- Mode of Application of Pelvic Floor 360   202
- Progressive Resistance Training System   206
- What are Home-used Devices for Pelvic Floor Rehabilitation? WOW-Woman   214
- Wow Vagina-Fit for Treatment   218
- Frequently Asked Questions   221
- Wow Vagina-Dilate Treatment   222
- Application Developed for the Home use   223

| Chapter 17. | Rehabilitation for Hypertonus Pelvic Floor Dysfunction (How to Treat Tight Pelvic Floor Muscle?) | 228 |

- Symptoms Associated with Hypertonus Pelvic Floor Muscle   228
- Different Rehabilitation Techniques and Protocols   229
- Modalities   233
- Exercise Training   235
- Het's Relaxation Protocol   242
- Het's Pelvic Floor Muscle Goals Scale for Hypertonus   244
- Hands On Training: PF 360 and Hypertonus Conditions   245

Contents | xxxi

Chapter 18. **Rehabilitation for Hypotonus Pelvic Floor Dysfunction (How to Treat Weak Pelvic Floor Muscles?)** 250
- Het's Pelvic Floor Muscle Goals Scale 250
- Sample Protocol 251
- Het's—Manual Muscle Testing (MMT) Grading—Pelvic Floor Muscles 252
- Het's Exercise Protocol For Pelvic Floor Dysfunction 253
- Het's Protocols 253
- Rehabilitation for Male Hypotonus Pelvic Floor Dysfunction 258
- Prostate Health and Pelvic Floor Muscle Rehabilitation 259
- Postprostatectomy Rehabilitation 259
- Postprostatectomy Protocol 261
- Rehabilitation for Erectile Dysfunction and PME: PFM Training and Prevention of Erectile Dysfunction 261
- Patient Education About Self-training 262
- Indirect Neuromuscular Re-education 263
- Erectile Dysfunction Treatment Options 265
- Premature Ejaculations 266
- Rehabilitation Principles for Urinary Incontinence 267
- Knack Technique for Stress Urinary Incontinence 267
- Hands On: PF360 and Hypotonus Conditions 268
- Het's BC Protocol for Male 269
- How to Customize Pelvic Floor Muscle Rehabilitation 269

Chapter 19. **Rehabilitation for Female Sexual Dysfunction (Woman's Sex Health and Rehabilitation)** 273
- Lifestyle Modifications 274
- Rehabilitation for Hypertonus Sexual Dysfunction 276
- Glazer's Pelvic Floor Rehabilitation Protocol 278
- Infertility and Pelvic Floor Rehabilitation 279
- Rehabilitation Guidelines for Hypotonus Sexual Health 279
- Hands On PF360 Guidelines for Female Sexual Dysfunction 281

Section 5: Medical and Surgical Management

Chapter 20. **Introduction of Medical and Surgical Management of Pelvic Floor Muscle Dysfunction** 285
- Treatment of Hypertonus Pelvic Floor Dysfunction in Females 287
- Treatment of Hypotonus Pelvic Floor Dysfunction in Females 291
- Treatment of Pelvic Floor Dysfunction In Males 293

Appendix 295

Resources and References 305

Index *323*

Section 1

Female: Pelvic Floor Dysfunction

"Feminism is not about making women stronger. Women are already strong. It is about changing the way the world perceives that strength."

—**GD Anderson**

"Pelvic floor strength" will change the way she perceives her own strength.

Woman's Life cycle effects "Pelvic Floor"

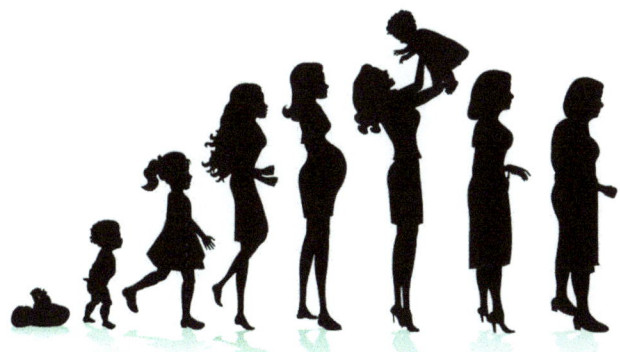

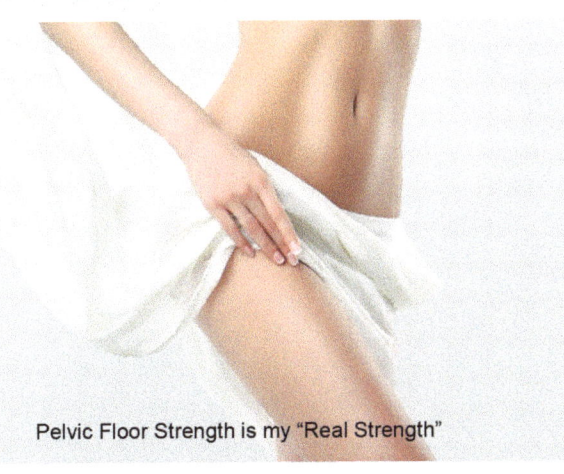

Pelvic Floor Strength is my "Real Strength"

Chapter 1

Quick Reminder: Functional Anatomy

INTRODUCTION

If pelvic floor is a huge ocean, surrounding organs are boats in the ocean. This chapter is a quick reminder of important points of functional anatomy. It will help you to recall—what you have already known. It covers some basic points about urinary tract, bladder, urethra, sphincter, and summary of process of the micturition along with basics of female reproductive system.

The female pelvis contains following pelvic organs:
- Bladder
- Urethra
- Uterus
- Vaginal canal
- Rectum
- Anal canal
- Pelvic floor muscles.

URINARY TRACT

Upper urinary tract contains pair of kidneys and ureters (Fig. 1).

BLADDER

It is a hollow muscular sac and the urinary bladder is located behind the pubic symphysis (Fig. 2). "Trigone" is the base of the bladder. It contains bladder sensory nerves and forms a funnel during voiding. The apex of the trigone is known as "bladder-neck", which is the junction where bladder and urethra meet. The base of the trigone receives the ureters from right and left kidneys. The bladder wall has three layers:
1. Outer fatty layer
2. Central muscular layer: It is made up of smooth muscles, known as detrusor muscles. These are involuntary muscles. During filling, bladder becomes distended as pressure inside increases. The smooth muscles lets the bladder stretch and expand as it fills with urine and then goes for reflexive contraction to expel urine.
3. Inner mucous layer.

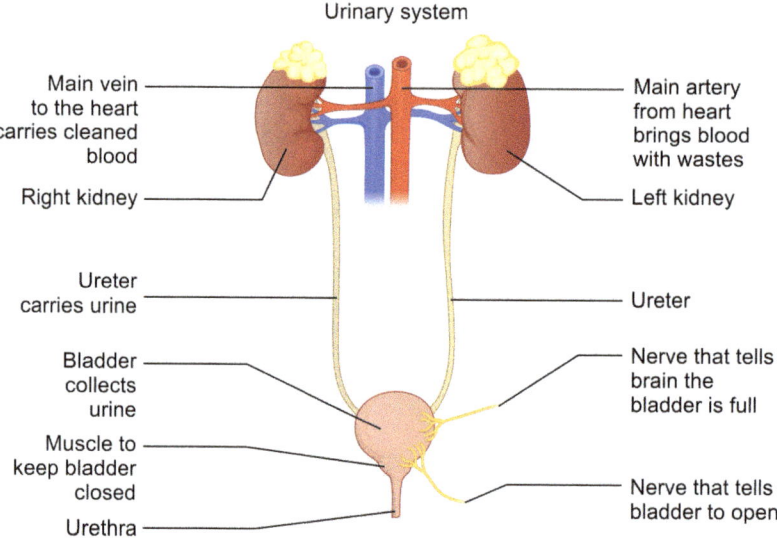

Fig. 1: Urinary system.

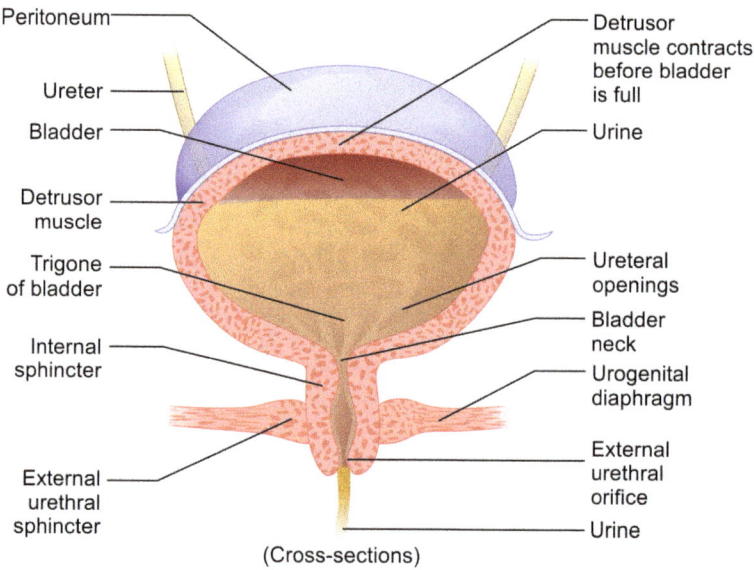

Fig. 2: The bladder (women).

Function of the Bladder

Bladder fills urine through ureter, stores urine and empties urine through the urethra.

Functional Capacity of Bladder

As compare to intestines, the capacity of the bladder is very small (360–480 mL). As a result it gives rise to frequent need of urination.

Elasticity

The bladder is not too elastic and as a result it stores urine at high pressure which ultimately contributes to urine leakage.

Key Bladder Reflexes

Muscle Guarding Reflexes

Muscle guarding of pelvic floor muscle (PFM) can happen during the filling stage of the bladder. The PFM guarding—contractions happen in progressively increasing magnitude. The increasing magnitude is directly proportional to the volume of the urine in the bladder, which helps to prevent leakage as the bladder becomes fuller.

Cough Reflex

Reflexive contraction of PFM happens with cough to prevent leakage with sudden raise in the intra-abdominal pressure.

Pelvic Floor Muscle—Bladder Reflex

The conscious contraction of PFM causes reflexive relaxation of the bladder. This reflex can be strengthened and used for patients with urgency incontinence.

■ URETHRA

Urethra is a tube that helps to empty urine from the bladder (Fig. 3). It starts from bladder and continues to outside the body with an opening known

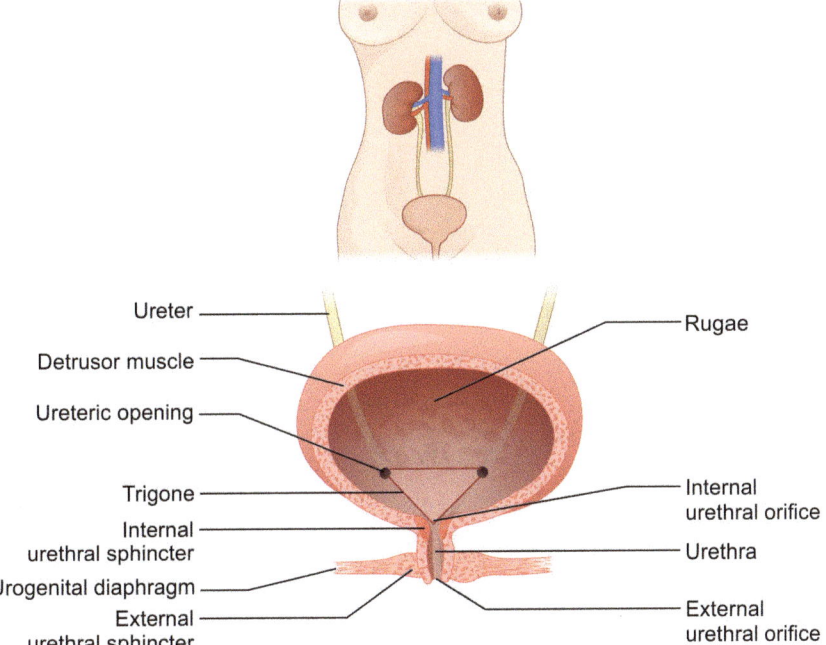

Fig. 3: Female urinary bladder and urethra.

as urinary meatus. It is made up of smooth muscles. In women, urethra is approximately 1.5 inches long which opens into vestibular area above vaginal orifice. It contains stratified squamous epithelium. During menopause, lack of estrogens leads to poor quality of collagen, skin tone, and muscles which can contribute to bladder disorders.

Sphincter

Urethral tube is collapsed and closed by internal and external sphincter muscles while not urinating.
- *Internal sphincter*: It is located at the bladder neck. It is made up of involuntary smooth muscles, innervated by autonomic fibers. It cannot be trained with active exercises as it is involuntary.
- *External sphincter*: It is made up of mainly slow-twitch muscle fibers and three small skeletal muscles. It maintains constant tone. It voluntarily contracts to prevent urine leakage during coughing, sneezing, and laughing-like activities where there is raised intra-abdominal pressure. It voluntarily relaxes to facilitate emptying of bladder.

Micturition (Fig. 4)

- *Filling phase*: The detrusor muscle will relax and the urethral sphincter and pelvic floor muscles will remain contracted.
- *First sensation*: Bladder is not completely full yet. First sensation to void is generated. However, urination is voluntarily inhibited until appropriate time.

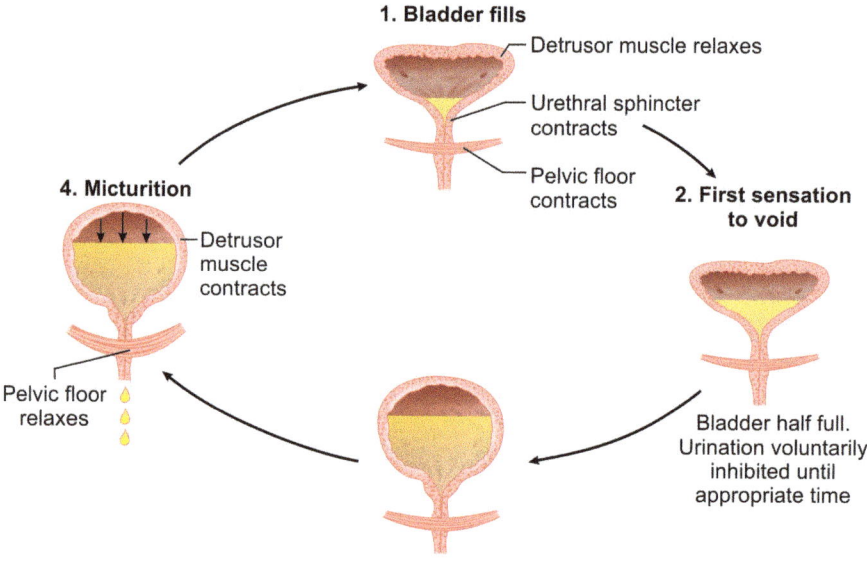

Fig. 4: Micturition.

- *Normal desire to void*: There is a normal desire to void urine which tells our brain to go to use the washroom.
- *Micturition*: The pelvic floor muscles and the sphincters were holding urine inside the bladder so far. The detrusor muscle contracts and pelvic floor muscles and sphincters relax at the time of micturition, which permits urine to expel from the body.

UTERUS

The uterus is the organ where fertilization occurs. It is an organ located between the bladder and the rectum. The lower part of the uterus is the cervix. A fertilized egg gets implanted on the uterine wall. The endometrium is lining of uterus, which nourishes the fertilized egg and helps with an environment for fetus development (Figs. 5A and B). There are three layers:
1. Endometrium
2. Myometrium
3. Perimetrium.

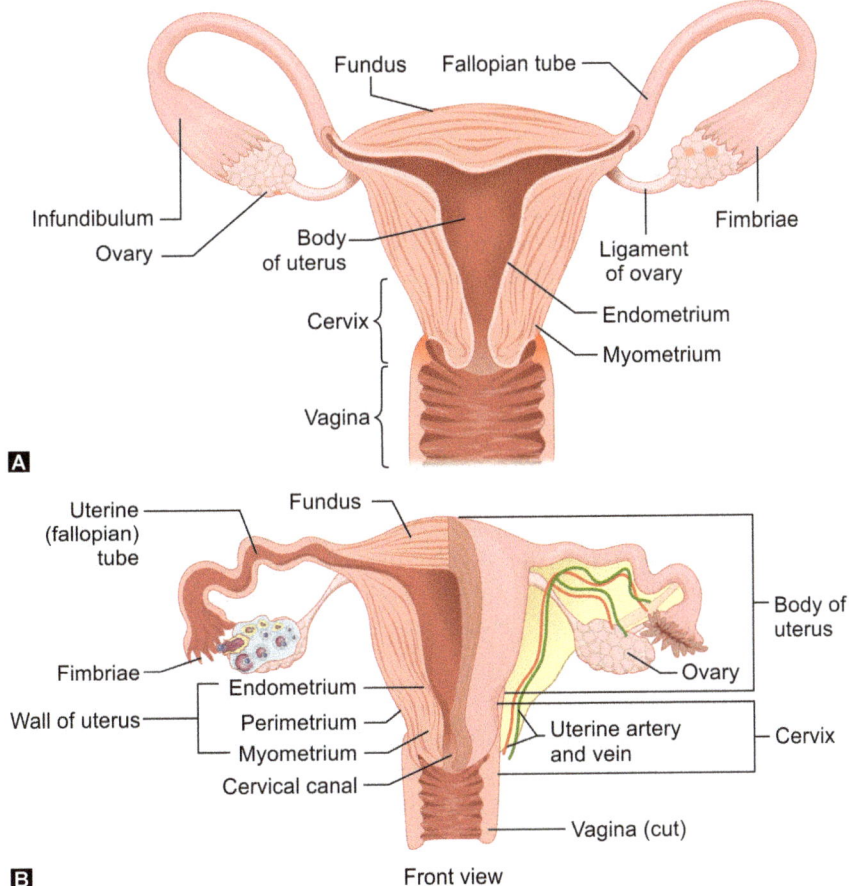

Figs. 5A and B: Female reproductive system.

Endometrium

The endometrium is a single-layered mucosa of the uterine body. This inner most layer of the uterus contains glycogen-secretory cells, with cilia and basal cells. The top layer of the endometrium has high amount of blood supply and it sheds off during each menstruation cycle. It also helps to alter the uterine glands by shedding its top layer for preparation of implantation. The blastocyst implants and placenta develops in the endometrium.

Myometrium

The myometrium is located between the endometrium and the perimetrium as a middle wall of the uterus. Its smooth muscle cells expand during pregnancy and make more room for support of the fetus. It helps to induce uterine contractions during labor. It also helps by contracting to push placenta out after birth. It also compresses blood vessels to reduce blood loss after labor.

Perimetrium

This outermost layer of the uterine wall helps to secrete fluid along the outside of the uterus. It helps to protect uterus from other organs that might rub against or bump into uterus.

Cervix

The little round structure at the end of the uterus is known as cervix. It is a boundary between the vagina and endometrium. The cervix dilates approximately 10 cm which helps baby to pass from the uterus into the vagina.

Orifices

The cervical orifice is a small hole at the top of the cervix that opens into the vagina.

OVARIES (FIG. 6)

The ovaries are small almond-sized organs located in the female pelvis. Their main function is to produce the ova. Ova are released from the ovaries during menstruation cycle. Ova travel through the fallopian tubes to the uterus. The ovaries are the main source of female hormones.

Ovum—Egg

The ovum is the female reproductive cell that develops into a fetus. The ovary releases an egg during the time of ovulation which travels into the fallopian tubes. The egg can be fertilized by a sperm cell. Fertilized egg moves down the

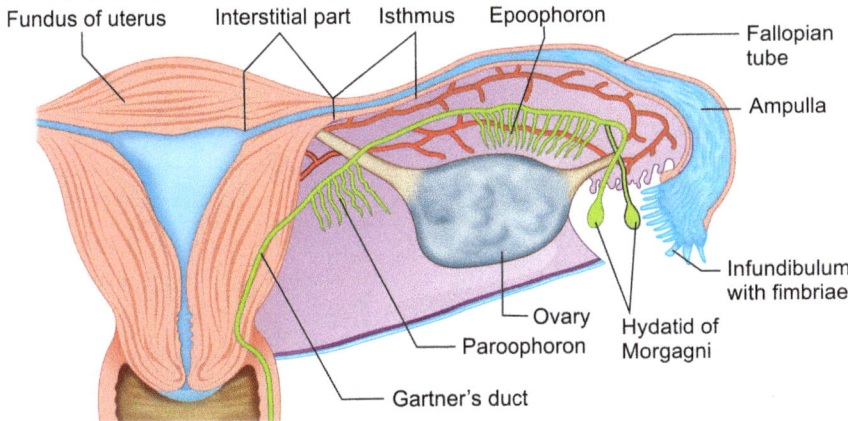

Fig. 6: Half of uterine cavity and fallopian tube of one side are cut open to show different parts of the tube. The vestigial structure in the broad ligament is shown.
Courtesy: DC Dutta's Textbook of Gynecology, Edited by Dr Hiralal Konar, New Delhi, Jaypee Brothers Medical Publishers, 2016; p8

fallopian tubes and implants on the wall of the uterus. Further development of embryo and fetus happens during pregnancy.

Corpus Luteum

It is a gland in the ovary. The ova sit there. It produces progesterone which helps to prepare uterus during pregnancy. The uterine lining grows. If the eggs remain unfertilized, the corpus luteum disappears and menstruation occurs.

FALLOPIAN TUBES

Two fallopian tubes carry the egg from the ovaries and take them to uterus during the menstruation cycle. Occasionally, the fertilized egg may also get implanted in the fallopian tube, causing ectopic pregnancy. It requires immediate medical assistance as it is very dangerous.

Fimbriae

Fimbriae are small extensions attached to the end of fallopian tubes. They help to transport egg from the ovaries to the uterus.

UTERINE LIGAMENTS (FIG. 7)

- Pubocervical ligament
- Cardinal ligament
- Uterosacral ligament
- Sacrospinous ligament.

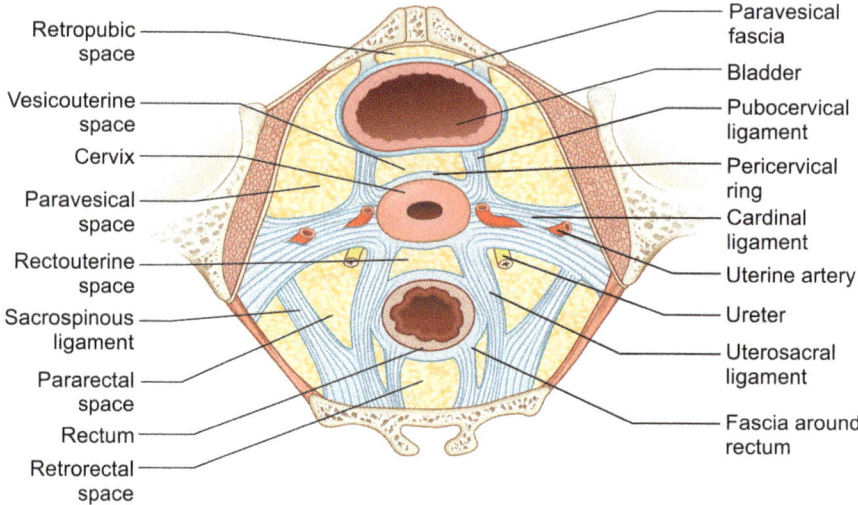

Fig. 7: The main supporting ligaments of the uterus viewed from above.
Courtesy: DC Dutta's Textbook of Gynecology, Edited by Dr Hiralal Konar, New Delhi, Jaypee Brothers Medical Publishers, 2016; p17

RECTUM (FIG. 8)

Rectum is a part of large intestine. It connects the colon to the anal canal. It holds the feces before it goes to anus to exit the body. Expansion of the rectal wall sends a signal to the brain to activate process of defecation.

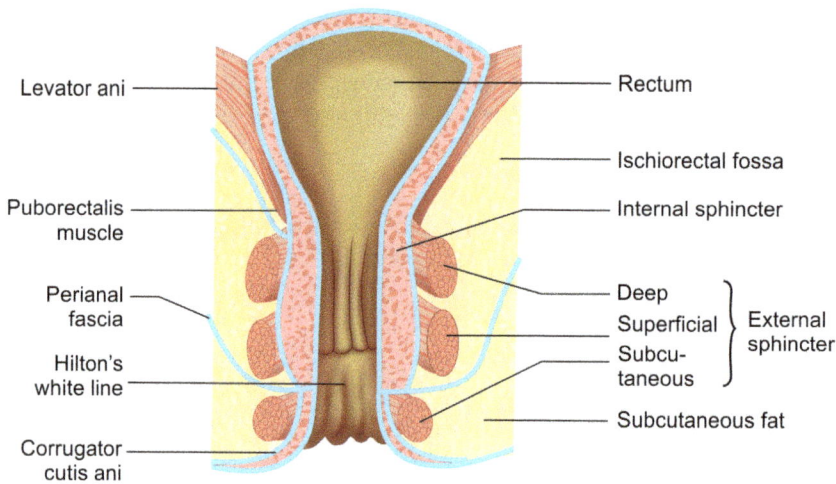

Fig. 8: Rectum and anal canal with anal structures.
Courtesy: DC Dutta's Textbook of Gynecology, Edited by Dr Hiralal Konar, New Delhi, Jaypee Brothers Medical Publishers, 2016; p13

ANUS

The anus is an opening that allows feces to exit the body.

Anal Sphincter

The anal sphincter is located around the anus which helps to hold the anus in a closed position. Opening of the anal sphincter allows the passage of feces.

By now we have revised the key points about functional anatomy. In the coming chapter we will discuss the details about pelvic floor muscles which serves as a base support for these organs.

OVERVIEW OF FEMALE REPRODUCTIVE SYSTEM

The female reproductive system is made up of external and internal sex organs. These organs work collectively for female sexual pleasure and reproductive abilities (Fig. 9).

VULVA (FIG. 10)

Overall term vulva consists of:
- Mons pubis
- Labia majora
- Labia minora
- Clitoral hood
- Clitoral glans
- Vestibule
- Urethral meatus
- Vaginal orifice
- Hymen.

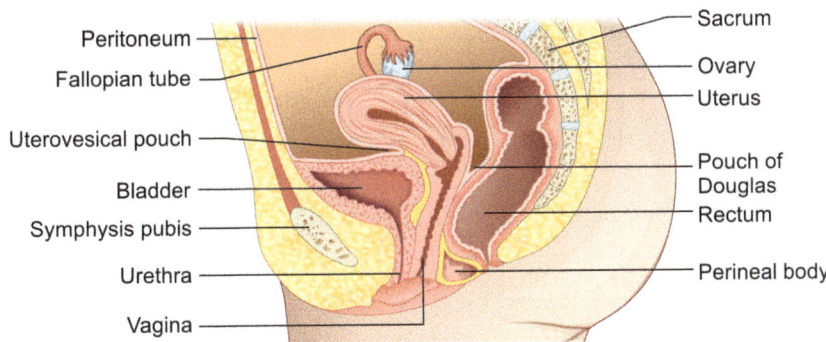

Fig. 9: Midsaggital section of the female pelvis showing relative positions of the pelvic organs.

Courtesy: DC Dutta's Textbook of Gynecology, Edited by Dr Hiralal Konar, New Delhi, Jaypee Brothers Medical Publishers, 2016; p4

Section 1: Female: Pelvic Floor Dysfunction

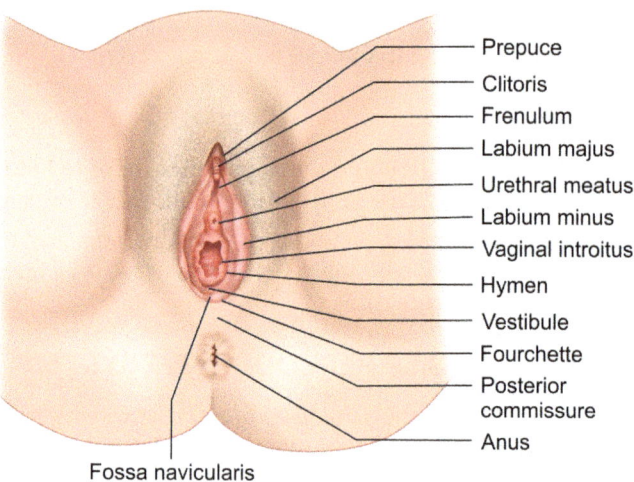

Fossa navicularis

Fig. 10: The vaginal vulva (external genitalia).
Courtesy: DC Dutta's Textbook of Gynecology, Edited by Dr Hiralal Konar, New Delhi, Jaypee Brothers Medical Publishers, 2016; p2

MULTIPLE CHOICE QUESTIONS

Q1. What consists of upper urinary tract?
 (a) Only kidney
 (b) Only ureter
 (c) Pair of kidney and ureter
 (d) None of the above

Q2. Detrusor forms the _____ layer of urinary bladder.
 (a) Outer layer
 (b) Middle layer
 (c) Inner layer
 (d) It forms all the three layers

Q3. How long is the female urethra?
 (a) 1.5 cm
 (b) 2.54 cm
 (c) 1 inch
 (d) 1.5 inches

Q4. Decreased level of which hormone during menopause leads to bladder disorder?
 (a) Estrogen
 (b) Luteinizing hormone
 (c) Relaxin
 (d) All of the above

Q5. Internal urethral sphincter is under voluntary control.
 (a) True
 (b) False

Q6. Anatomical position of the uterus is _____
 (a) Posterior to rectum
 (b) Below the urinary bladder
 (c) Posterior to urinary bladder and anterior to rectum
 (d) Just posterior to symphysis pubis

Q7. Which layer of uterus sheds during menstrual cycle every month?
 (a) Endometrium
 (b) Myometrium
 (c) Perimetrium
 (d) All of the above

Q8. How much is the functional capacity of urinary bladder?
- (a) 2,000 mL
- (b) 360–480 mL
- (c) 800 mL
- (d) 200 mL

Q9. Which hormone prepares the uterus for pregnancy?
- (a) Luteinizing hormone
- (b) Progesterone
- (c) Estrogen
- (d) Follicle stimulating hormone

Q10. Transportation of ovum from ovaries to uterus is done by?
- (a) Fimbriae
- (b) Fallopian tubes
- (c) Both (a) and (b)
- (d) None of the above

ANSWERS

1: (c) Pair of kidney and ureter
2: (b) Middle layer
3: (d) 1.5 inches
4: (a) Estrogen
5: (b) False
6: (c) Posterior to urinary bladder and anterior to rectum
7: (a) Endometrium
8: (b) 360–480 mL
9: (b) Progesterone
10: (c) Both (a) and (b)

Chapter 2

Pelvic Floor Muscles and Functions

INTRODUCTION

The pelvic floor is hammock-shaped group of muscles extending from the base of the spine to the pubic bone. Pelvic floor muscles (PFMs) are interconnected and work together as a unit and collectively help with tightening loose vagina, urine control, supporting pelvic organs, and to enhance intimate health. PFM are divided into three layers (Fig. 1):
1. Superficial layer or urogenital and anal triangle
2. Middle layer or urogenital diaphragm
3. Deep layer or pelvic diaphragm.

PELVIC FLOOR MUSCLE LAYERS

First Layer: Urogenital Triangle and Anal Triangle

It is mainly responsible for continence and sexual functions. It helps levator ani but is not directly responsible for support.
- *Superficial transverse perineal (STP) muscle*: It arises from ischial tuberosity to perineal body. It helps action of deep transverse perineal muscles to stabilize perineal body.

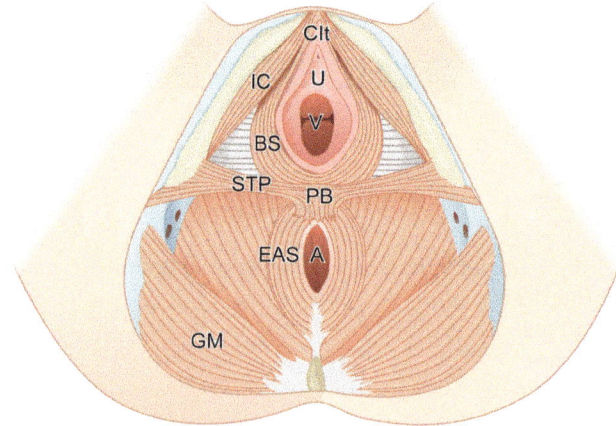

Fig. 1: Pelvic floor muscles.
(Clt: clitoris; U: urethra; V: vagina; IC: ischiocavernosus; BS: bulbospongiosus; STP: superficial transverse perineal; PB: perineal body; A: anus opening; EAS: external anal sphincter; GM: gluteus maximus).

- *Bulbocavernosus (BC) muscle or bulbospongiosus*: This muscle arises from perineal body to bulb of vestibule, perineal membrane, body of clitoris, and corpus cavernosum. In women, it contracts during orgasm and helps with the erection of clitoris and moves blood from attached parts to the clitoris.
- *Ischiocavernosus (IC)*: It arises from ischial tuberosity to clitoris. It helps to move blood from body of crura into the body of clitoris. In women, it erects the clitoris.
- *Anal sphincter*: It arises from anal canal; it anchored to perineal body and anococcygeal body. Loops around the anus to provide continence.

Second Layer or Middle Layer or Urogenital Diaphragm (Fig. 2)

This muscle has different parts as per direction:
1. *Deep transverse perineal (DTP):* Muscles from ischial ramus to perineal body. It stabilizes position of perineal body. Consists of additional fibers like sphincter urethra which loops around urethra and helps with continence. Its under voluntary control can be activated and trained.
2. *External urethral sphincter* also called *sphincter urethera* are circular fibers from inferior pubic arch to anterolateral walls of vagina and trigonal ring surrounding the urethera. It constricts and relax the urethera and assists in the continence mechanism, can be trained as under voluntary control.
3. *Compressor urethrae* (in women only) from ischiopubic ramus to anterior surface of urethra and vaginal wall. Compress the urethral wall and helps in continence.

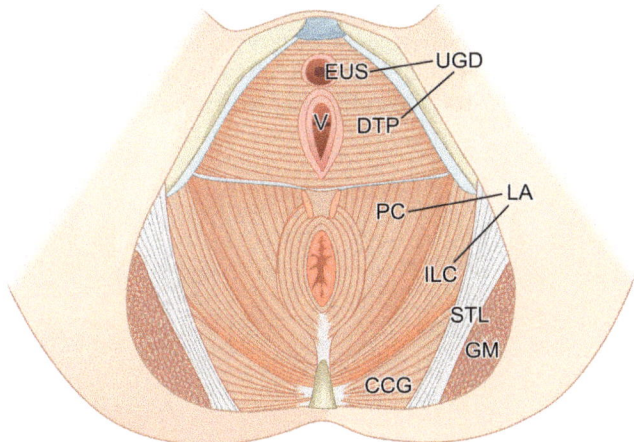

Fig. 2: Middle layer muscles.
(EUS: external urethral sphincter; DTP: deep transverse perineal; UGD: urogenital diaphragm; V: Vagina; PC: pubococcygeus; ILC: iliococcygeus; STL: sacrotuberous ligament; GM: gluteus maximus; CCG: coccygeus)

Third Layer or Deep Layer or Inner Most Layer (Fig. 3)

Levator ani muscle: Pelvic diaphragm is made up of levator ani, which is the most important supportive muscle. Its a hammock like between the pubic bones infront and coccyx behind. The difference between levator ani and other skeletal muscle is higher resting tone. Main function of levator ani is to provide support to pelvic organs and to provide continence at night. It is innervated by pudendal nerve. Advanced contractions are required to maintain continence during coughing, sneezing, laughing, jumping, etc. This muscle has approximately 70% slow twitch and 30% fast twitch muscle fibers.

This muscles has different parts as per direction.

- **Pubococcygeus (PC) muscle:** From the pubic bones to coccyx. It lies lateral to the vagina on both the sides. It feels like band above hymenal ring. It can be felt during an intravaginal examination. It has again 3 parts:
  1. Pubovisceral most anterior part and only in women. Loops around the urethera.
  2. Pubovaginalis: Only in women. Loops around the vagina.
  3. Puborectalis muscle from pubic bone to anococcygeal body, slings around the junction of rectum and anal canal, loops around rectum. It pulls the rectum forward during contraction, towards pubic symphysis to assist fecal continence.
- **Iliococcygeus:** From coccyx to each of the ischial tuberosity. Mainly supportive work, not much contribution on lifting anus.
- **Coccygeus muscle:** From ischial spine to coccyx. Contributes with stability of sacroiliac joint. It lies close to iliococcygeus muscles. Supports pelvic viscera and pulls coccyx forward after defecation.

Endopelvic Fascia

It is made up of smooth muscle fibers, ligaments, nerves, blood vessels and connective tissue. It supports the bladder, the inner organs like intestines and uterus in women. It also connects to the lumbar spine and the symphysis pubis. This muscle layers cannot be exercised. However, one can improve back pain by training inner layer of pelvic diaphragm which increases support of the bladder and uterus and reduces strain over ligaments. Training them can also reduce

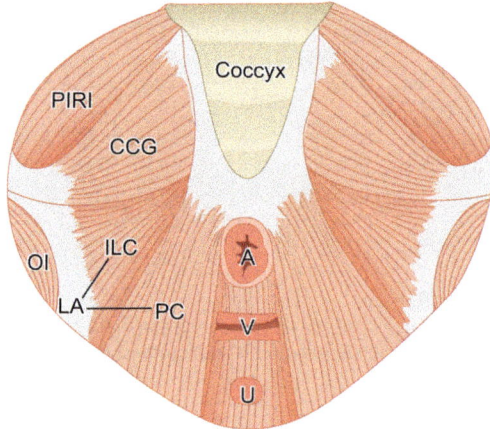

Fig. 3: Inner layer muscles.

(PIR: piriformis; CCG: coccygeus; ILC: iliococcygeus; PC: pubococcygeus; OI: obturator internus; LA: levator ani; A: anus; V: vagina; U: urethra)

the strain on the ligaments. Strengthening pelvic floor muscles can increases visceral support also in a patient who has sustained tear of endopelvic fascia during child birth or other injury.

Other Key Muscles

- *Obturator internus*: It arises from pelvis to greater trochanter of femur. Lateral rotation of extended hip and abduction of flexed hip (L5-S1).
- *Piriformis*: This muscle arises from sacrum to greater trochanter of femur. Lateral rotation of extended hip and abduction of flexed hip.

Key Ligaments

Cardinal or MacKenrodt or transverse cervical ligament: Anchor for vagina at the level of cervix
Broad ligament: Anchor for the uterus, ovaries and fallopian tubes
Round ligament: Anchor for the uterus and inserts into labia majora
Uterosacral ligament: Anchor for uterus to the sacrum posteriorly
Pubovesical ligament: Anchor for bladder to pubic bone
Nerve supply: The pudendal nerve
Blood supply: The pudendal arteries.

FUNCTIONS OF PELVIC FLOOR MUSCLES (FIG. 4)

The PFMs have 5 key functions. Stronger PFMs help to carry these functions in proper manner. The functions of pelvic floor muscles are as follows:
1. Supportive
2. Stabilization
3. Sphincteric
4. Sexual
5. Lymphatic.

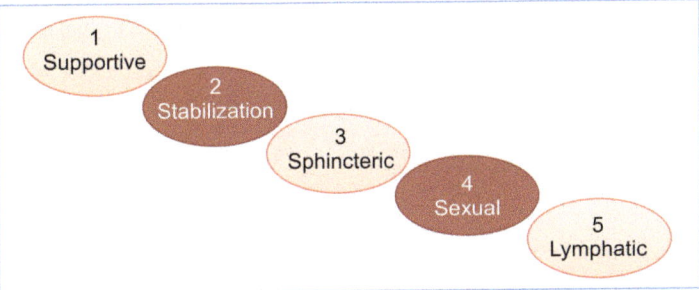

Fig. 4: Major functions of pelvic floor muscles.

Supportive

Pelvic floor muscle works together to provide a muscular sling or support to pelvic organs like bladder, uterus, rectum, intestines, etc. Especially levator ani muscle has constant resting tone to support pelvic viscera. It can also be

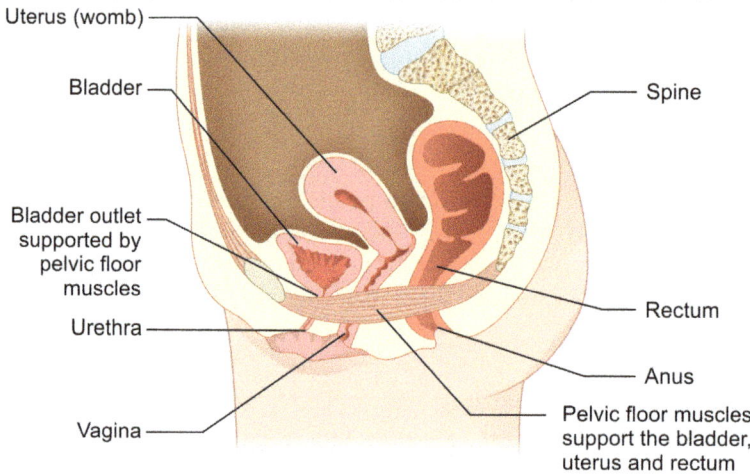

Fig. 5: Supportive function of pelvic floor muscle.

trained and contracted to create stronger pelvic floor closure during increase in intra-abdominal pressure. PFMs provide muscular net for the bladder, uterus, and rectum (Fig. 5).

Stabilization

Pelvic floor muscles work with other core muscles to maintain lumbopelvic stability. Pelvic floor helps other core muscles like transverses abdominis, multifidus, and diaphragm in compressing the abdominal and pelvic content during forced expiration, coughing, etc. It also helps in trunk fixation during upper limb movements (Fig. 6).

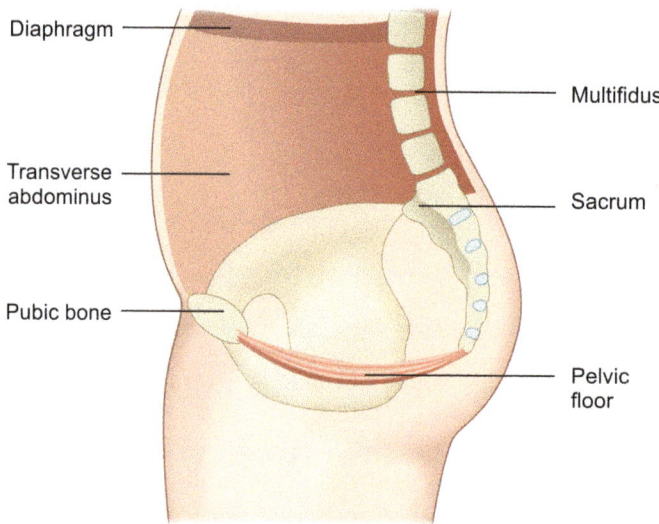

Fig. 6: Stabilization function of pelvic floor muscle.

Pelvic Floor Muscles and Functions

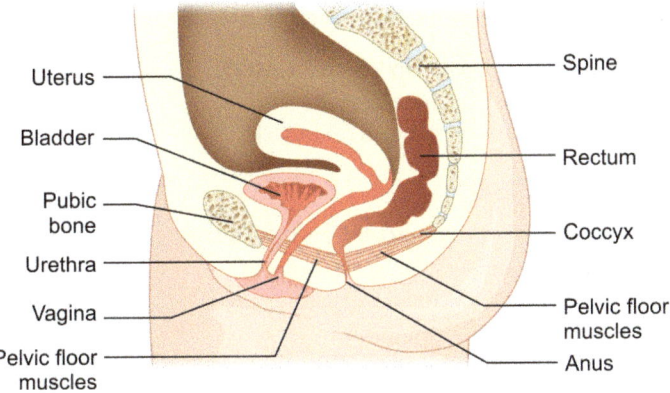

Fig. 7: Sphincteric function of Pelvic floor muscle.

Sphincteric

Pelvic floor muscle helps to maintain urinary and fecal continence. Especially levator muscles interdigitate with the vaginal and rectal canal and encircle them to provide the tone and pressure to close the sphincters (Fig. 7).

Sexual

Pelvic floor provides a foundation of proprioceptors in the canals. Also, muscles like bulbospongiosus and ischiocavernosus, helps to improve blood circulation and assist the erection of clitoris in women. It also helps to increase sexual sensation and intensity of orgasm.

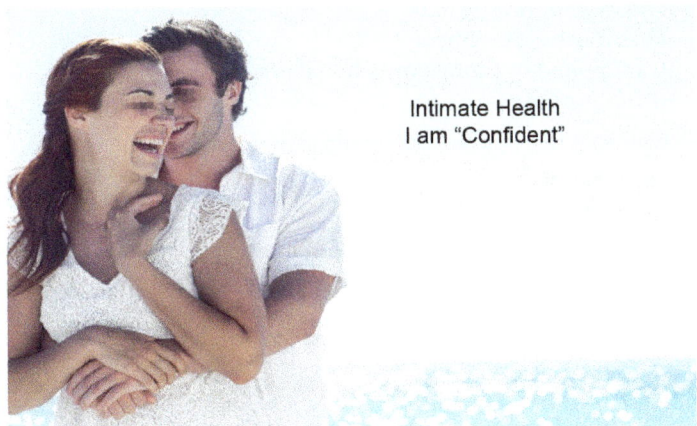

Intimate Health
I am "Confident"

Lymphatic

Along with diaphragm, it helps to create a mechanical pump for the lymph vessels and venous sinuses in the pelvis.

Section 1: Female: Pelvic Floor Dysfunction

MULTIPLE CHOICE QUESTIONS

Q1. Sphincter urethra is formed by which muscles?
(a) Deep transverse perineal muscle
(b) Superficial transverse perineal muscle
(c) Bulbospongiosus
(d) Ischiocavernosus

Q2. Which muscle works to stabilize the perineal body?
(a) Superficial transverse perineal muscle
(b) Deep transverse perineal muscle
(c) Levator ani muscle
(d) None of the above

Q3. What is the action of bulbospongiosus and ischiocavernosus muscles in females?
(a) Support to pelvic organs
(b) Opening and closing of urethra
(c) Both (a) and (b)
(d) Erection of clitoris and increasing blood supply to clitoris during sexual activity

Q4. The attachment of anal sphincter is _____
(a) Perineal body to anococcygeal body
(b) Anococcygeal body to coccyx
(c) Perineal body to coccyx
(d) Anococcygeal body to pubic symphysis

Q5. What is the main function of levator ani group of muscles?
(a) Sphincteric control
(b) Sexual role
(c) Both of the above
(d) Supportive role

Q6. How does the levator ani muscles are different from other skeletal muscles?
(a) It has higher resting tone
(b) It has more motor fibers
(c) It is supplied by more than 1 spinal nerve
(d) All of the above

Q7. Which nerve supplies levator ani group of muscles?
(a) Pelvic nerve
(b) Perineal nerve
(c) Pudendal nerve
(d) Iliac nerve

Q8. The levator ani group of muscles have almost _____% of slow twitch muscle fibers.
(a) 50%
(b) 30%
(c) 70%
(d) 80%

Q9. The levator ani group of muscles have almost _____% of fast twitch muscle fibers.
(a) 50%
(b) 30%
(c) 70%
(d) 80%

Q10. Which muscle helps in defecation?
- (a) Urethral sphincter
- (b) Pubococcygeus
- (c) Puborectalis
- (d) Iliococcygeus

Q11. Muscle which contributes for maintaining stability of sacroiliac joint is.
- (a) Coccygeus
- (b) Iliococcygeus
- (c) Pubococcygeus
- (d) Obturator internus

Q12. Which layer of pelvic floor muscle should be trained for treating the patients with back pain?
- (a) Layer of superficial transverse perineal muscles
- (b) Layer of levator ani group of muscles
- (c) Endopelvic fascia
- (d) Only the layer of deep transverse perineal muscles

Q13. Which ligament supports the uterus?
- (a) Broad ligament
- (b) Round ligament
- (c) Pubovesical ligament
- (d) Uterosacral ligament

Q14. Which part of urethra and urinary bladder is most commonly affected during radical prostate surgery?
- (a) External urethral sphincter
- (b) Trigone of bladder
- (c) Internal urethral sphincter muscles
- (d) Fundus of bladder

ANSWERS

1: (a) Deep transverse perineal muscle
2: (b) Deep transverse perineal muscle
3: (d) Erection of clitoris and increasing blood supply to clitoris during sexual activity
4: (a) Perineal body to anococcygeal body
5: (d) Supportive role
6: (a) It has higher resting tone
7: (c) Pudendal nerve
8: (c) 70%
9: (b) 30%
10: (c) Puborectalis
11: (a) Coccygeus
12: (b) Layer of levator ani group of muscles
13: (d) Uterosacral ligament
14: (c) Internal urethral sphincter muscles

Chapter 3

Pelvic Floor Muscles Dysfunction and Types

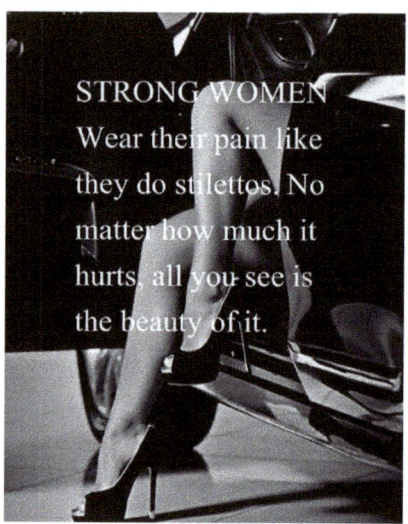

PELVIC FLOOR MUSCLES DYSFUNCTION

In the previous chapter, we have understood the functions of pelvic floor muscle (PFM), how they can help with woman's urinary health, pelvic organ support, and intimate health.

Pelvic floor muscles can become too loose, too tight or incoordinated. They can fail to continue with their normal functions, which is known as pelvic floor dysfunction (PFD).

Causes of Pelvic Floor Muscle Dysfunction (PFMD)
- Pregnancy
- Labor
- Childbirth
- Emergency C section (where patient has already gone through straining of PFMs)
- Planed C section (has less odds to damage PFM as labor and vaginal birth trauma or straining is not there; however we cannot overlook the fact of weight gain during pregnancy which strains PFM)

- Menopause
- Weight gain
- Poor posture
- Sedentary lifestyle
- Diabetes
- Use of tobacco
- Steroid use
- Disuse atrophy
- Too much passive stretching (too thick male genital organs) through sexual overactivity
- Pelvic organ pathologies
- Pelvic trauma
- Perineal trauma or burns.

Types of Pelvic Floor Muscle Dysfunction (Figs. 1A to C)

For clinical use, we can make it even simpler to learn and understand about PFD. For best functioning of PFM it is very important to maintain delicate balance between stability, mobility, and usability. Too much stability leads to tightness, hypertonus dysfunction or spams of PFM. Too much mobility, loosening, or weakness leads to vaginal laxity.

According to American Physical Therapy Association (APTA)

American Physical Therapy Association has classified PFMs dysfunction into four types.

Four basic types of pelvic floor dysfunction:
1. Hypotonus dysfunction
2. Hypertonus dysfunction

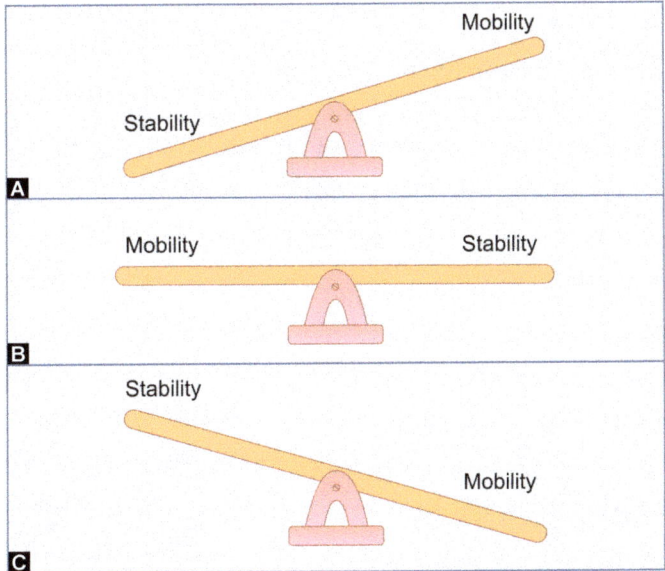

Figs. 1A to C: (A) Hypertonus pelvic floor dysfunction; (B) Fit pelvic floor; (C) Hypotonus pelvic floor dysfunction.

3. Incoordination dysfunction
4. Visceral dysfunction.

According to Het's classification of PFD:
1. Hypertonous PFD
2. Hypotonous PFD
3. Incoordination/combined PFD
4. Visceral PFD
5. Nonfunctional PFD.

Hypertonus—vaginal spasm dysfunction:
This is the type of PFD where PFM becomes overactive, which means too tight PFMs do not let the organs fully expand due to adhesions, tissue changes, surgical scars, and conditions like endometriosis. Generally, it is present with absence of voluntary PFM complete or partial relaxation. Patients may present with spasms, pressure, pain, constipation, urinary frequency, dyspareunia, and urethral syndrome. Hypertonus or spasmodic PFMs create impairment of muscle isolation, contraction, and relaxation. Pain may be localized to the suprapubic area, vaginal area, coccyx, lower sacrum, rectum, and pelvic areas. In summary, either PFMs do not know how to relax completely or they contract or spasm when full relaxation is necessary, e.g. central precocious puberty (CPP) conditions.

Hypotonus—vaginal laxity dysfunction: In hypotonus type of PFD, PFMs fail to maintain normal tone. They fail to create a strong contraction when it is necessary. It is due to too weak PFMs. Generally happens due to pregnancy, childbirth, birth trauma or age. It can lead to perineal pressure, pelvic heaviness, incontinence, reduced sexual sensation, and pelvic organ prolapse (POP) like cystocele, rectocele, enterocele, etc. (Fig. 2).

Other Classification of Pelvic Floor Dysfunction

Incoordination/Combined Dysfunction

- Difficulty to create proper or complete sequencing of pelvic floor or abdominal muscles contraction and relaxations or it can be present with combination of two or more types of PFD. It can be due to neurological, functional or habitual causes.

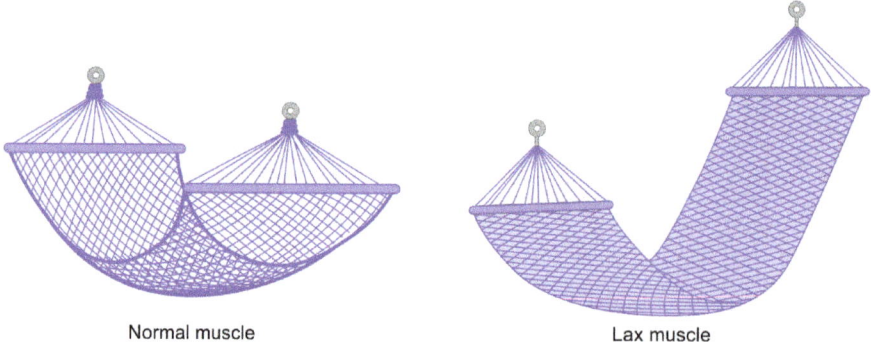

Normal muscle | Lax muscle
Fig. 2: Hypotonus pelvic floor dysfunction.

- For example, you might provide strength training for patient with stress urinary incontinence (SUI), patient might demonstrate objective improvements in muscle strength and endurance. However, they may not show much improvement with incontinence. This might be because of incoordination dysfunction. Patient has gained strength in PFM. However, patient is not trained to use it in coordination with functional needs like coughing, sneezing, etc. Proper coordination training is helpful to generate reflexive activity of the PFM.

Visceral Dysfunction

Dysfunction of PFMs due to visceral pathology like interstitial cystitis, irritable bowel syndrome (IBS), endometriosis, etc. is known as visceral dysfunction.

Nonfunctional Dysfunction

Nonpalpable PFM contraction and relaxation can be categorized as nonfunctional dysfunction.

MULTIPLE CHOICE QUESTIONS

Q1. Which type of pelvic floor dysfunction will occur if the pelvic floor muscles are too loose?
   (a) Incoordinated
   (b) Hypotonus
   (c) Hypertonus
   (d) Visceral

Q2. If a patient comes to your clinic having complains of low back pain along with long history of constipation and pain in the perineal area, what type of pelvic floor dysfunction will you suspect?
   (a) Hypertonus
   (b) Incoordinated
   (c) Visceral
   (d) None of the above

Q3. A patient with good pelvic floor strength but still has complains of urine leak during activities like sneezing or coughing. Good strength but no reflexive control, this can be a sign of which type of pelvic floor dysfunction?
   (a) Hypertonus
   (b) Hypotonus
   (c) Incoordinated
   (d) Visceral

Q4. A 45-years-old female having two normal deliveries is having a complain of urine leak during high impact activities and her gynecologist has diagnosed her as having pelvic floor organ prolapse, in this case what is your provisional diagnosis?
   (a) She has an incoordinated type of pelvic floor dysfunction
   (b) She has hypertonus dysfunction
   (c) She has hypotonus dysfunction
   (d) Insufficient information

Q5. Arrange the type of deliveries from most damaging to less damaging way (the way they affect the pelvic floor muscles).
   (a) Planned cesarean section
   (b) 18 hours long labor with normal delivery
   (c) Unplanned cesarean section
   (d) 15 hours long labor with episiotomy

Section 1: Female: Pelvic Floor Dysfunction

Q6. Any visceral pathologies like endometriosis or interstitial cystitis when affect the pelvic floor muscles it can be termed as visceral dysfunction of pelvic floor muscle but it can be treated by using same protocol like we use for _____.
(a) Hypertonus dysfunction
(b) Hypotonus dysfunction
(c) Both the protocol can be used simultaneously
(d) We cannot treat this type of dysfunction.

ANSWERS
1: (b) Hypotonus
2: (a) Hypertonus
3: (c) Incoordinated
4: (c) She has hypotonus dyfunction
5: (d) (b) (c) (a)
6: (a) Hypertonus dyfunction

Chapter 4

Assessment of Pelvic Floor Muscles

■ INTRODUCTION

When it comes to pelvic floor dysfunction (PFD), each patient is a teacher. Thorough examination and detailed assessment is very important to find out the exact problem and will help in proper treatment and plan of care (POC). The therapist should take proper:
- Subjective history
- Objective history

Subjective	Objective

• Age
• Habits
• Lifestyle or occupation
• Chief complaints of:
  – Pain
  – Discomfort
  – Heaviness
• Past history of:
  – Injury or trauma
  – Childbirth
  – Sex life
  – Surgeries
  – Pelvic organ prolapse (POP)
	• Assessment of posture
	• Vulvar or perineal observation
	• Vaginal and rectal examination
	• External palpation of urogenital triangle/anorectal triangle
	• Internal palpation of deep pelvic floor muscle
	• Pelvic ultrasonography
	• Electromyography (EMG)
	• Anorectal manometry or rectal balloon expulsion
	• Perineometer

■ SUBJECTIVE HISTORY

It is very important to take detailed subjective history. Following parts of history taking are essential to understand type of PFD:

Chief complaints: Exact complaint in patient's own words would easily be able to provide a signal toward type of PFD.
- Take detailed history of childbirth, type of childbirth, number of pregnancies, number of children, age of the youngest or oldest child, any complications during pregnancy or childbirth, history of cesarean section (C-section) or laparotomy, tear, episiotomy, etc.
- *Urinary leakage*: Detailed history about types of activities that create leakage, number of times of leakage, ability to hold urine for prolonged

time, e.g. while traveling, amount of leakage, need to wear or change pads, urine leakage during sexual intercourse, etc.
- *Pelvic organ prolapse*: Detailed history about pelvic pain, heaviness, ball-like sensation, deep pressure, something coming out of vagina, sitting on a ball kind of sensation, something falling down, difficulty walking, etc.
- *Sexual health or pelvic pain*: Detailed history about pain, discomfort, diminished sensation or reduced pleasure during sex, pain during penetration, spasms, tightness or looseness, reduced intensity of orgasms, reduced frequency of sexual intercourse, reduced libido, couple distress. Female sexual function index (FSFI) is a good form for subjective history and progress measurement.

Other Medical History

- Back pain, postural dysfunction, referred pain, leg pain, other related musculoskeletal syndromes, particularly in around the lumbopelvic junction.
- Conditions like diabetes.
- Respiratory conditions like cough, allergies, sneezing.
- Gastrointestinal (GI)–bowel dysfunctions: Vomiting, irritable bowels, fecal incontinence, constipation, hemorrhoids, or inability to control flatus, rectal pain, etc.
- Neurological conditions.
- Psychosocial issues that may alter outcomes including affect, understanding about condition, compliance, marital or sexual status, etc.
- Activities of daily living (ADLs): Factors contributing to symptoms like heavy lifting, prolonged standing, sitting.
- Exercise history: Past and current exercise techniques utilizing Valsalva or high impact that may be exacerbating symptoms, etc.
- Dietary issues: Weight gain, fiber intake, other.
- Smoking, alcohol or any other form of addiction.

OTHER KEY POINTS IN PELVIC FLOOR EVALUATION

Health History Specific to This Diagnosis

- Present illness:
  - Onset of symptoms
  - Patient's chief complaints (functional problems)
  - Patient's perception of the severity of condition.
  - Past or present treatment for this condition
  - Effectiveness of past treatment
  - Patient's primary goals for physical therapy.
- Urinary symptoms:
  - Number of accidents per day
  - Quantity of urine loss
  - Number and type of pads used per day

- Bladder volume, number of voids per day
- Causes or triggers of incontinence: Cold, bladder irritants, cough, laugh, sneeze, giggle, orgasm, other urgency, frequency
- Frequency of nocturia, enuresis
- Difficulty level: Starting urination, dribbling after urination
- Fluid intake: Amount in relationship to age, activity and medical condition.

Medications

- Hormone replacement therapy
- Diuretics
- Bladder drying agents
- Pain medications
- Antidepressants, etc.

Obstetrical History

- Number of pregnancies and deliveries
- Type of deliveries, vaginal or C-section.
- Birth weight of babies
- Duration of labor
- Birth trauma (episiotomy, lacerations, forceps)
- Postpartum problems
- Back pain prenatal or postpartum.

Gynecological History

- Gynecological surgeries like bladder suspensions, hysterectomy, myomectomy, laparoscopic surgery, repair of prolapsed organs, and other abdominal surgeries
- Hormonal status; hormone replacement therapy, menopausal issues and pelvic pain syndromes: Nature and location of the pain, related to muscle or organ dysfunction. Pain intensity
- Fibroids, cysts, warts, human papillomavirus (HPV).

Sexual Activity

- Change in sexual feeling
- Pain with intercourse, at penetration or deep
- Problems with lubrication
- History of sexual abuse. Patient may not be comfortable to share this at the first visit but may share after a relationship has been established with the therapist
- Other or miscellaneous relevant informations which are significant in the rehabilitation outcome of this patient.

Diagnostic Tests
- Het's MMT
- Ultrasonography
- Electromyography.

Others: Perineometer, etc.

External Observation
- Gait pattern
- postural assessment
- Feet: Pronation, supination
- Lumbar ROM or other symptoms radiating from lumbar spine
- Thoracic spine or lumbopelvic mobility or other symptoms.

The Pelvic Girdle
- Bony landmarks
- Pelvic alignment
- Sacral alignment pubic symphysis
- Sacroiliac joints
- Level of anterior superior iliac spine (ASIS) and posterior superior iliac spine (PSIS).

Most Commonly Affected Muscles and their Symptoms
- Pelvic girdle:
    - Adductors
    - Hamstrings
    - Psoas
    - Quadratus lumborum
    - Glutes
    - Piriformis
    - Coccygeus
    - Obturator internus
    - Other
- Soft tissue assessment:
    - Trigger points—extra pelvis
    - Scars: Mobility and/or pain
    - Fascial restrictions
    - Connective tissue assessment

Assessment of Pelvic Floor Muscles | 31

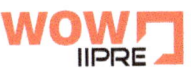

PELVIC REHAB CLINIC

M.ID   :
Date   :
Patient Name :
Age   :

Consulted by   :
Chief Complain :
Referred by   :

■ OBJECTIVE ASSESSMENT

Perineum Observation/Palpation
- Static:
- Dynamic:
  use of accessary muscles.
- Responses of perineum to cough:
                            Inward/outward.

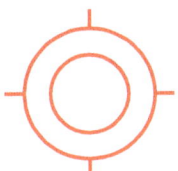

Het's SERF

	S	E	R	F
Goal	-3 |+3	10 sec	10	10
Current				

Het's RR scale/level :_____
Het's FMT Scale :
- Vagina-Fit/Level :
- Vagina-Dilate/level :

Type of PFD

Sessions required:

Het's MMT

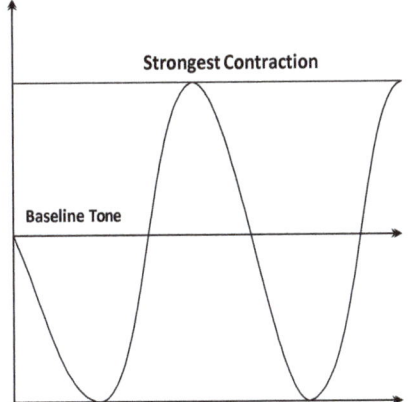

■ ADVICE

Section 1: Female: Pelvic Floor Dysfunction

GENERAL QUESTIONS

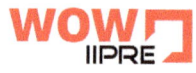

- Do you have regular periods cycle?
  a. Yes ☐   b. No ☐
- Do you suffer from any gynaec problem?
  a. Yes ☐   b. No ☐
- Are you using any birth control measure?
  a Yes ☐   b. No ☐
- Are you pregnant?
  a. Yes ☐   b. No ☐
- Pregnancy history
  a. Number of Pregnancy_____
  b. Number of deliveries_____
  c. Mode of deliveries_____
- Are you aware of any episiotomy or incision during delivery?
  a. Yes ☐   b. No ☐
- What was the weight of your kids during delivery? _____
- How long was your labour? _____
- Have you gone through menopause?
  a. Yes ☐   b. No ☐
- From how long? _____

BLADDER HEALTH SAMPLE ASSESSMENT

1. Do you smoke/consume alcohol?
2. Have you ever had /have:
   a. Cough
   b. Severe vomiting
   c. Constipation
   d. Any Urinary infection
   e. Pain

Please specify your symptoms
1. Do you have urine leakage?
   a. Yes   b. No
   On a scale of 0-10, 10 being excessive, how much_____
2. When have you experienced urine leakage?
   a. Coughing   b. Sneezing
   c. Laughing   d. Exercising
   On a scale of 0-10, 10 being excessive, how much_____
3. How much urine leakage happens?
   a. None   b. Few drops
   c. Approx. one Table spoon   d. Large amount
4. Do you have leakage with sexual intercourse? If Yes
   a. Sometime   b. More often
   c. Frequently   d. Always
   On a scale of 0-10, 10 being excessive, how much_____

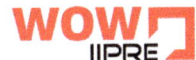

5. Did you have urine leakage during pregnancy? If yes which trimester
   a. First   b. Second
   c. Third
6. Did you ever have urine leakage in childhood? If yes, when
   a. During sleep   b. During daytime
7. Do you feel strong urge of voiding/passing urine but you can control?
   a. Yes   b. No
8. Do you feel strong urge of voiding/passing urine but cannot control?
   a. Yes   b. No
9. Do you have to put strain/pressure during the starting of urination?
   a. Yes   b. No
10. Do you feel any pain/ irritation while passing urine?
    a. Yes   b. No
    On a scale of 0-10, 10 being excessive, how much _____
11. Do you feel your bladder does not get completely empty?
    a. Yes   b. No
    On a scale of 0-10, 10 being excessive, how much _____
12. Do you feel drops of leakage /dribbling even after urination?
    a. Yes   b. No
    On a scale of 0-10, 10 being excessive, how much _____
13. Do you feel like going again immediately after urination?
    a. Never   b. Sometimes
    c. Always
14. Do you feel you have to go frequently for urination again after passing urine?
    a. Never   b. Sometimes
    c. Always
15. Do you urinate more than 8 times a day?
    a. Never   b. 10 times
    c. 15 times   d) 20 times
    e. More than 20 times
16. Do you have to wake up multiple times to urinate at night?
    a. Never   b. Sometimes
    c. Often   d. Frequently
17. Did you ever have any episodes of urine leakage at night?
    a. Never   b. Sometimes
    c. Often   d. Frequently
18. Do you wear pad/Diaper if yes, how many in a day?_____
19. Does your problem affects your daily routine (any functional activity)?
    If yes how much on a scale of 1 to 10 where 10 being most affected._____
20. Since when are you suffering from this problem?_____
21. Have you ever had any treatment for the same problem?
    a. Yes   b. No
22. If answer to the above question is yes than, from the scale of 1 to 10, 10 being most effective. What was your success rate?_____
    Please specify your fluid intake in 24 hours
No. of glass of water _____   No. of cup of tea _____
No. of cup of coffee _____   No.of any other fluid intake _____

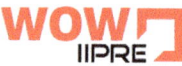

SAMPLE FORM FOR VAGINAL LAXITY AND PELVIC ORGAN PROLAPSE

- Are you feeling looseness down their?
  a. Yes ☐   b. No ☐
  c. Sometimes ☐
- Do you feel like you are sitting on a ball?
  a. Yes ☐   b. No ☐
- Do you feel like something is coming/dropping out of the vagina?
  a. Yes ☐   b. No ☐
  c. Sometimes
- If yes then, is it affecting your sexual life?
  a. Yes ☐   b. No ☐
  c. Sometimes
- Do you have urine leakage with sexual intercourse?
  a. Never ☐   b. Sometime ☐
  c. More often ☐   d. Frequently ☐
  e. Always ☐
- If yes then, is it affecting your sexual life?
  a. Yes ☐   b. No ☐
  c. Sometimes ☐
- Since when are you suffering from this problem? _____
  Is it affecting your social life?
  a. Yes ☐   b. No ☐
- Confidence level
  a. Yes ☐   b. No ☐
- Have you taken any treatment before for this problem?
  a. Yes ☐   b. No ☐

If the answer to the above question is yes, then on a scale of 0-10 where 10 being the most effective. What was your success rate? _____
Please describe your problem in your own words_____

HET'S FSF SCALE (PAIN-HYPERTONUS)
(Female Sexual Function)

- Are you sexually active?
  a. Yes ☐   b. No ☐
- If yes, what is your current frequency of sexual intercourse?
  _____/week
  _____/month
- What was your past frequency of sexual intercourse?
  _____/week
  _____/month

Pain, Tightness and Discomfort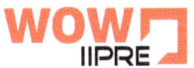

- Are you able to have sexual penetration?
  - a. Yes ☐   b. No ☐   c. Sometimes ☐
- Do you feel any pain, tightness or discomfort during intercourse?
  - a. Yes ☐   b. No ☐
- If yes, how frequently do you feel pain, tightness or discomfort during intercourse?
  - a. Always ☐   b. Sometimes ☐   c. Rarely ☐
- What is your level of pain, tightness and discomfort during penetration?
  - a. Intense ☐   b. Moderate ☐   c. Mild ☐
- Are you able to complete intercourse even with pain?
  - a. Yes ☐   b. Most of the time ☐   c. Have to stop ☐
- If there is pain, does it lasts even after intercourse?
  - a. Yes ☐   b. No ☐   c. Sometimes ☐
  - For how long_____
- Which is the most painful or uncomfortable position for sexual intercourse?
  _____
  Which is the most comfortable/pain free position for sexual intercourse?
  _____
- Do you have any history of sexual abuse or misconduct?
  - a. Yes ☐   b. No ☐
  - If yes, then when_____

1. Please rate how comfortable and pain free your sexual intercourse is.

0	1	2	3	4	5	6	7	8	9	10

Very uncomfortable and painful   Comfortable and pain free

Sexual Desire

- What is the level of your sexual desire or interest?
  - a. High ☐   b. Moderate ☐   c. Low ☐
- Do you find yourself fantasising or thinking about sexual intimacy?
  - a. Yes ☐   b. No ☐   c. Rarely ☐
- How will you rate your desire to have sex compared to past or before pregnancy?
  - a. More Intense ☐   b. Same ☐   c. Less ☐
- Do you feel receptive towards partner's initiation?
  - a. Yes ☐   b. No ☐
- If yes, how often do, you feel receptive towards partner's initiation _____/10

2. Please rate your overall desire to have sex.

0	1	2	3	4	5	6	7	8	9	10

No desire   High desire

Sexual Arousal

- Do you feel that getting sexually aroused is easy for you?
  - a. Yes ☐   b. No ☐   c. Sometimes ☐

Section 1: Female: Pelvic Floor Dysfunction

WOW IIPRE

- Do you feel that you always have enough foreplay to be aroused?
  - a. Yes ☐
  - b. No ☐
  - c. Sometimes ☐
- How satisfied you are with your arousal during sexual intercourse?
  - a. Very satisfied ☐
  - b. Somewhat satisfied ☐
  - c. Dissatisfied ☐
- Are you able to maintain sexual excitement throughout the intercourse?
  - a. Yes ☐
  - b. No ☐
  - c. Sometimes ☐
- How would you rate you confidence level for sexual arousal?
  - a. High ☐
  - b. Average ☐
  - c. Low ☐
- How would you rate your sexual excitement compared to past?
  - a. More Intense ☐
  - b. Same ☐
  - c. Less Intense ☐

3. Please rate your overall ability to get aroused during sexual intercourse

0	1	2	3	4	5	6	7	8	9	10

Inability   Best ability

Lubrication

- Do you feel like you are well lubricated for penetration during sexual activities?
  - a. Yes ☐
  - b. No ☐
  - c. Sometimes ☐
- How frequently do you feel lubricated during sexual activity/intercourse?
  - a. Always ☐
  - b. Sometimes ☐
  - c. Never ☐
- Do you feel any difficulty in achieving or maintaining lubrication throughout your sexual intercourse?
  - a. Yes ☐
  - b. No ☐
  - c. Sometimes ☐
- How much lubrication you feel compared to past?
  - a. Same ☐
  - b. Less ☐
  - c. More ☐

4. Please rate your overall ability to get lubricated.

0	1	2	3	4	5	6	7	8	9	10

No lubrication   Best lubrication

Orgasm

- How frequently do you experience orgasm?
  - a. Always ☐
  - b. Sometimes ☐
  - c. Never ☐
- How intense is your orgasm?
  - a. High ☐
  - b. Moderate ☐
  - c. Low ☐
- Do you feel that you find difficulty/delay in reaching orgasm?
  - a. Yes ☐
  - b. No ☐
  - c. Sometimes ☐
- Are you satisfied with orgasm you reach during sexual intercourse?
  - a. Yes ☐
  - b. No ☐
  - c. Sometime ☐

5. Please rate your overall orgasmic experience.

0	1	2	3	4	5	6	7	8	9	10

No orgasm   Best orgasm

Other Questions

- How well is your emotional bonding with your partner?
  - a. Good ☐
  - b. Average ☐
  - c. Bad ☐
- How well is your intimate bonding with your partner?
  - a. Good ☐
  - b. Average ☐
  - c. Bad ☐
- Do you feel that emotional distress negatively affects your sexual life?
  - a. Yes ☐
  - b. No ☐
  - c. Sometimes ☐
- Do you feel that you get distracted due to some negative thoughts during sexual intercourse?
  - a. Yes ☐
  - b. No ☐
  - c. Sometimes ☐
- How do you feel about your overall sexual life?
  - a. Very satisfied ☐
  - b. Somewhat satisfied ☐
  - c. Not satisfied ☐
- Does your sexual well-being negatively affects other aspect of your life?
  - a Yes ☐
  - b. No ☐

  Please answer these questions:
  Since when are you suffering from this problem? _____
- Have you ever had any treatment for this problem?
  - a. Yes ☐
  - b. No ☐

  If the answer to the above question is yes (specify), what was your success rate?
  _____

  Please describe your problem in your own words.
  _____

HET'S FSF SCALE (LAXITY-HYPOTONUS)
(Female Sexual Function)

- Are you sexually active?
  - a. Yes ☐
  - b. No ☐
- If yes, what is your current frequency of sexual intercourse?
  - _____/week
  - _____/Month
- What was your past frequency of sexual intercourse?
  - _____/week
  - _____/month

Sexual Desire:

- What is the level of your sexual desire or interest?
  - a. High ☐
  - b. Moderate ☐
  - c. Low ☐
- Do you find yourself fantasising or thinking about sexual intimacy?
  - a. Yes ☐
  - b. No ☐
  - c. Rarely ☐
- How will you rate your desire to have sex compared to past or before pregnancy?
  - a. More intense ☐
  - b. Same ☐
  - c. Less ☐
- Do you feel receptive towards partner's initiation?
  - a Yes ☐
  - b. No ☐
- If yes, how often do, you feel receptive towards partner's initiation.
  - _____/10

Section 1: Female: Pelvic Floor Dysfunction

1. Please rate your overall desire to have sex.

0	1	2	3	4	5	6	7	8	9	10

No desire   High desire

Sexual Arousal

- Do you feel that getting sexually aroused is easy for you?
  - a. Yes ☐   b. No ☐   c. Sometimes ☐
- Do you feel that you always have enough foreplay to be aroused?
  - a. Yes ☐   b. No ☐   c. Sometimes ☐
- How satisfied you are with your arousal during sexual intercourse?
  - a. Very satisfied ☐   b. Somewhat satisfied ☐   c. Dissatisfied ☐
- Are you able to maintain sexual excitement throughout the intercourse?
  - a. Yes ☐   b. No ☐   c. Sometimes ☐
- How would you rate you confidence level for sexual arousal?
  - a. High ☐   b. Average ☐   c. Low ☐
- How would you rate your sexual excitement compared to past?
  - a. More intense ☐   b Same ☐   c Less intense ☐

2. Please rate your overall ability to get aroused during sexual intercourse.

0	1	2	3	4	5	6	7	8	9	10

Inability   Best ability

Lubrication

- Do you feel like you are well lubricated for penetration during sexual intercourse?
  - a. Yes ☐   b. No ☐   c. Sometimes ☐
- Do you feel any difficulty in achieving or maintaining lubrication throughout your sexual intercourse?
  - a. Yes ☐   b. No ☐   c. Sometimes ☐
- How frequently do you feel lubricated during sexual intercourse?
  - a. Always ☐   b. Sometimes ☐   c. Never ☐
- How much lubrication you feel compared to past?
  - a. More ☐   b. Same ☐   c. Less ☐

3. Please rate your overall ability to get lubricated.

0	1	2	3	4	5	6	7	8	9	10

No lubrication   Best lubrication

Orgasm

- How frequently you experience orgasm?
  - a. Always ☐   b. Sometimes ☐   c. Never ☐
- How intense is your orgasm?
  - a. High ☐   b. Moderate ☐   c. Low ☐

- Do you feel that you find difficulty/delay in reaching orgasm?
  a. Yes ☐   b. No ☐   c. Sometimes ☐
- Are you satisfied with orgasm you reach during sexual intercourse?
  a. Yes ☐   b. No ☐   c. Sometime ☐

4. Please rate your overall orgasmic experience.

| 0 | 1 | 2 | 3 | 4 | 5 | 6 | 7 | 8 | 9 | 10 |

No orgasm   Best orgasm

- Sexual Dysfunction and Vaginal laxity: Do you feel Vaginal Looseness?
  a. Yes ☐   b. No ☐
- Do you feel reduced sensation during sexual intercourse?
  a. Yes ☐   b. No ☐   c. Sometimes ☐
- Do you feel like you are having sensation of urine leakage during sexual intercourse?
  a. Yes ☐   b. No ☐   c. Sometimes ☐
- Do you feel like passing of air (vaginal flatulence) during sexual intercourse?
  a. Yes ☐   b. No ☐   c. Sometimes ☐
- Does your partner complains about feeling bulge during sexual intercourse?
  a. Yes ☐   b. No ☐   c. Sometimes ☐

5. Please rate your ability to grip the penis during sexual intercourse.

| 0 | 1 | 2 | 3 | 4 | 5 | 6 | 7 | 8 | 9 | 10 |

Very weak grip   Very strong grip

Other Questions

- How well is your emotional bonding with your partner?
  a. Good ☐   b. Average ☐   c. Bad ☐
- How well is your intimate bonding with your partner?
  a. Good ☐   b. Average ☐   c. Bad ☐
- Do you feel that emotional distress negatively affects your sexual life?
  a. Yes ☐   b. No ☐   c. Sometimes ☐
- Do you feel that you get distracted due to some negative thoughts during sexual intercourse?
  a. Yes ☐   b. No ☐   c. Sometimes ☐
- How do you feel about your overall sexual life?
  a. Very satisfied ☐   b. Somewhat satisfied ☐   c. Not satisfied ☐
- Does your sexual well-being negatively affects other aspect of your life ?
  a. Yes ☐   b. No ☐
  Please answer these questions:
  Since when are you suffering from this problem? _____
- Have you ever had any treatment for this problem?
  a Yes ☐   b. No ☐
  If the answer to the above question is yes (specify), what was your success rate?
  _____

  Please describe your problem in your own words.
  _____
  _____

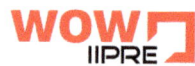

Interpretation of Het's FSF Scale

The Het's FSF scale is designed to find the sexual score of a patient suffering from Female Sexual Dysfunction.
The scale is divided into two parts (pain–hypertonus and laxity–hypotonus).
The pain—Hypertonus scale deals with the patients who are suffering from fsd due to hypertonus pelvic floor muscle dysfunction.
Hypotonus/laxity scale deals with the patients who are suffering from fsd due to hypotonus pelvic floor muscle dysfunction.

The scale has 5 components, out of which the questions for desire, arousal, lubrication, orgasm and psychology are same for both the dysfunctions but the hypertonus dysfunction form has questions related to pain, tightness and discomfort and the hypotonus dysfunction form has questions related to vaginal laxity.
The last question in all the component except for psychological factors has a score from 0-10, so the maximum score of the whole scale will be 50.

The initial questions in all the component are not used to find the score they are designed mainly for clinical understanding and to check the progress.
Only the last questions score will give the value.

Result:- Score interpretation
0-25 is poor sexual health
25-40 is average sexual health
40-50 is good sexual health
(0 is worst and 50 is best female sexual health).

The accurate cause of FSD can be diagnosed by seeing the individual score of the 5 components.

Component	Minimum score	Maximum score	Patient score
Pain or Laxity	0	10	
Desire	0	10	
Arousal	0	10	
Lubrication	0	10	
Orgasm	0	10	
Total score	_____	50	

Relation of the components to Pelvic Floor Dysfunction:

- **Laxity:**
  Any pelvic organ prolapse can cause mechanical obstruction and associated discomfort during sexual intercourse. Urine leakage during intercourse leads to emotional distress and psychological withdrawal from sexual activities due to smell and embarrassment. Even asymptomatic vaginal laxity may negatively affect sensations and ability to grip the penis.

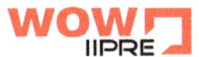

- Desire:
  Overall desire means either self driven desire or receptive to partner's initiation.
  Too tight pelvic floor muscles can lead to pain, tightness or discomfort during sexual activity which can create unpleasant experience and reduced desire.
  Too loose pelvic floor muscles can lead to reduced sensation and pleasure during sexual intercourse which can ultimately lead to reduced desire.
- Arousal:
  Too tight pelvic floor muscles can lead to anticipation of pain due to past experience which can affect arousal or sexual excitement. Too loose pelvic floor muscle can lead to reduced clitoral activation and reduced pumping of Bulbocavernosus and Ischiocavernosus along with other pelvic floor muscles thus leading to difficulty in attaining and maintain arousal.
- Lubrication:
  Note: Less lubrication or vaginal dryness can be because of the factors like aging menopause, hormonal imbalance, psychosomatic dysfunctions, etc. however addressing the lubrication issue along with pelvic floor rehab may greatly enhance the sexual well-being of the patient.
- Orgasm:
  Too tight pelvic floor muscles will lead to pain, tightness or discomfort during intercourse. As a result patient will experience reduced, delayed or even absence of orgasm.
  Too loose pelvic floor muscles specially (PC) will fail to hold the penis tightly which leads to reduced sensation and will also fail to perform rhythmic forceful contractions at the time of orgasm which will compromise intensity, frequency and duration of orgasm.
- Psychological factors:
  Any psychological factors like relationship issues, low self-esteem, emotional distress other health issues, partners sexual health issues, etc. can also greatly lead to compromised sexual well-being.
  Treating sexual dysfunction is not only about pelvic floor rehab specialists, the role of pelvic floor experts is to make sure that pelvic floor functioning is normal. Simultaneously patient should also be referred to other medical specialists like psychiatrists, psychologists gynecologists, urogynecologists, sexologists, etc.
  In this scale the unrelated questions to pelvic floor are kept with a purpose of better clinical understanding so the patients can be referred to appropriate medical specialist for the complete treatment.

Important note: On the scale of Het's MMT (-3/-3) that is complete relaxation and (+3/+3) that is complete contraction can greatly enhance overall sexual well-being of the patient, provided psychological and other medical factors are simultaneously addressed.

Please visit www.visionwowgroup.com" to download the forms.

OBJECTIVE HISTORY

- Posture examination
- Self-examination—Het's self test: Finger test
- Het's manual muscle testing (MMT)
- Perineum observation
- Transvaginal pelvic floor examination
- Electromyography (EMG)
- Specialized sonography: Suprapubic view.

Assessment of Posture

Chronic Pelvic Pain Posture

- Increased lumbar lordosis
- Anterior pelvic tilt
- Lordosis-kyphosis
- Reduced spinal range of motion (ROM)
- Thomas test positive

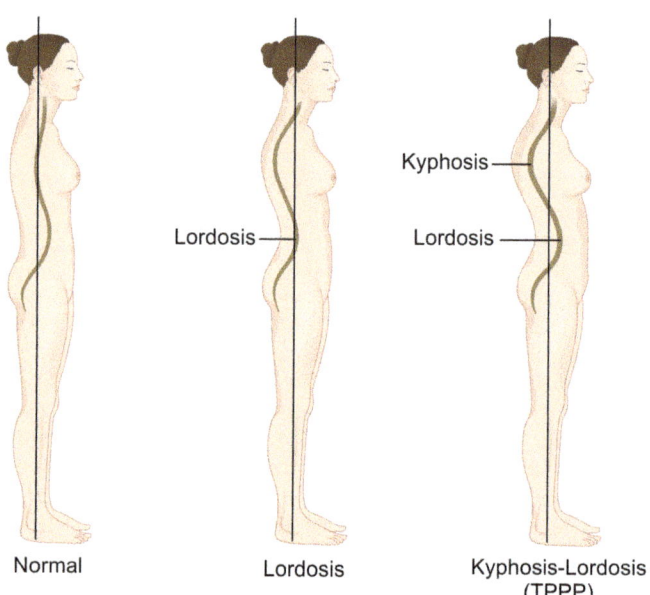

Common Posture with Pelvic Floor Dysfunction

Prolonged sitting can lead to over flexion of the coccyx, which can create disturbance in PFM alignments.

Any other form of changes in the frequent static and dynamic biomechanics of lumbopelvic junction can lead to overstretched or over compressed PFMs dysfunctions. It fails to maintain normal tone of PFMs which can lead to trigger point formation and hypertonus dysfunction as per Lukban, 2002. Even the presence of any kind of sacroiliac joint dysfunction at any stage can lead to trigger point development of PFMs.

Het's MMT GRADE FOR PELVIC FLOOR MUSCLES

- Het's MMT is a unique transvaginal/ transrectal manual muscle testing scale exclusively designed for evaluation of pelvic floor muscles.
- Most of the doctors all over the world have been using Oxford scale for assessment of pelvic floor muscles. However, there has been a huge limitation with Oxford assessment scale.
- Oxford scale (from 0 to 5 grades) can help medical and paramedical professionals to assess only contractile component of pelvic floor muscles. There is no evidence to rate relaxation ability of pelvic floor muscles. Relaxation ability of pelvic floor muscles is equally important, if not more.
- Inability to relax pelvic floor muscles can lead to multiple pathological conditions like vaginismus, dyspareunia, chronic pelvic pain etc. Therefore it is extremely important to assess relaxation ability along with contraction ability of pelvic floor muscles. Oxford scale will measure only strength component which is not sufficient for doctors to complete the evaluation of pelvic floor muscles.
- Het's MMT offers a way to evaluate relaxation component of pelvic floor muscles along with contractile component. So one scale can provide complete evaluation of pelvic floor dysfunctions.
- Het's MMT is very simple to understand and easy to use.
- Het's MMT can help the doctors to measure the strength and relaxation of pelvic floor muscles for all hypotonus, hypertonus and incoordination types of dysfunctions in female and male.
- Het's MMT will not only help the doctors for initial evaluation of patients, but it will also help to design more precise plan of care and assess progress of the patients after the treatment.
- Het's MMT scale will be a revolutionary approach to evaluate and revaluate any condition of pelvic floor dysfunctions.
- Het's MMT Grading scale is so simple and easy to use that even patient can be taught and they can perform self-test as well.

Het's—MANUAL MUSCLE TESTING (MMT) GRADING— PELVIC FLOOR MUSCLES

Het's—manual muscle testing grading—PFM has been described here.

CONTRACTION	Grade 3	Strong upward and inward pull against resistance
	Grade 2	Grip with complete circumference
	Grade 1	Mild contraction (from any side)
0	Grade 0	Baseline tone
RELAXATION	Grade -1	Inability to penetrate
	Grade -2	Symptomatic penetration (pain, tightness, discomfort or any other symptom)
	Grade -3	Asymptomatic penetration (easy penetration)

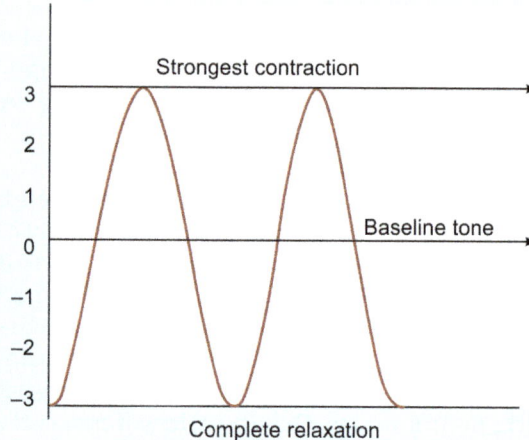

Disclaimer: Professional Responsibility

- Check with state, national and international practice act. Any suggestion or material from this book is not liable if you fail to be compliance with legal or regulatory body of your state, country.
- Use of correct terminology like—transvaginal or internal examination of PFMs versus vaginal examination.
- Practitioner should have undergone specific training for transvaginal PFM examination.
- Respect patient privacy and comfort.
- Patient always has a choice to opt in or out for internal examination.
- Patient always has a choice to proceed or terminate during any phase of examination.
- Chaperone by regional standards and business policy is very important.
- Verbal and written consent is must.
- Very important to identify yourself and support staff with their name tags.

Self–Transvaginal Pelvic Floor Examination

If patient is not comfortable with transvaginal exam, you may teach following Het's MMT test as a self test.

Self Vaginal Examination of Pelvic Floor Muscle

- If you are a provider who is still not certified for pelvic floor transvaginal or transrectal examination or you have patient who is not comfortable with transvaginal or transrectal self-examination.

Assessment of Pelvic Floor Muscles

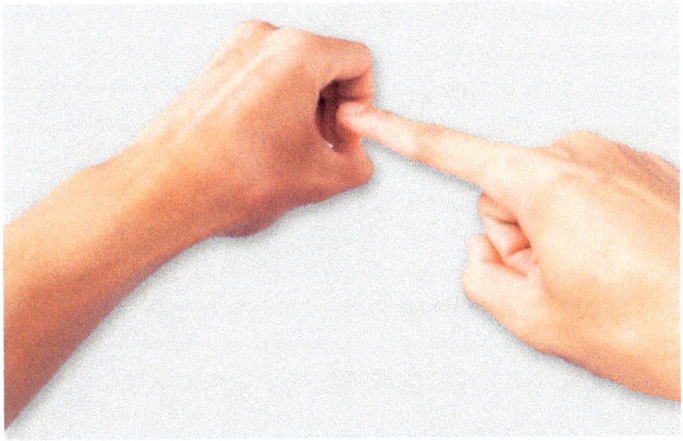

- You can simply suggest your patient to perform Self vaginal examination of PFM.
- Where patient can examine herself in her own privacy and report results to you.
- Suggest her to lie down on her back with no clothes waist down.
- Suggest her to keep her knees and hips bend.
- Ask her to use pillows under her neck and shoulder to relax back. That also enables her to reach down.
- Teach her to insert a clean finger inside the vagina and try to feel inside the vagina.
- Ask her to squeeze her PFM (as if she is trying to hold urine) and hold her own finger as hard as possible.
- Teach her about Het's MMT scale
- Document what she reports.

WOW VAGINA-FIT

- **Test and train intimate muscles**
- **Pelvic floor (-vaginal) muscles**
- WOW Vagina-Fit is a unique device (pelvic floor exerciser) which is biomechanically designed to objectively test and train (proprioceptive and resistive) the pelvic floor muscles which are located surrounding vaginal orifice.
- **Disclaimer:** Vagina-Fit is not a medical device and should not be used for any illegal purpose. It is a pelvic floor muscle exerciser.
- It can be used as an objective self-test which can be carried out by the female patients directly. It is a single user device. The Vagina-Fit is conical in shape and has three parts—a head, body (ridges) and a tail. The tail is made up of rod. The purpose of body/ridges is very scientific, it will help the medical practitioner or the patient to objectively assess the severity of downward and outward displacement in case of vaginal laxity. The device is openable to add the weights (resistance) for testing and training. (Fig. 1)

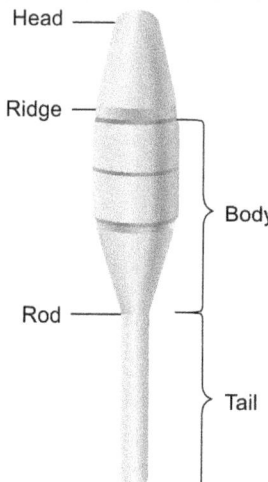

Fig. 1: Vagina-Fit device.

Testing the Pelvic Floor Muscle Strength

Directions to Use

- Wash the device thoroughly with nonperfumed soap and water. Make sure the device is completely hygienic for vaginal penetration. Suggest patient to empty the bladder and bowel and clean her hands appropriately for self-insertion of Vagina-Fit transvaginally.
- The test can be done at any time depending upon the comfort of the female patients in a comfortable room after taking the lowers off or after shower. Before using in standing position, insert the device in supine position to get comfortable with the Vagina-Fit if necessary.
- Once the patient is familiar and comfortable with the device in supine position, start the test in standing position. Patient will be in standing position with legs apart and she will insert the head part of the device into the vaginal opening in the similar way of inserting tampon where the tail of the device stays out, (if necessary, have the patient use water based lubrication to make the penetration easier, however please be careful as too much lubrication might lead to false results of the test) and instruct the patient to hold the device by squeezing her pelvic floor (-vaginal) muscles as if she is trying to stop the urine flow. Also instruct the patient to try to prevent any outward or downward displacement of the device by squeezing pelvic floor muscles with best of their ability. Then the patient has to perform 3 functional activities (10 coughs, 10 squats and 10 jumps) while keeping the device intravaginally and hold it by doing pelvic floor muscles contraction.
- At the same time educate the patient to prevent any use of accessory muscles like gluteus, hip adductors and lower abdominals. Also make sure that the patient breathes normally.
- The result of this test will give you the Het's functional grade of the pelvic floor muscles. (Table 1)

Assessment of Pelvic Floor Muscles

TABLE 1: Het's FMT grades for hypotonus PFM Vagina-Fit.

Description	Het's FMT Grade	Interpretation
Inability to hold Vagina-Fit in standing position while patient is trying to hold Vagina-Fit by contracting PFM it falls out before beginning or before completion of all 3 functional activities	C (Falls out)	Extremely weak pelvic floor muscles (severs laxity)
Inability to complete all 3 functional activities while patient is trying to hold Vagina-Fit by contracting PFM (it may slide/displace downward or outwards)	B	Weak pelvic floor muscles (mild to moderate laxity)
Ability to complete all functional activities without any downward or outward displacement of Vagina-Fit while patient is trying to hold Vagina-Fit by contracting PFM	A	Strong pelvic floor muscles (no vaginal laxity)
Three functional activities are: 10 coughs, 10 squats and 10 jumps		

- If the device slips out, gets pushed out or falls out; in other words, if the patient is unable to hold the device intravaginally in standing position then it will be Het's FMT grade "C" which will indicate severe laxity.
- If the device is not slipping (falling) out, then the patient has to perform 3 functional activities (10 coughs, 10 squats and 10 jumps) while keeping the device intravaginally and hold it by doing pelvic floor muscles contraction. If the device falls out before completion of the functional activities then also it is grade "C".
- If the device does not falls out completely but the patient is unable to hold it firmly and it shows any downward or outward displacement, then it will be Het's FMT grade "B" which will indicate mild to moderate vaginal laxity.
- If the patient is able to do all three functional activities without any downward displacement by holding the device through pelvic floor muscle contraction then it is grade Het's FMT grade "A".
- If the patient shows the strength of grade "A" then repeat the test after rest period of 24 hours and ask the patient do all the functional activities by using the device with the given weights.
- If the patient is able to do all three functional activities without any downward or outward displacement by holding the Vagina-Fit (with all the given weights) then the grade is "A+".
- Every woman including the women who are planning for pregnancy, postpartum women, postmenopausal women or suffering from any type of hypotonus conditions—vaginal laxity can have a goal of ATLEAST STRENGTH LEVEL "A" preferred "A+".

Interpretation

- The patient with a functional grade of "C" or "B" might have moderate to severe form of pelvic floor muscle weakness and she should start the pelvic floor rehab/strengthening exercises.

- The patient with a functional grade of "A" demonstrates a good pelvic floor muscle strength and should progress towards "A+" which is even better (for further information on strengthening please refer Chapter no 16)

Before checking the Het's FMT grades, it is necessary to check the Het's MMT grade because:
- Het's MMT can empower a doctor with better understanding of the isolated muscle strength of the right and left side. There is a possibility where right side might be stronger than left or vice versa. Het's MMT can help the medical practitioner to precisely customize the rehab plan.
- Het's MMT will help the therapist to more efficiently differentiate isolated action of pelvic floor muscles and the accessory muscles.
- Het's MMT is also helpful to make the patient comfortable with the therapist which is needed for the Ring Clock Assessment and even customized planning of the treatment.

Indications

- Stress incontinence
- Urge incontinence
- Mixed incontinence
- Vaginal laxity
- Grade 1 pelvic organ prolapse
- Prepregnancy strengthening
- Postpregnancy strengthening
- Presurgical patients
- Postsurgical patients (with the advice of your doctors).

Contraindications

- Severe vaginitis
- Severe vestibulitis
- Vaginismus , infections
- Any type of pain, tightness or discomfort on insertion
- Hypersensitivity to the material
- Before or after coital activity (intercourse)
- Pregnancy and postpartum (till the time of doctor's clearance)
- Lower urinary tract infection
- During menstrual cycle
- Grade 2 or more pelvic organ prolapse
- In case of intrauterine device
- Transrectal
- Any other medical contraindication

WOW VAGINA-DILATE

- Unique all in one vaginal dilator
- The vaginal dilator is a unique all in one dilator which is scientifically designed in such a way that a single dilator can serve the purpose of different diameter dilator. It's a One Size Fits All dilator (Fig. 2).

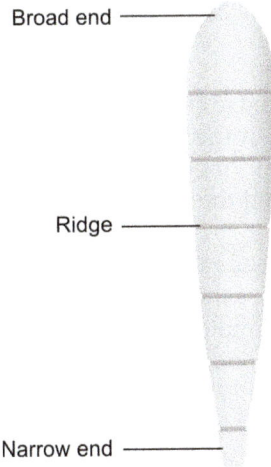

Fig. 2: Vagina-Dilate device.

Unique Features

- It is all in one, one size fits all dilator as it has a progressive increase in its diameter.
- Its smallest diameter provides an easy penetration for severe cases.
- It also provides comfortable progressive penetration as there is no need to pull out the dilator. This also helps to eliminate apprehensive spasms which might be triggered by regular dilator. Different sized dilators needs to be pulled out completely and requires reinsertion of larger diameter which might lead to apprehensive spasm or tightness of pelvic floor muscles.
- The ridges can be used to provide a short-term achievable goal for the patient and hereby gives satisfaction to the patient.
- The broader end enables to improve functional outcomes in patients with FSD for conditions like vaginismus, dyspareunia.
- This dilator is very convenient to carry as it is a single piece dilator.
- It is also cost effective.

Indications

- Vaginismus
- Pain while intercourse
- Dyspreunia.

Contraindications

- Severe vaginitis
- Severe vestibulitis infections
- Hypersensitivity to the material
- Any other medical contraindication.

Testing The Pelvic Floor Muscle Relaxation Ability

Directions to Use

- The vaginal dilator is used to check the relaxation ability of the pelvic floor muscles. It can be used by the patient as objective self-test.
- This test should be performed in a private and comfortable room. The dilator should be washed thoroughly with soap and water taking care of vaginal hygiene.
- The dilator should be used by putting condom over it and lubricating gel can also be used to reduce the friction.
- The patient should be completely relaxed and in crook lying position with legs apart; if needed supported by pillows on both the side. Ask the patient to slowly and gently palpate her vaginal opening and then try to gently slide the dilator into the vaginal opening on her own to prevent apprehensive spasms.

Interpretation

- If the patient is not able to slide even the narrow end of the dilator into her vaginal opening then her **Het's FMT grade is "C"** (Table 2)
- If the entry of narrow end or the broad end is possible but it is symptomatic (pain, tightness or discomfort) then it will be **Het's FMT grade is "B"**. However, the medical practitioner can motivate the patient by showing the progression by measuring the number of ridges inserted on narrow end. When patient progresses from narrow end to broad end indirectly it reflects the progression towards grade "A".
- If the broad end has a complete pain free in and out entry and exit then it is **Het's FMT grade "A"**.

Note: If on transvaginal examination the examiner finds a grade of -1 on Het's MMT then it is not advisable to go for objective test using vaginal dilator. Pelvic rehab specialist might customise the care by combining manual therapy and use of WOW Vagina-Dilate at home.

TABLE 2: Het's FMT grade for hypertonus PFM (Vagina-Dilate).

Description	Grade	Interpretation
Inability to penetrate even with narrow end	C	Extremely tight pelvic floor muscles
Symptomatic penetration of narrow or broad end (pain, tightness or discomfort)	B	Tight pelvic floor muscles
Easy and pain free penetration of broad end	A	Completely relaxed pelvic floor muscles

Perineum Observation

Before you conduct transvaginal PFM examination, take time for perineum observation which will be helpful (Fig. 3).

Assessment of Pelvic Floor Muscles

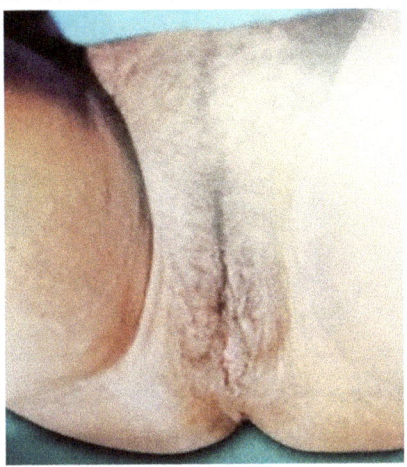

Fig. 3: Inspection of vulva in dorsal position.

Identify structures and symmetry of tissues.
- Scar
- Episiotomy
- Skin condition
- Scars at perineal body
- Excursion
- Contraction
- Relaxation
- Bulge or drop or distend without Valsalva
- Anus winks
- Perineal body draws up and in, clitoral nodes
- Observation of PFM during coughing
- How perineum reacts to increase in intra-abdominal pressure?

Observation		Sensation test
Static observation	Dynamic observation	Sensation check
<ul><li>Skin condition</li><li>Identify structures and symmetry of tissues positions</li><li>Scars at perineal body</li><li>Edema</li><li>Redness</li><li>Episiotomy</li><li>Excursion and ROM</li><li>Bulge/drop/distend without Valsalva</li></ul>	<ul><li>Contraction of PFM and perineal lift</li><li>Relaxation of PFM and perineal release</li><li>The perineal body draws up and in, clitoral nodes</li><li>The anus winks</li><li>Observation of PFM during coughing</li><li>Bulge/drop/distend with Valsalve</li></ul>TEACHING "KNACK"<ul><li>How perineum reacts to increase in intra-abdominal pressure?</li><li>Visual—mirror biofeedback</li><li>Biofeedback tools</li></ul>	With the help of cotton bud over the:<ul><li>Pubic symphysis</li><li>Labia majora</li><li>Labia minora</li><li>Vestibular area</li><li>At sides of vaginal opening</li></ul>

Transvaginal Pelvic Floor Muscle Examination

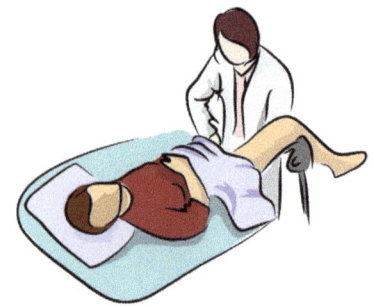

Indications

Pelvic floor dysfunction and conditions like:
- Vaginal laxity
- Incontinence
- Pelvic pain
- Pelvic organ prolapse
- History of sexual dysfunction.

Contraindications

State, Federal or National Law's Restrictions or Professional Body's Restrictions.
- Lack of consent
- Six week postpartum and postsurgery
- Severe vaginitis and infection
- During menstruation and pregnancy
- Pregnancy
- Sexual abuse
- Severe pelvic pain
- Age less than 18 and pediatric patients
- Absence of patient's written consent
- Physician's restrictions and surgery, recent radiotherapy.

PROCEDURE: DURING TRANSVAGINAL EXAMINATION

APTA—Transvaginal Pelvic Floor Muscle Examination

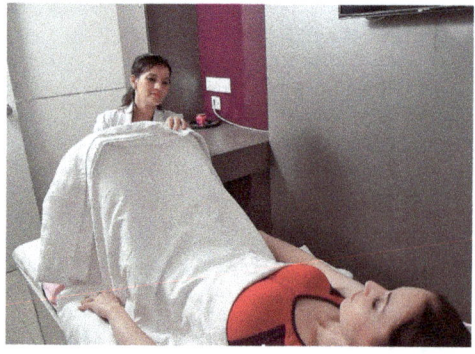

Internal examination of PFMs is valid way for physical therapists to assess and treat PFD. The American Physical Therapy Association (APTA)—"examination of the PFMs is consistent with physical therapy practice. It complies with national physical therapy policies requiring the performance of tests and measurements of neuromuscular function as an aid to the evaluation and treatment of a specific medical condition."

Position of Patient

- Patient should be in supine position with hip and knee flexed with heel elevated on pillows for transvaginal examination. Patient should be in left lateral position and relaxed for transrectal examination.
- Therapist should be seated on the side.
- Maintain eye contact and check body language of the patient.
- Place the nonexamining hand on patient's knees or legs.
- Verbally explain the examination or procedure before you initiate, to your patients.
- How you will insert your finger or fingers, what you will expect when you ask for PFC, how you will palpate by putting pressure.
- How you will turn your fingers inside to access different areas.
- Tell them about trigger points, sweet spot and how you will need patients feedback.
- Tell them how much pressure you intend to put and what level of discomfort patient may experience.
- Tell them if you plan to apply quick stretch or ischemic pressure technique.
- Tell them if you want them to squeeze finger inward and upward.
- Tell them on how you might ask them to approximate fingers by squeezing their PFMs.

VAGINAL PELVIC FLOOR MUSCLE EXAMINATION—ONE OR TWO FINGERS?

Single Finger versus Two Fingers for Examination

Dr Kegel's suggestion: It is a good idea to at least start with one-finger examination. Two fingers can create a mild stretch to muscle spindle, and reflex facilitation of muscle which can misguide reading or palpation. However, if vagina is too much laxity, where there is least possibility of muscle spindle stretch you can perform with two, index and middle finger.

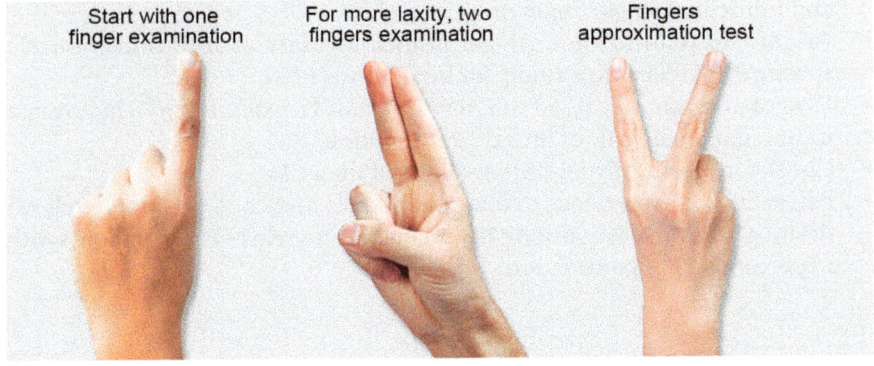

Start with one finger examination | For more laxity, two fingers examination | Fingers approximation test

Hands on: Transvaginal Pelvic Floor Muscle Exam (Fig. 4)

We strongly suggest to keep it mandatory to have a chaperone during any intravaginal or intrarectal examination.

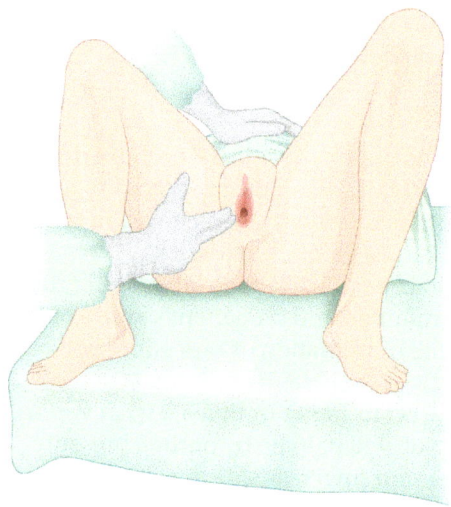

Fig. 4: Transvaginal pelvic floor muscle exam.

Courtesy: DC Dutta's Textbook of Gynecology, Edited by Dr Hiralal Konar, New Delhi, Jaypee Brothers Medical Publishers, 2016; p84

Palpation of PFM can be performed transvaginal or transrectum. Supine position is generally preferred position as it allows the examiner to evaluate muscle bulk, muscles resting tone, contractile strength, relaxation ability, sensation deficit, tenderness, pain and reflex response to cough or Valsalva maneuver.

- Most of the time, detailed subjective history of the patient will give you a clear idea about what you are going to encounter during transvaginal PFM examination.
- When you get the patient comfortable for examination, pay attention to patients body language. If patient is adducting her legs or anticipating pain due to PFM examination, means it is likely to be hypertonus PFM.
- In that case, examiner can assure the patient of keeping the examination pain-free and taking extra care to be extremely gentle while inserting gloved and lubricated single finger only.
- Palpate for painful spot, trigger points, myofascial adhesions, muscle spasm, PFM relaxation ability for hypertonus PFM.
- First of all examiner need to know Het's MMT exam before she initiate transvaginal pelvic floor muscle examination.
- Check for voluntarily relaxation ability of the PFM.
- Pelvic floor muscle needs to relax completely and contract completely on desire. However, it is common to find inability to relax PFM in patients with hypertonus PFM contraction.

- It definitely depends on length of your finger as well and individual anatomy of patients. This is just general guideline for approximate ideas.
- Weak muscles bands—may be poorly or indistinguishable from surrounding tissues.
- Pubococcygeus (PC) muscle—it is felt as 1-2 cm band palpated at lateral vaginal wall. Location of the PC muscle can be found 3-5 cm beyond the vaginal introitus.
- Ask your patient to contract her PFM as hard as possible and ask her to try to squeeze examiner's finger together and lift it inward and upward direction.
- Ask the patient to do the same PFM contraction while the index and middle fingers are spread laterally so that right and left side can be palpated simultaneously.
- As mentioned before, use of two fingers for the examination should only be performed if the provider feels the laxity and no chance to activate muscle spindle by inserting second finger.
- The strong muscles will be felt as a thick, firm 3-5 cm band of muscles, compared with weak or loose muscles which can feel thin and flabby in indistinguishable from surrounding tissues.
- Transvaginally one can also palpate rectum by posterior pressure and rectal contents can be found.
- Examiner can use her other hand to palpate for use of accessory muscles like hip adductors, abductors, lower abs, etc. by using other hand externally to palpate those muscles.
- Palpate the ability and time duration to hold PFM contraction before reduction of any strength.
- Suggest patient to KNACK technique—try to cough artificially while trying to hold PFM without losing the grip on examiner's finger.
- Also, examine coordination by asking patient to do deep breathing exercises (DBE) while holding PFM or by asking patient to move her legs or bend and straighten knees while holding examiner's finger by PFM.
- Ask patient to create submaximal contraction to access control. Examine eccentric strength and control of the muscles by slowly releasing the fully contracted muscles by 10% progressively.
- Make sure to maintain the eye contact with patient throughout transvaginal examination. Assess body language to figure out patient's cooperation and comfort level is also very essential.

Het's RING CLOCK ASSESSMENT

Between first layer (almost externally palpated) and second layer of pelvic floor:
- When you insert your finger imagine an oval circle of first layer of pelvic floor muscles (Fig. 5)
- When you go little deeper there will be an oval circle of second layer of pelvic floor muscles (Figs. 6 and 7)
- Imagine a clock in oval circle of both area
- Palpate individually, from 12 o'clock to 3 o'clock area; 3 o'clock to 6 o'clock area; 6 o'clock to 9 o'clock area; 9 o'clock to 12 o'clock area

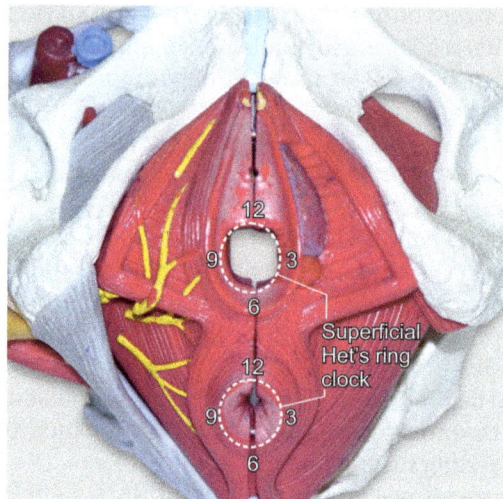

Fig. 5: Showing the orifice of superficial Het's ring clock, at transvaginal and transrectal opening in females only.

- Then ask patient to do pelvic floor exercise and measure palpable contractions and relaxation ability in above mentioned all areas
- You might notice one area different than other. It might be inability to contract or relax. It could be trigger points. It could be hypotonus or hypertonus muscles."
- This detailed examination will help you create plan of care in much more efficient way
- It will help you plan treatment with PF360 and manual therapy.

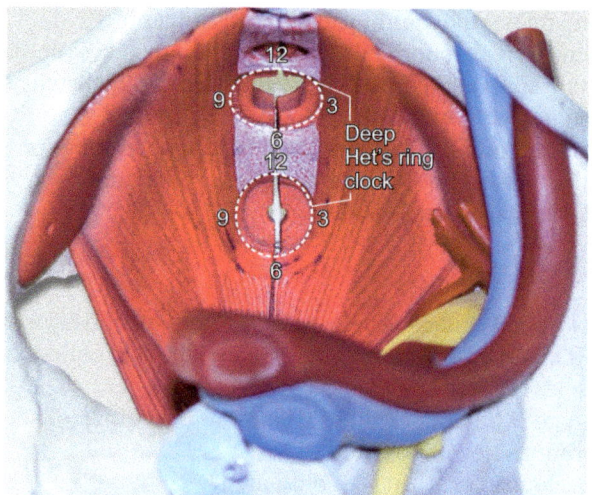

Fig. 6: Showing the orifice of deep Het's ring clock, at transvaginal and transrectal opening in females only.

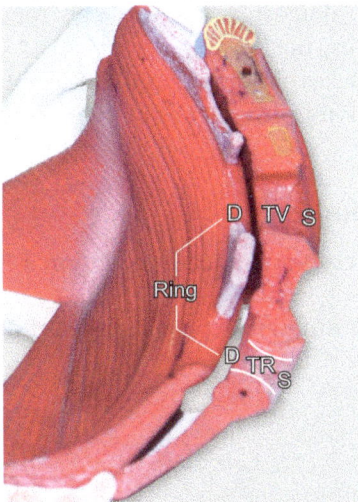

Fig. 7: Side section of Het's ring (skeletal muscle ring).

Assessment of Pelvic Floor Muscle Coordination

- Pelvic floor muscle coordination can be assessed by asking the patient to contract and relax quickly and slowly.
- Checking ability to relax quickly and completely.
- Checking for the time to reach maximum firm contraction, not sluggish, can also help to access coordination of PFMs and provides information about timing for fast twitch muscle fibers to respond.
- Progressive reduction of this timings (time taken to reach from completely relaxed state of PFM to completely firm state of squeezed PFM) on coughing like activities can help to gain better continence.

Urethrovesical Junction

Palpation periurethral muscles on each side of the urethra in 11 o'clock and 1 o'clock position can help to assess contractility and symmetry of the urethrovesical junction.

Transrectal Pelvic Floor Examination

- Preferred position for transrectal examination is left-lateral position. It enables examiners to perform transrectal examination and easily palpate puborectalis and external anal sphincter at rest and during PFM contraction.
- Properly lubricated index finger is introduced 3–4 cm through the anus to the rectum.
- Suggest patient to squeeze the finger as if she is trying to stop passing of gas. Sling-like puborectalis pulls the examiner's finger anteriorly.
- The puborectalis muscle swings around the anorectal junction, it pulls the junction forward. It is expected that both puborectalis and anal sphincter

to be relaxed during defecation and while instructing the patient to relax as if they are emptying the bowel.
- When the patient relaxes pelvic floor muscles examiner should feel opening of anal sphincter along with release of puborectalis posteriorly towards coccyx.

Ultrasound Examination

- You may also access your patient or client's PFM with ultrasound machine.
- Figures 8 and 9 are different types of state of PFM through abdominal sonography.

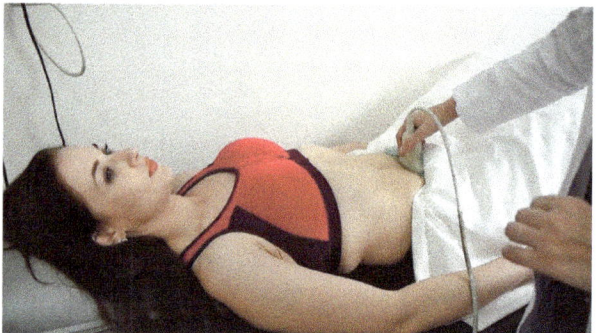

Fig. 8: Ultrasound of contracted versus relaxed muscles.

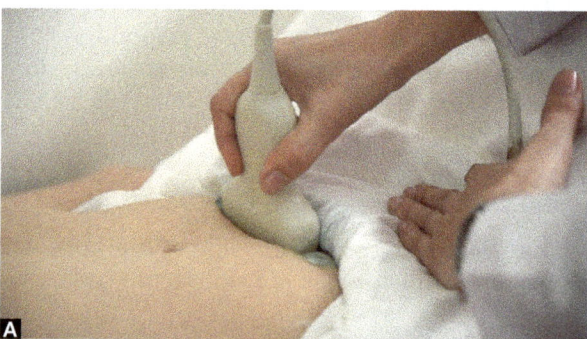

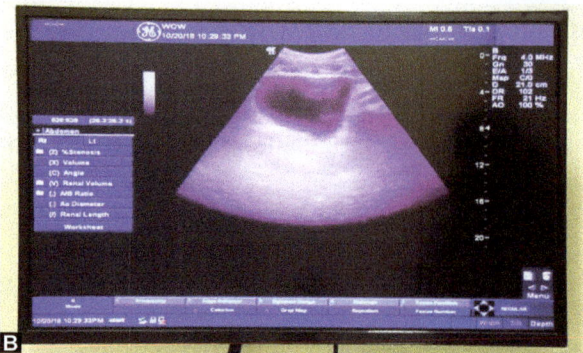

Figs. 9A and B: Ultrasonic pelvic floor muscle examination.

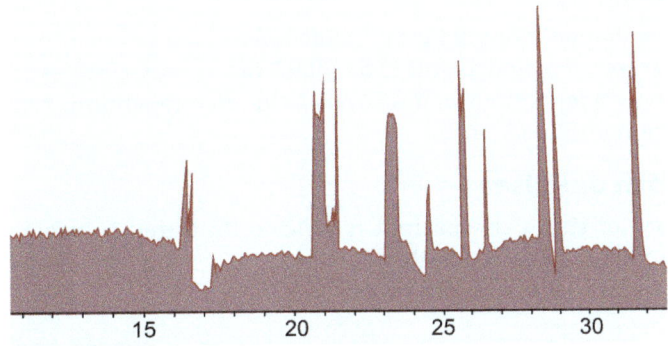

Fig. 10: EMG, patient—contracted muscles versus relaxed healthy muscles.

Electromyography Assessment

- EMG, patient—contracted muscles versus relaxed healthy muscles.
- You can also use EMG assessment of PFM by using surface electrodes at perianal junction, vaginal or rectal electrode.
- Provider can use EMG display to differentiate between too much or too less tone. However, it could be misguided due to sensitivity of EMG especially from use of accessory muscles (Fig. 10).

Het's ULTIMATE GOAL: FULL CURVE (FROM −3 TO 3, FROM COMPLETE RELAXATION TO COMPLETE CONTRACTION)

Het's SERF assessment scale.

- S Strength and relaxation: 3/-3
- E Endurance: 10 sec hold/relax
- R Repetition: 10/10 counts
- F Fast twitch: 10 pulses as fast as possible

Strength

- Ability to completely contract and completely relax
- Graph from 3 to −3
- It could be applied for contraction and relaxation both
- Suggests complete strength and relaxation of PFM.

Endurance

- Ability to hold PFM contraction for number of seconds (at the same strength level)
- For example, if muscle strength is 2/3; patient can hold it for 7 seconds. But the strength becomes 1/3 after first 4 seconds.
- Then the documented hold time should be 4 seconds only 4/10
- Suggest slow twitch muscle fibers.

Repetitions
- Number of repetitions at best possible hold.
- For example, if patient is able to do total 5 repetitions. However. She is able to do only 3 repetitions of 4 seconds hold, then repetitions range should be documented as 3/10.

Fast Twitch or Pulses
- Number of times the patient is able to do quick 1-2 seconds hold contractions as fast as possible.
- Suggests fast twitch muscle fibers.

Het's ASSESSMENT LEVEL FOR PELVIC FLOOR MUSCLE

Het's reflexive result scale (Het's RR scale)

Het Levels/Stages	Diagnosis	Current status of patient
1	Unintentional—unable	• Patient is unaware of PFM • Patient is unable to do proper PFM contractions
2	Intentional—unable	• Patient is aware about PFM • Patient is trying to do correct PFM contractions or relaxation. But unable to do
3	Intentional—partially able	• Patient is aware about PFM • Patient is trying her best to perform PFM complete contraction or relaxation. But can only do partial contractions or relaxation of PFM
4	Intentional—completely able	• Patient is aware about PFM • Patient is completely able to do isolated complete PFM contractions and relaxations • But cannot use them properly during functional activities
5	Intentional—functionally able	• Patient is aware to use PFM in functional activities and patient intentionally uses PFM contraction and relaxation during functional movements • But still it is not automatic yet
6	Final goal—reflexive activation/relaxation	• Patient automatically uses PFM contraction or relaxation during related functional activities. • Patient does not to try to do PFM activity intentionally. • However, later on patient realizes that they did it. In other words, now it has become subconscious reflexive behavior to use PFM

Het's assessment level–final goal: Reflexive activation.

Final goal: Reflexive activation of PFM—
- Patient automatically uses PFM contraction or relaxation during related functional activities
- Patient does not try to do PFM activity intentionally
- However, later on patient realizes that they did it. In other words, now it has become subconscious reflexive behavior to use PFM.

OTHER SCHOOL OF THOUGHTS

Harvard or Oxford Scale

- 0: No palpation
- 1: Trace
  - Flicker or feels like a pulsation
  - Not visible on inspection of perineum.
- 2: Poor
  - Asymmetrical muscle contraction on both sides.
  - Very slight pressure on examiner's finger.
- 3: Moderate
  - Symmetrical
  - Displacement of part of the finger in upward and forward direction
  - Visible on perineal surface.
- 4: Good
  - Symmetrical and circular pressure can be felt on examiner's finger
  - Elevation against slight resistance
  - Displacement of whole finger in upward and forward direction
  - Two fingers, index and middle placed laterally in the vagina and separated each side, contraction can squeeze them together—only without any resistance.
- 5: Strong
  - Symmetrical and circular pressure
  - Solid grip of full circumference compression of whole finger along with inward pull
  - Strong resistance can be given against elevation of the postvaginal wall
  - Approximation of index and middle fingers against vigorous resistance.

LAYCOCK QUANTITATIVE ASSESSMENT SCALE (PERFECT)

P = Power:
- Ask your patient to squeeze PFM trying to hold your finger inside.
- Based on oxford grading system from grade 0 to 5.
- Power is contributed by both fast and slow twitch muscle fibers.

E = Endurance:
- Ask your patient to hold PFM and measure hold time in seconds for which maximal vaginal contraction can be maintained up to 10 seconds.
- Measure number of seconds a patient can hold for PFM contraction before a drop of 50% of strength.
- Mainly reflects the activity of slow twitch muscle fibers.

R = Repetitions:
- Ask the patient to contract PFMs and hold the contractions for as long as possible.
- Repeat the contraction as many times as possible with limited rest in between.

- If the hold time decreases or power of the contraction is reduced by 50%, it is the time to stop assessment and number of repetitions should be recorded.

  For example, if patient can hold it for 6 seconds for maximal contraction of grade 4 and ask her to repeat the contractions. Now let us say she reaches 10 repetitions and the 11th repetition is either less than 6 seconds or less than grade 2, then her successful repetitions for that assessment are considered as 10 repetitions.
- HEP will greatly depend on number of good repetitions that are performed during PFM.
- If your pelvic floor rehabilitation (PFR) goal is to get 80 repetitions/day then for above-mentioned example you can teach patients to do Kegel exercises for 10 repetitions and 8 times a day.

F = Fast contractions:

- Mainly measures contractility of fast-twitch muscle fibers.
- Generally this stage of assessment is performed after 2 minutes of rest.
- Ask the patient to perform fast or quick PFM exercises.
- Hold for 1 or 2 seconds. Find the number of repetitions and record it.

Every Contraction Timed

- It is a reminder for provider to measure time for every contraction of PFMs.
- Adapted from Laycock and Jerwood, 2001.

MULTIPLE CHOICE QUESTIONS

Q1. All are the indications for transvaginal examination *except?*
- (a) Vaginal laxity
- (b) Incontinence
- (c) Prolapse
- (d) Severe pelvic pain

Q2. Excessive flexion at coccyx can commonly lead to _____ type of pelvic floor dysfunction.
- (a) Incoordination
- (b) Hypotonus
- (c) Hypertonus
- (d) Visceral

Q3. After how many weeks of surgery or delivery transvaginal examination is allowed?
- (a) 6 weeks
- (b) 1 week
- (c) 4 weeks
- (d) 6.5 weeks

Q4. What will be the Het's MMT grade of the pelvic floor muscle if it is able to partially relax or partially contract due to the presence of pain?
- (a) –1
- (b) 1
- (c) –2
- (d) 2

Q5. Assume that your pelvic floor are like elevator and this elevator is stuck between ground floor and basement and is unable to reach basement, what grade will it be on Het's MMT?
- (a) 0
- (b) –1
- (c) 1
- (d) –2

Q6. The grade of MMT according to Het's protocol ranges from_____.
   (a) 0 to 5
   (b) –3 to 0
   (c) 0 to 3
   (d) –3 to 3

Q7. What is the full form of SERF?
   (a) Strength and relaxation, endurance, repetition, fast twitch
   (b) Strength, endurance relaxation fast, twitch
   (c) Slow twitch, endurance, repetition, fatigue
   (d) Strength and relaxation, endurance, resting, fast twitch

Q8. When you are checking the endurance of the pelvic floor muscle by using Het's assessment scale, how much second hold will you expect to term it as a good endurance?
   (a) 1 seconds
   (b) 5 seconds
   (c) 8 seconds
   (d) 10 seconds

Q9. During transvaginal examination where is the pubococcygeus muscle palpated?
   (a) 3–5 cm beyond the vaginal introitus
   (b) Just inside the vaginal introitus
   (c) 1–2 cm beyond the vaginal introitus
   (d) 8 cm beyond the vaginal introitus

Q10. What is the final goal for pelvic floor rehab according to Het's assessment level?
   (a) Patient should be intentionally able to do activation of pelvic floor muscle
   (b) Patient is able to do reflexive activation of pelvic floor muscle
   (c) Both (a) and (b)
   (d) None of the above.

ANSWERS

1: (d) Severe pelvic pain
2: (c) Hypertonus
3: (a) 6 weeks
4: (c) –2
5: (b) –1
6: (d) –3 to 3
7: (a) Strength and relaxation, endurance, repetition, fast twitch
8: (d) 10 seconds
9: (a) 3–5 cm beyond the vaginal introitus
10: (b) Patient is able to do reflexive activation of pelvic floor muscle.

Chapter 5

Hypertonus Pelvic Floor Dysfunction (Vaginal Spasm and Health Issues)

"Give your stress wings and let it fly away."
—**Terri Guillemets**

"Are they too tight? Relax PFM."

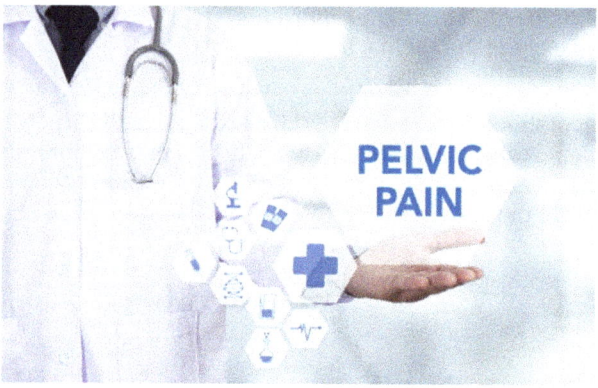

As discussed before if pelvic floor muscles tone becomes too high, spasmodic or if the muscles fail to relax, the condition is known as hypertonus type of pelvic floor muscle (PFM) dysfunction. Following are some of the conditions which can lead to increase in the tone of pelvic floor muscles spasms and tightness.

▮ PUDENDAL NEURALGIA

Pudendal nerve originates from sacral plexus with sensory and motor fibers. Neuralgia of pudendal nerve can lead to pain or irritation and leads to spasms of muscles. Sensory symptoms may extend in the groin, abdomen, legs and buttocks. Patient presents with pelvic pain in sitting but reports improvement with standing or sitting on toilet seat. Patient might also experience discomfort with tight clothing, frequent urination, dyspareunia, spasms after orgasm, etc.

▮ TENSION MYALGIA

Pain in the lower abdomen or pelvic area associated with back pain and heaviness in the perineum area. Presents with trigger points in pelvic floor, abdomen, back and hip or leg region.

COCCYDYNIA

Pain at the coccyx or tail bone. It may refer to pain and trigger points in pelvic floor, the coccygeus muscle and gluteus maximus muscles. Pain localized to coccyx and lower sacrum. It can also present spasm of levator ani and coccygeus. Ultimately, it can lead to pelvic floor muscle spasms.

LEVATOR ANI SYNDROME

Patient presents with history of childbirth injury, surgical trauma, lumbar disc surgery, pelvic infection, inflammation and habitual and postural pattern. Over activity of levator ani muscles from injury, disease or surgery. Patients present with pain, ache or pressure in the sacrum, coccyx, rectum, and pelvic diaphragm that may increase during sitting, urination, defecation, constipation and sexual intercourse. Pain may refer to the thigh, coccyx, sacrum, or gluteus region. Pain, pressure or discomfort in the region of rectum, sacrum and coccyx may be associated with pain in the gluteal region and thighs. History of pain for at least 12 weeks in last 12 months, chronic or recurrent rectal pain or aching and duration of pain 20 minutes or longer helps to diagnose levator ani syndrome.

PROCTALGIA FUGAX

Patient of proctalgia fugax presents with pain due to spasm of the anal sphincter/puborectalis. Patient may experience relief by sitting on the toilet and bearing down as if voiding feces. This type of bearing down can trigger the relaxation of PFM which can relax the anal sphincter.

HEMORRHOIDS

Hemorrhoids/piles: Swellings containing enlarged blood vessels found inside or around the bottom (rectum and anus) patient may present with bleeding after passing a stool—the blood is usually bright red itchy, anal area—a lump hanging down outside of the anus which may need to be pushed back in after passing a stool, a mucus discharge after passing a stool—soreness, redness, pain and swelling around anus.

Pelvic floor muscle weakness, constipation, straining during bowel movements and even straining during childbirth can also cause hemorrhoids.

ANISMUS

Spasms of external and internal anal sphincters which lead to inability to perform the rectal exam. It leads to difficult voiding and finally severe constipation.

PELVIC INFLAMMATORY DISEASE

Pelvic inflammatory disease means inflammation in the pelvic cavity. It can create scaring around fallopian tubes, which can lead to infertility and pelvic pain.

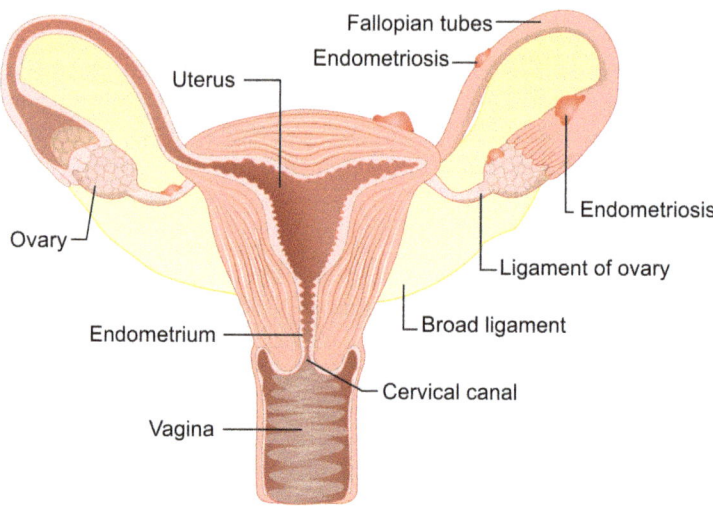

Fig. 1: Endometriosis.

ENDOMETRIOSIS

Definition: Endometriosis is the presence of functioning endometrium in the sites other than uterine mucosa (Fig. 1).

Tissues similar to uterine tissue is found outside the uterus, in the ovaries and fallopian tubes or surrounding the uterus. Adhesions are created from surgery, cesarean section (C section) or laparoscopy. Adhesions can be present on the bowel, intestines, bladder, colon, appendix and rectum. It can also be found inside vagina, cause is unknown. It can be exacerbated by estrogen. Patient presents with pelvic pain, dyspareunia, fatigue, painful periods, infertility, painful urination, abdominal cramps and severe spasm of pelvic floor muscles.

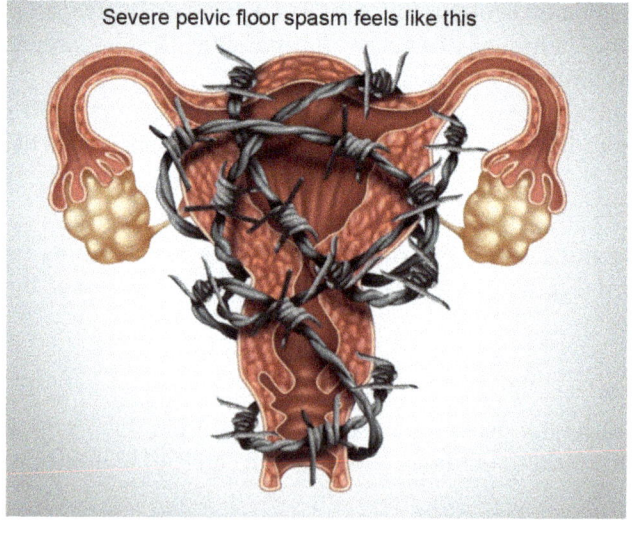

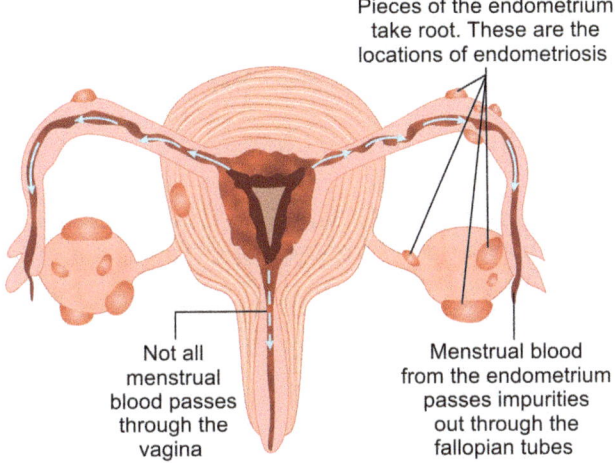

Fig. 2: The occurrence of endometriosis.

Abnormal bands of fibrous tissue lead to pelvic floor and organs stick together, resulting in bad environment for pelvic floor (PF), decreased circulation, tight muscles, myofascial adhesions and trigger points in abdominal and pelvic floor (Fig. 2).

COCCYGEUS-LEVATOR SPASM SYNDROME

Associated with pelvic floor muscle spasm along with rectal pain, tenderness on ischial spines and coccyx which can include involvement of musculofascial, ligamentous, and tendinous structures.

VULVODYNIA

Patient presents with burning, irritation, dryness, pain, dyspareunia and chronic vulvar discomfort due to pelvic floor muscle spasm. Inability to penetrate vaginal opening. Patient presents with low libido, difficulty inserting a tampon or speculum and reluctant to transvaginal exam. History of atrophic vaginitis, fistula or fissure and vulvar vestibulitis. Dehydrated vaginal tissues, less elastic vaginal tissues, pale vulvar tissues, surface electromyography (sEMG) resting above 2 mV.

VULVAR VESTIBULITIS

Patients present with severe pain, irritation and spasm localized to on vestibular touch or vaginal entry along with erythema in the vestibule and and bartholi's gland openings. It is associated with pelvic floor muscle spasm.

Definition: Friedreich's criteria. On internal vaginal exam, pain at vestibule 3–9 o'clock position; 2, 4, 6, 8 o'clock position; pain with vaginal penetration, erythema, dyspareunia, skin irritation and inflammation, increased urinary urgency and frequency; high resting surface (sEMG)—more than 2 mV multiple trigger points—in bulbocavernosus, superficial transverse perineal, levator ani, obturator internus.

INTERSTITIAL CYSTITIS

Also known as painful bladder syndrome (PBS) presents with pain or discomfort in the bladder and surrounding pelvic region. Chronic or severe inflammation of bladder wall.

Causes

1. Bladder trauma or over distention
2. Pelvic floor muscle dysfunction
3. Autoimmune disorders
4. Primary neurogenic inflammation
5. Spinal cord trauma
6. Genetics or heredity
7. Allergy.

Symptoms

Patient presents with urinary urgency, frequency, retention, dyspareunia, back pain, suprapubic pain, abdominal pain, nocturia; pain before, during or after urination and incontinence. Pain in pelvis or between the vagina and anus in women. Pain between the scrotum and anus in men (perineum) and chronic pelvic pain. A persistent, urgent need to urinate. Frequent urination often of small amounts, throughout the day and night (up to 60 times a day). Pain or discomfort while the bladder fills and relief after urinating. Pain during sexual intercourse and flexed posture. Hypertonus pelvic floor muscles and myofascial restrictions.

URETHRAL SYNDROME

Patient presents with urethral pain, burning and sensitivity which can be associated with spasm of pelvic floor muscles.

URGENCY-FREQUENCY SYNDROME

Patient presents with urinary frequency, retention, urgency, with or without pain in urethra, bladder, abdomen and pelvis. It can result in irritation and development of trigger points in pelvic floor which can lead to shortening and tightening of pelvic floor muscles which creates even intense pain and irritation along with muscle imbalance. Patient can get an urge to frequently go for urination due to irritation and ultimately patient tries to "hold it in" which results in tightening of the pelvic floor muscles. Even the muscles around the bladder tighten and produce the urge even when the bladder is not full. Hypertonous pelvic floor creates a vicious cycle of pain and tightness.

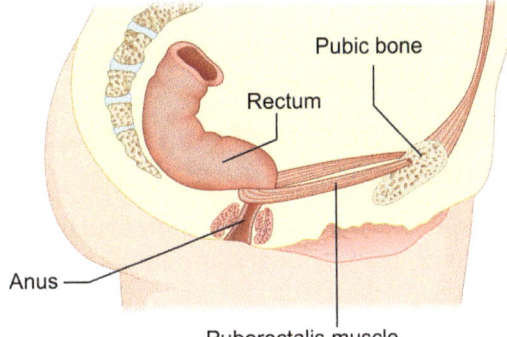

Fig. 3: Too tight puborectalis muscle can lead to pain and or constipation.

HYPERTONUS PELVIC FLOOR MUSCLE

- Difficulty starting urine stream
- Weak stream
- Incomplete emptying of the bladder
- Overactive bladder symptoms
- Constipation, hemorrhoids, fissures
- Dyspareunia.

CONSTIPATION

Too tight or too weak pelvic floor muscles dysfunction can lead to constipation. Abdominal trigger point release can help (Fig. 3).

INFLAMMATORY BOWEL DISEASE

Crohn's disease is an inflammation of the digestive tract located between mouth and anus. Mostly affects small intestine, ileum. Ulcerative colitis is an inflammation of thin lining of the large intestine, colon and rectum. It can result in ulcer. Patient presents with abdominal pain, rectal bleeding, diarrhea, fever, weight loss, and arthritis and skin problems.

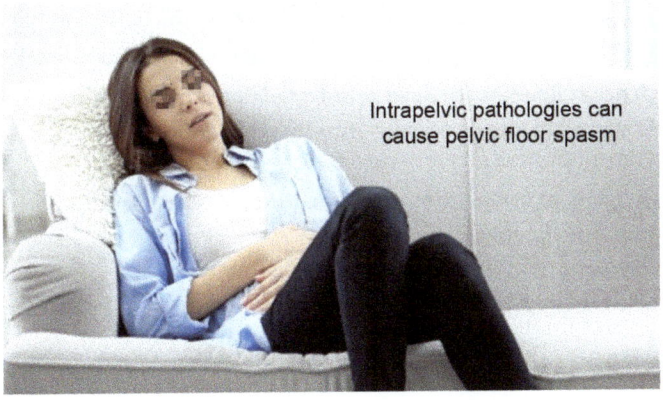

Intrapelvic pathologies can cause pelvic floor spasm

IRRITABLE BOWEL SYNDROME

Patients present with abdominal pain, bloating, gas, frequent bowel movements, diarrhea and/or constipation.

VICIOUS CYCLE: PELVIC FLOOR MUSCLE PAINFUL TIGHTNESS AND ANXIETY

- Too tight PFM creates pain during penetration as they fail to relax.
- When it happens repeatedly, patient starts anticipating pain even before penetration.
- As a result, emotional anxiety of anticipation of pain can cause more spasms or tightness of PFM.
- Similarly, spasmodic or over tight PFM creates more pain and causes more anxiety.
- This becomes vicious cycle.
- Proper patient education, PFM relaxation training, anxiety management, improved PFM blood circulation helps to break this vicious cycle.

SUMMARY

All above mentioned pathologies can lead to chronic irritation or reflexive spasm of pelvic floor muscles due to increased toxins in the gut. In a long run, multiple trigger points are created, which leads to increase spasms of pelvic floor muscles. Pain and spasm of pelvic floor might refer to low back, leg and buttock area. Chronic tightness, multiple trigger points, myofascial adhesions and spasm of PFM leads to inability for them to relax.

MULTIPLE CHOICE QUESTIONS

Q1. Which neuralgia causes hypertonus pelvic floor dysfunction?
- (a) Iliac neuralgia
- (b) Pudendal neuralgia
- (c) Meralgia paresthetica
- (d) Pelvic neuralgia

Q2. The sensory symptoms of pudendal neuralgia can extend up to_____.
- (a) Groin, buttocks, abdomen
- (b) Groin, buttocks, left hand
- (c) Groin, buttocks, right foot
- (d) Groin, abdomen, left thigh

Q3. Which pelvic floor muscles can get affected due to coccydynia?
- (a) Levator ani and coccygeus muscle
- (b) Gluteal muscle
- (c) Obturator internus muscle
- (d) Piriformis

Q4. Which ligament divides the greater sciatic and lesser sciatic foramen?
- (a) Inguinal ligament
- (b) Sacrospinous and sacrotuberous ligaments
- (c) Iliofemoral ligament
- (d) Supraspinous ligament

Q5. Presence of functioning endometrium at places other than uterine mucosa is known as:
  (a) Endometriosis
  (b) Interstitial cystitis
  (c) Vestibulitis
  (d) Vulvodynia

Q6. If the patient has complaint of frequent urination (50–60 times a day) along with complain of pain during and after urination and also has perineal pain at the area between vagina and anus it can be due to:
  (a) Endometriosis
  (b) Interstitial cystitis
  (c) Vestibulitis
  (d) Coccydynia

Q7. If a patient complains of hemorrhoids and has longstanding constipation most probably them might be suffering from:
  (a) Incoordination
  (b) Hypotonus dysfunction
  (c) Hypertonus dysfunction
  (d) All of the above

Q8. What is the other name of spasm of puborectalis which can even lead to rectal pain and painful defecation?
  (a) Proctalgia fugax
  (b) Vestibulitis
  (c) Anismus
  (d) Levator ani syndrome

Q9. Irritable bladder syndrome if present for a long time can result into which type of pelvic floor dysfunction?
  (a) Hypotonus
  (b) Hypertonus
  (c) Incoordination
  (d) All of the above

ANSWERS

1: (b) Pudendal neuralgia
2: (a) Groin, buttocks, abdomen
3: (a) Levator ani and coccygeus muscle
4: (b) Sacrospinous and sacrotuberous ligaments
5: (a) Endometrosis
6: (b) Interstitial cystitis
7: (c) Hypertonus dysfunction
8: (a) Proctalgia fugax
9: (b) Hypertonus

Chapter 6

Hypotonus Pelvic Floor Dysfunction (Vaginal Laxity and Health Issues)

"I bet you're worried. I was worried. I was worried about vaginas. I was worried about what we think about vaginas, and even more worried that we don't think about them."

—**Eve Ensler**

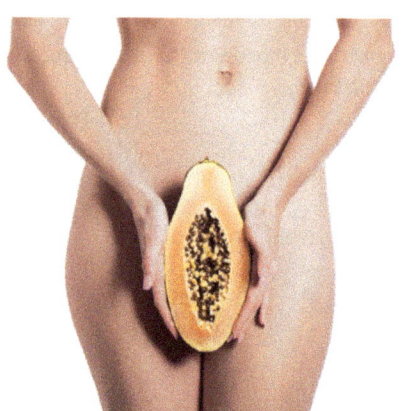

Vaginal laxity may start postnatal

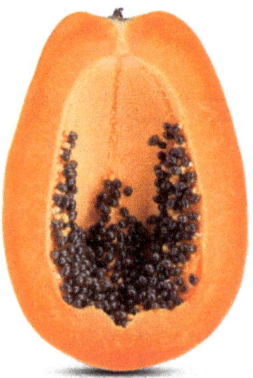

With age, it keeps getting worst..

Hypotonus Pelvic Floor Dysfunction (Vaginal Laxity and Health Issues)

INTRODUCTION

Hypotonus pelvic floor muscle (PFM) is too loose, weak, or overly stretched PFM.

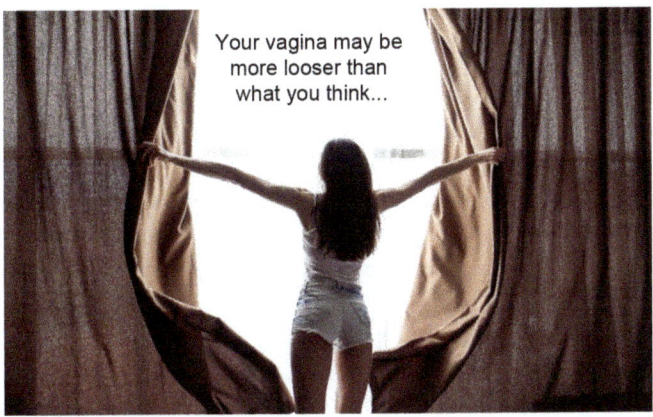

CAUSES OF HYPOTONUS PELVIC FLOOR MUSCLE

Most of the women are not aware that their vagina becomes weak, loose, or dysfunctional. Following are the reasons which can cause hypotonus pelvic floor muscles (Fig. 1):
- Inadequate—under use of these muscles/disuse atrophy
- Vaginal laxity after pregnancy and childbirth
- Change in hormones due to menopause
- Decreased muscle tone due to aging

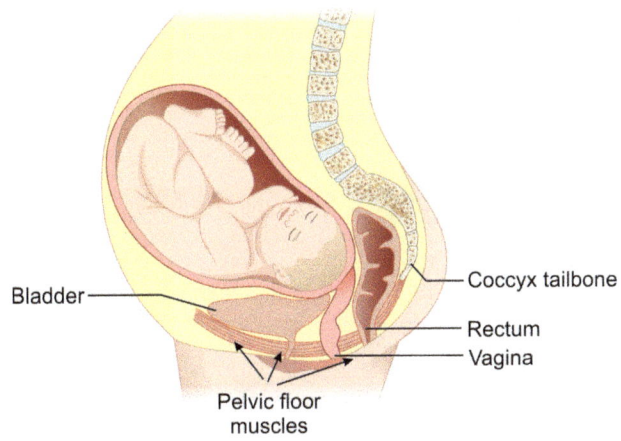

Pregnancy takes a toll on the vagina and the pelvic floor muscle causing a weakening in the pelvic msucles and vaginal loosening

Fig. 1: Location of pelvic floor muscle.

- Straining because of chronic constipation
- Straining associated with a chronic cough
- Overweight or obesity
- Diseases or surgery in pelvic region
- Pregnancy
- Labor
- Childbirth
- Emergency cesarean section (C-section) (where patient has already gone through straining of pelvic floor muscles)
- Planned C-section (has less odds to damage PFM as labor and vaginal birth trauma/straining is not there; however we cannot overlook the fact of weight gain during pregnancy, which strains PFM)
- Overweight/weight gain
- Poor posture
- Sedentary lifestyle
- Too much passive stretching, (too thick male genital organs) through sexual activity.

PREGNANCY, LABOR, CHILDBIRTH, AND VAGINAL LAXITY (FIGS. 2A AND B)

What happens to pelvic floor muscle (PFM) during pregnancy, labor, and childbirth?

- Pregnancy
- Vaginal delivery
  - *Perineal tear*: First degree to fourth degree
  - Episiotomy:
    - Midline incision
    - Mediolateral incision
- Obstetric fistula
- C-section:
  - Planned C-section
  - Emergency C-section

(C-section: cesarean section)

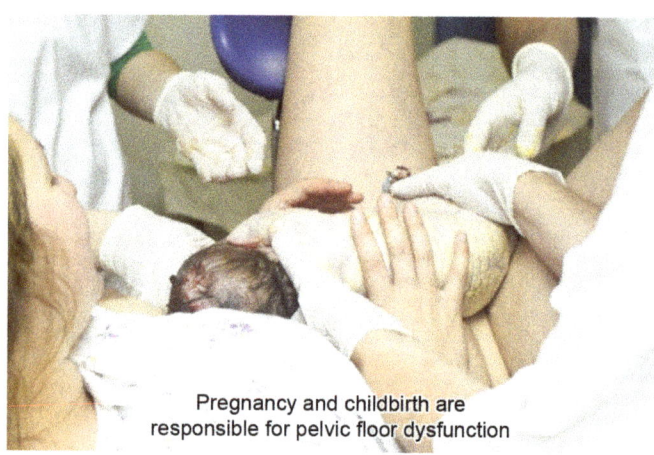

Pregnancy and childbirth are responsible for pelvic floor dysfunction

Hypotonus Pelvic Floor Dysfunction (Vaginal Laxity and Health Issues)

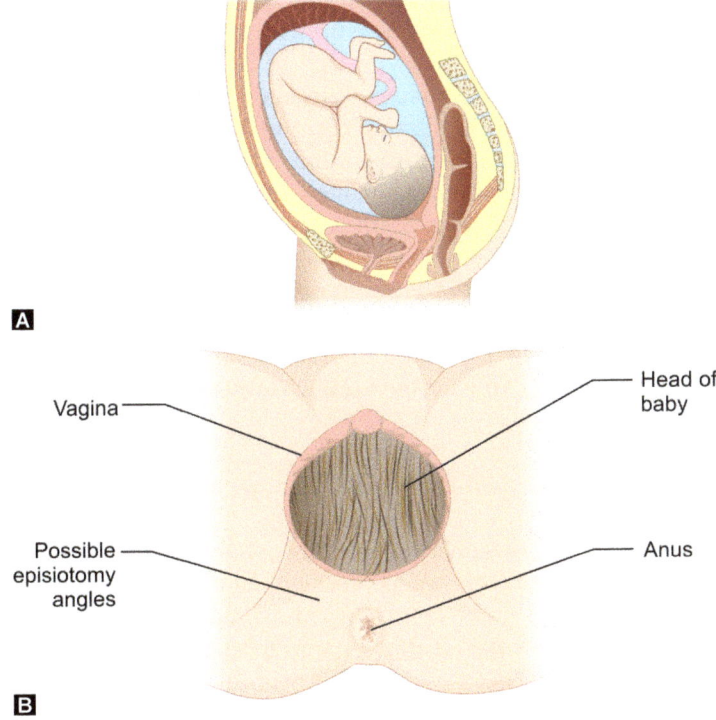

Figs. 2A and B: Pregnancy, childbirth can lead to vaginal laxity.

What Happens to PFM During Pregnancy, Labor, and Childbirth?

- *Pregnancy and labor:*
  - Pregnancy leads to maternal weight gain, anterior tilt of pelvis, complete change of body posture, hormonal changes, laxity of ligaments, and too much pressure on PFM.
  - High progesterone level during pregnancy helps to reduce the tone in ureters, bladder, and urethra as it helps to relax the smooth muscles.
  - Relaxin hormone modifies connective tissue to allow for appropriate stretching during vaginal birth.
  - These specific hormonal changes allow dense connective tissue to soften
  - About 85% women suffer from urinary incontinence during pregnancy.
  - If you stretch an elastic rubber for 9 months, it will be loose and might lose its elasticity; similar is true with PFM.
  - During labor, a woman is likely to spend hours pushing and straining PFM.
  - Prolonged labor is damaging to PFM.
- *Vaginal delivery:*
  - The fetal head descends through the curve of sacrum and coccyx, and reaches pelvic floor.

- The pressure dilates vagina and stretches the perineum.
- The skull of baby and resistance from mother's pelvic bone can really crush PFM and soft tissue.
- The PFM, connective tissues, and even nerves undergo vigorous stretching, straining, and trauma during delivery.
- Vaginal delivery can be most traumatic event to the PFM. Different degree of vaginal tear during delivery could be even more traumatic.
- It also separates the levator ani muscle and displaces it on the sides and downward.
- Snooks et al., 1984 and Sorensen et al., 1988 suggested that stretching and straining PFM, especially forceps delivery, can damage the innervations of PFMs, which ultimately can lead to urinary or fecal incontinence. It can lead to vascular damage, overstretched or torn muscle fibers.

Perineal tear:
- Many times, perineal tissues are torn, which may lead to multiple degrees of tear.
    1. *First-degree tear*—involves only mucosa and skin, e.g. the fourchette.
    2. *Second-degree tear*—affects some or all of the superficial perineal muscles. Tear may extend up to one or both side of vaginal wall.
    3. *Third-degree tear*—all above + anal sphincter.
    4. *Fourth-degree tear*—more severity of third-degree tear extending through rectal mucosa.
- Research says that a mother demonstrates 50% of reduction of strength of PFM after childbirth.
  Postnatal larger diameter of vaginal opening and weaker PFM is very obvious. Vagina becomes looser and more open. In other words, postnatal vaginal laxity is very obvious.

Episiotomy:
- An incision of the perineal body and vagina with a purpose to enlarge the vaginal opening and facilitate childbirth.
- **Midline incision:**
    » The incision is made through the central tendinous portion of the perineal body.
    » The incision is also made through bulbocavernosus (BC) muscles.
    » It can increase the risk of third- or fourth-degree tears in spontaneous delivery and PFD.
- **Mediolateral incision:**
    » Incision is made through BC, transverse perineal muscle, and levator ani muscles.
    » Risk of extensive tear is reduced but can lead to poor healing and PFD. The severe pain due to episiotomy can lead to dyspareunia, hypertonus type of PFD.
    » Sometimes episiotomy is required to avoid uncontrollable tears. No doubt, postepisiotomy or postsuturing, the vaginal tissues and PFM can heal completely but it does not get stronger on its own.

- **Obstetric fistula:**
  - It is also known as obstructed labor, where the head of the baby constantly pushes against the pelvic bone of mother during contractions. It prevents blood flow to the pelvis and causes a tissue death and hole between the vagina and the bladder or vagina and the rectum. It is known as "fistula". It leads to severe urinary and bowel incontinence.
- **C-section:**
  - Cesarean section is a surgical method of delivering baby under epidural or general anesthesia.
  - There can be two categories of C-sections:
    1. *Planned C-section*: If C-section is previously planned, it is likely to reduce strain of PFM due to prolonged labor. However, still patients might present with PFD due to all body changes and load bearing during pregnancy.
    2. *Emergency C-section*: If patient undergoes prolonged labor and C-section is done as an emergency, prolonged pushing and straining are likely to cause more damage to PFM. Almost like vaginal delivery.

SUMMARY

In summary, pregnancy, labor, and childbirth can create overstretching, tearing, compression, and crushing of PFM, which can lead to vaginal laxity or different types of PFD. They can heal on its own over the period of time. However, they do not get stronger on its own. There is a big difference between healing and getting stronger. Healing could be a natural body response. But PF Rehab has a vital role to get them stronger.

- According to Lien et al., pubococcygeus (PC) muscles, especially the most medial part of it, bear the largest stretching up to 3.26 times its original length.
- C-section is also not a solution to prevent PFD. It can reduce the risk of PFD but cannot totally prevent it.
- It is also believed that muscle stretching in combination of additional weight of the baby, increased body mass index, and hormonal changes can significantly lead to PFM laxity. However, further research is needed.
- Antenatal exercises can help to reduce postpartum stress urinary incontinence.
- Obese or overweight women are at higher risk of PFD or urinary incontinence during pregnancy and during postpartum.

VAGINAL LAXITY

Vaginal laxity is more common and more intense than what we can imagine. Our research says: Nine out of ten mothers face vaginal laxity. Progressively, it worsens with age. Vaginal laxity is misnomer and it is most commonly misunderstood. Vaginal laxity is not caused by an intrinsic problem within the vagina. Vaginal laxity is caused by weakened PFM which fails to provide optimal vaginal support or vaginal grip. Real terminology of vaginal laxity should be PFM laxity.

Causes

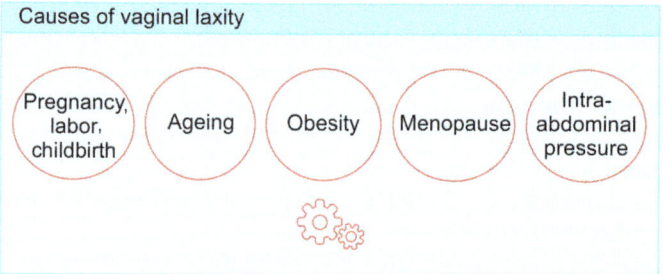

Causes of vaginal laxity

- Pregnancy, labor, and childbirth
- Obesity
- Disuse PFM
- Passive stretching of PFM
- Too much or too long sexual activities in multiple positions that can lead to mechanical stretching
- Sexual activities with sexual partner who has obese penis (thicker penis) or penetration from multiple angles. For example, if a male partner has obese penis and the size of the pelvis of female partner is small-to-medium.
- Constipation or bearing down activities.

Clinical Features

Laxity of superficial PFM between the vagina and anus. These muscles become flabby, weak, and atrophied. PFM at anorectal junction might remain strong. In other words, patient might not have any problems with fecal incontinence, etc. Only PFM at urogenital triangle might be looser compared to anorectal triangle.
- Vaginal laxity leads to widened and loose vaginal opening
- Decreased distance between vagina and anus
- Change is vaginal axis (normally, vaginal angulation should be downward toward the sacrum, in many cases the vaginal angulation becomes upward oriented).
- Looseness of vagina
- Gapping in vagina
- Less satisfying intercourse compared to before
- Difficult or delayed orgasms compared to before
- Reduced vaginal sensations
- Difficulty in retaining tampons
- Difficulty in holding penis tightly during intercourse: With vaginal laxity, vagina only provides surroundings to the penis friction, instead of holding penis tightly, which negatively affects sensations.
- *Vaginal flatulence*: Sometimes the air enters the vagina due to vaginal/PFM laxity. It can create noise and can be very embarrassing situation.
- Low self-esteem and low confidence.

Consequences of Vaginal Laxity

Vaginal laxity or PFM weakness leads to following women's health issues:
- Urinary incontinence

- POP—pelvic organ prolapse
- FSD—female sexual health issues

Urinary Incontinence (Figs. 3A and B)

Urinary incontinence (UI) is involuntary and unwanted loss of urine. More than 17 million adult American suffer from it. Cost to manage UI is approximately around $28 billion per year.

Definition: Urinary incontinence is involuntary loss of urine, which is objectively demonstrable and can cause hygienic, personal, or social inconvenience for activities of daily living.

Pathophysiology of Urinary Incontinence

- The rise of the intravesical pressure over that of maximum pressure of urethra. It could be due to trauma, surgery, childbirth, aging, weak pelvic floor muscles, and overactive detrusor.

Types of urinary incontinence

- SUI—stress urinary incontinence
- UUI-OAB—urge urinary incontinence–overactive bladder
- MI—mixed urinary incontinence
- OI—overflow incontinence.

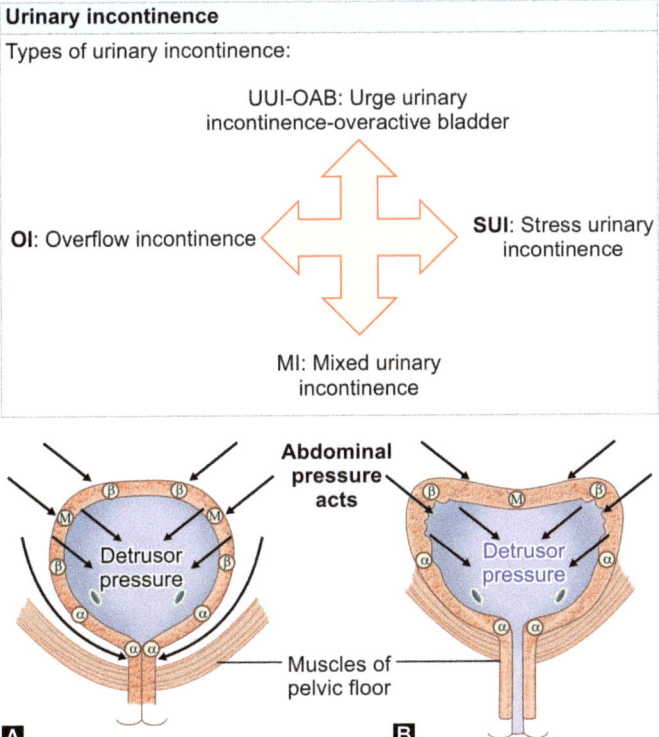

Figs. 3A and B: Urinary incontinence (UI).

Courtesy: DC Dutta's Textbook of Gynecology, Edited by Dr Hiralal Konar, New Delhi, Jaypee Brothers Medical Publishers, 2016; p328

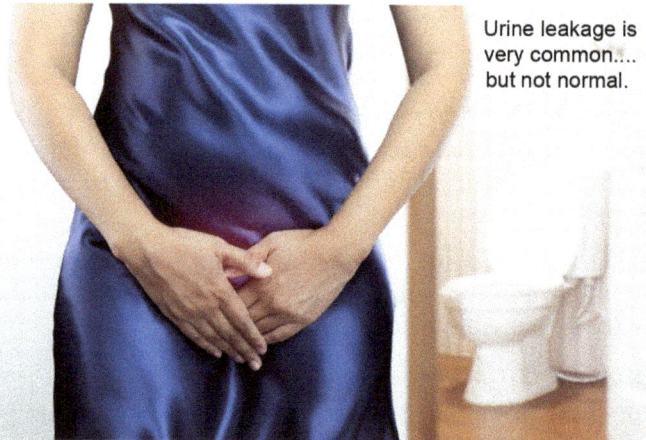

Stress Urinary Incontinence

- Stress urinary incontinence is involuntary loss of urine due to increase in intra-abdominal pressure.
- Primary cause is weakness of pelvic floor muscles which could be caused by multiple childbirth, estrogen deficiency, or trauma to external urinary sphincter during childbirth.

Clinical features: Urinary incontinence during coughing, laughing, sneezing, lifting, exercise, and physical exertion.

Genuine Stress Incontinence (Fig. 4)

- According to International Continence Society (ICS), GSI is defined as involuntary urethral loss of urine when the intravesical pressure exceeds the maximum urethral pressure in the absence of detrusor activity.
- Incidence is as high as 40% in association with pelvic organ prolapse.

Mechanics: Normally, the bladder neck and the proximal urethra are intra-abdominal located above the pelvic floor muscles in standing position. The

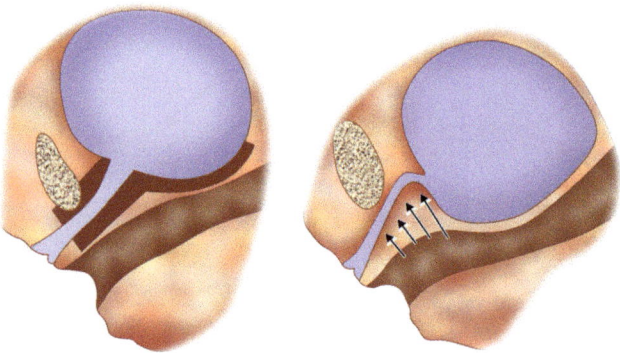

Fig. 4: Kinking of the urethra during stress pulling the bladder neck upward and forward.
Courtesy: DC Dutta's Textbook of Gynecology, Edited by Dr Hiralal Konar, New Delhi, Jaypee Brothers Medical Publishers, 2016; p328

urethral pressure is more than the intravesical pressure. Descent of the bladder neck and the proximal urethra leads to rise in the intraurethral pressure in standing.

Risk Factors
- Childbirth trauma to pelvic floor muscles
- Developmental weakness
- Functionally raised progesterone due to pregnancy
- Trauma to pubic symphysis
- Postmenopausal estrogen deficiency
- Body mass index (BMI): More than 30 indicated obesity
- Aging
- Genuine stress incontinence is closely associated with urethral hypermobility and urethral diverticulum.

Clinical Features
- Urinary incontinence during coughing, sneezing, laughing, jumping, and exercising
- Symptoms are not associated with urge
- Rarely occurs during sleep or supine position mainly in standing.

Tests
- Stress test: Small amount of urine loss from external urethral meatus when patient is asked to cough. Urine loss may not happen during supine, but happens in standing position.
- Pad test:
  - Patient is suggested to wear sanitary pad for an hour, drink about 500 mL water, and rest for 15 minutes. Then let patient perform exercise like walk or stair climb for 30 minutes. Then get them do activities like coughing, jumping, and bending for 15 minutes. Weigh the sanitary pad after the period of 1 hour. An increase in weight by 1 g means significant UI.
- Bladder diary: Suggest patients to record her fluid intake, output, leakage episodes in relation to time and activity. Do it for 3 days which will give an idea about daily urine output, frequency, and bladder capacity.

Grades of Genuine Incontinence
- Grade 1—incontinence on cough or sneeze
- Grade 2—incontinence with mild exercise
- Grade 3—incontinence even by changing posture.

Urge incontinence—Urinary Incontinence:
Urinary incontinence (UI) is urge incontinence because of detrusor muscle overactivity, especially common in elderly group. There are two major types of urge incontinence:
1. OAB—overactive bladder—detrusor overactivity
2. Sensory urge incontinence.

Urge urinary incontinence–overactive bladder (detrusor overactivity): Urge urinary incontinence (UUI) is a urine loss associated with sudden and strong desire to void. It can be provoked by involuntary bladder spasms. The International Continence Society has defined OAB as "bladder contracts spontaneously or on provocation during filling phase while patient is attempting to inhibit micturition."

Cause:
- *Hyper-reflexia of detrusor muscles*: Overactivity of detrusor muscles which can be due to central nervous system (CNS) disorders like stroke, Parkinson's disease, Alzheimer's disease, brain tumor, aneurysm, spinal cord injury, or conditions like cystitis, urethritis, tumors, stones, atrophic vaginitis, outflow obstruction, urinary tract infection (UTI), impaired bladder contractility, etc.
- Psychosomatic origin related to anxiety and stress
- Idiopathic
- Postsurgical
- Movement-associated hyperactivity of detrusor even stimulated by movements like sit to stand or transfer activities.

Pathophysiology: Possible increase in alpha-adrenergic activities which causes increased detrusor activities; it creates identical situation of normal micturition which means relaxation of pelvic floor and urethral muscles followed by detrusor contractions.

Reflex incontinence: Older adults may have overactive bladder, but they do not empty their bladder completely which causes chronic urine retention which leads to decreased urge sensation.

Clinical features:
- Loss of urine before getting to bathroom.
- Urgency—sudden urge and unintentional voiding before reaching bathroom.
- Frequency—more than ten times in 24 hours.
- Nocturia—awakening in night more than one or more times due to urge.
- Nocturnal enuresis—incontinence during sleep, volume of urine loss in a few hundred milliliters, incontinence in any position.
- Generally, urge leads to incontinence which is triggered by events like sound of running water or cold weather. "Key in the lock" or "garage door syndrome"—strong urge as soon as coming home even if the bladder was recently emptied.

Types of Urinary Incontinence

1. *Overactive bladder:*
    - Urinating approximately eight times daily and twice a night or more.
    - *PFM—bladder reflex*: Voluntarily.
    - The bladder muscles are relaxed during urine storage and urinary sphincters and PFM are contracted.

Hypotonus Pelvic Floor Dysfunction (Vaginal Laxity and Health Issues)

- The bladder muscles contract and the PFM relax during emptying.
- *PFM*: Bladder reflex creates relaxation of the bladder muscles when a person voluntarily contracts the PFM.

2. *Sensory UI:*
   - Urinary incontinence at strong urge.
   - It is not associated with detrusor contraction until urinary contraction is initiated.
   - It occurs without any anatomic descent of bladder neck or urethra.

Tears shed for self are tears of weakness, but tears shed for others are a sign of strength.
—**Billy Graham**

Tears shed down your pants when you laugh hard are a sign of pelvic floor weakness.

Hypermobile urethra:
- Weak PFM and connective tissues fail to provide adequate support to the urethra.
- As a result, urethra gets pushed down and out of position at times of sudden rise in intra-abdominal pressure, which is known as urethral hypermobility.
- Approximately 2% of women report SUI during 3rd month of pregnancy and 50% of women at full-term.
- Pelvic floor muscle rehabilitation can improve urethral support and diminish urethral hypermobility.

Urethral diverticulum:
- A small sac—like out-pouching from the urethra is known as urethral diverticulum. It can fillup with urine and leak during activities.

Difference between UUI and SUI.		
Points	UUI	SUI
Volume	UUI—large volume of leakage	SUI—reasonably small amount of leakage happens
Associated with	UUI is associated with strong urgency	SUI is associated with increased intra-abdominal pressure
Causes	UUI—involuntary bladder contractions	SUI—weak pelvic floor and weak support of urethra
Predictability	UUI is more unpredictable	SUI is somewhat predictable
For mixed	SUI +	UUI—manage major problem first

Mixed urinary incontinence: Mixed UI is combination of UUI and SUI.

Overflow incontinence (OI): It is urine incontinence due to overdistended bladder because of obstruction of the urethra. Bladder can not empty completely because of obstruction, which leads to urine retention. Bladder becomes overdistended, which results in OI. It could be urinary dribbling or constant leakage of small amount of urine.

That happens due to:
- Cystocele
- Bowel impaction
- Urethral stricture
- Hypotonicity of detrusor muscles in patients with diabetes mellitus or spinal cord injury.

Clinical features:
- Incontinence in small amounts
- Suprapubic tenderness
- Reduced urine stream
- Palpable bladder
- Interrupted urine flow
- Postvoid dribbling
- Difficulty or straining to void
- Sensation of incomplete voiding
- Sensation of bladder fullness.

RESEARCH AND STATISTICS FOR URINARY INCONTINENCE

Research: One out of two every young moms, as young as 25 years, is likely to have vaginal laxity. Vaginal laxity is to be most common physical concern discussed with obstetrician-gynecologist (ob-gyns) after childbirth.
- Vaginal laxity can occur naturally with aging.
- Good pelvic floor tone, strength, and ability to contract this muscle can improve vaginal sensations during intercourse including feelings of tightness, orgasmic response, and the pleasure for both partners.

Vaginal looseness and urine leakage (infographics):
- Research says that "urinary incontinence affects more than 30 million American adults" which means it is not only you who suffers from urine leakage.
- According to research "one in two women over age of 18 experiences involuntarily urine leakage. Urge urine leakage happens more frequently in women than in men, especially in women age 44 or older. and, there is a marked rise in urge incontinence in women 64 and older. It is opposite to stress incontinence, which is more common in women under 50."
  That means every other woman you meet is likely to be having urine leakage problems.
- One-third of women age 30–70 have experienced loss of bladder control at some time in their life.
- As per research "on an average, women wait for six and a half years until they start any form of treatment". That means most women just try to ignore the problem. They wait till the time it gets worse before they look for solution!
- Research says "two-thirds of women who have experienced loss of bladder control do not use any form of treatment", which means they just try to learn to live with the problems instead of looking for the solution.

One study showed that, "on an average, women with urine leakage spend more than $1,000 per year on diapers, pads, laundry, etc." "Once, cost of urinary incontinence just in America was $19 billion", which means most women spend all this money just to hide or cover up the problem instead of treating them.

- "American Academy of Family Physician declared that urinary incontinence is more prevalent issue than even diabetes or asthma for primary care physicians" which means its a huge quality of life conern. However, most women suffer silently.
- "Overweight and obesity" make it more challenging for urine control. Loosing only 5% of body weight can significantly improve symptoms of urinary leakage.
- According to study by the National Institute of Health, "women who lost 8% of body weight, or about 17 pounds of weight, reduced their leakage by 50%", which means more you loose extra body fat, more you are likely to keep a good urine control.
- According to research, "urine leakage problem affects 33% of women aged 45-64 years and 24% of women aged 25-44 experience urinary incontinence", which means women of all ages are at risk of urine leakage.
- Sooner you start treating urine leakage problems, faster you get success with the treatments.
- According to agency of healthcare research and policy, "eight out of ten women with urinary incontinence, symptoms can be improved", which means if you try to treat urine leakage, you are likely to get fantastic results.
- According to research, "pelvic floor muscle is often suggested as an effective and highly recommended first-line of treatment for women with stress incontinence", which means training vaginal muscle for tightening should be the priority for every woman and mother.
- Studies show that "pelvic floor muscle retraining alone has an average cure rate of 73%, if combined with other conservative therapies, the average cure rate is very high up to 97%".
- Research suggests that "women who follow pelvic floor muscle retraining program correctly and faithfully have much higher success rate than women who do not", which means success of urine leakage problem depends on your consistent efforts.
- According to research by American Urogynecologic Society, biofeedback cured 22% of women with urinary incontinence and decreased the symptoms for 43% of the women.
- Research says that conservative treatments are highly effective in treating urge incontinence. However, sooner treatments are more effective later. Because of the effects of aging, gravity and behavioral issues worsen with time.
- According to NOBLE (National Overactive Bladder Evaluation) study, more than 50% of women with overactive bladder leak urine.
- Research says that "at least 70% of women report an improvement of urge incontinence symptoms from Kegel and other physical rehabilitation programs", which means surgery is not the only option or priority.

- The American Urogynecologic Society states that biofeedback is generally effective in improving urinary incontinence for 43% of women.

PELVIC ORGAN PROLAPSE (*SEE* FIG. 8)

- *Think about it*: According to evolution theory, we were evolved over the period of time from four legs to two legs. In other words, PFMs were built by God to function in elimination of gravity. When we evolved to two legs of standing position, PFMs are required to work against gravity in order to function and provide supportive functions (Fig. 5).
- Many different types of physical activities lead to increased abdominal pressure. It generates intense downward pressure against pelvic floor muscles (Fig. 6).
- Increased downward pressure along with gravity in the presence of vaginal laxity or weakness of PFM increases the risk of POP (Fig. 7).

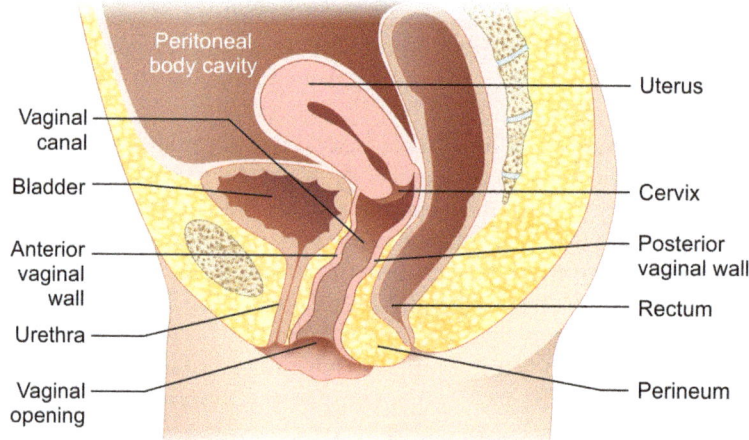

Fig. 5: Anatomy of female.

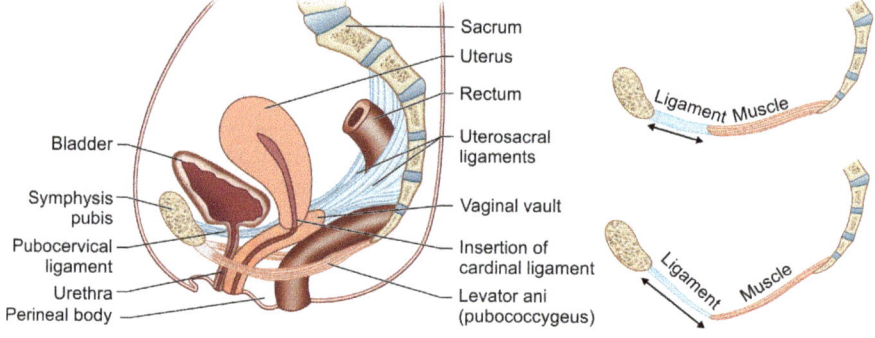

Fig. 6: Pelvic floor weakness, stretched ligaments and prolapse.

Courtesy: DC Dutta's Textbook of Gynecology, Edited by Dr Hiralal Konar, New Delhi, Jaypee Brothers Medical Publishers, 2016; p167

Hypotonus Pelvic Floor Dysfunction (Vaginal Laxity and Health Issues)

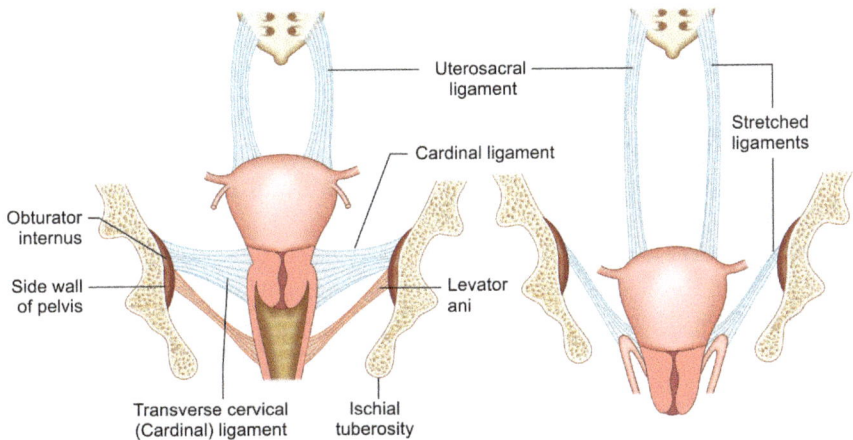

Fig. 7: Weak pelvic floor muscles along with stretched ligaments can lead to prolapse.
Courtesy: DC Dutta's Textbook of Gynecology, Edited by Dr Hiralal Konar, New Delhi, Jaypee Brothers Medical Publishers, 2016; p166

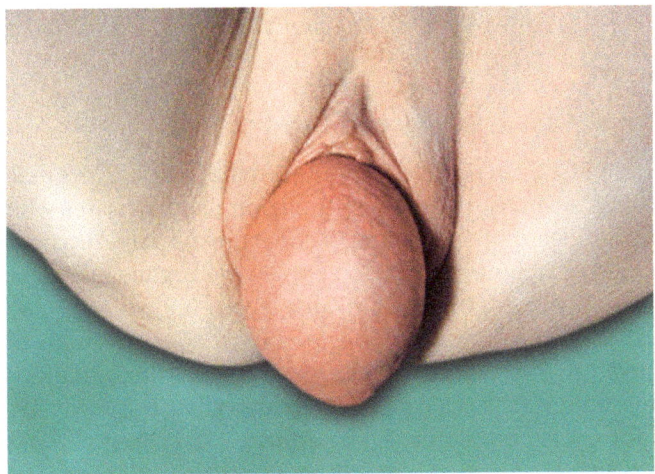

Fig. 8: Pelvic organ prolapse.
Courtesy: DC Dutta's Textbook of Gynecology, Edited by Dr Hiralal Konar, New Delhi, Jaypee Brothers Medical Publishers, 2016; p170

- Approximately, two-thirds of the women with the history of vaginal childbirth are likely to get POP. Up to 20% of these women may need to undergo surgical procedures (Fig. 8).

Clinical Features
- Vaginal bulge
- Sense of organs falling out
- Popping out sensations
- Increased vaginal pressure
- Painful intercourse

- Reduced sexual sensations and difficulty achieving orgasms
- Sensory deficit (women with POP have lesser sensitivity to temperature and vibration than normal women).

Causes of Prolapse

- Stretching, compressing, tearing, or crushing of PFM during vaginal deliveries
- Vaginal laxity
- Menopause
- Hysterectomy
- Obesity
- Aging
- Asthma, bronchitis, and emphysema, or seasonal allergies that lead to increased abdominal pressure
- Constipation
- Repetitive lifting
- Connective tissue disorder
- More than 10% of women after hysterectomy require second surgery for POP.

Pelvic Floor Muscle Laxity can Lead to POP

Intact and fit pelvic floor muscles can support the organs of the pelvis without tension on their suspensory ligaments. Imagine a boat in water, where water is pelvic floor muscles, which supports the boat means pelvic organs; moorings mean suspensory ligaments help to support the organs by suspension and stabilization. Now imagine when water is taken away, it puts way more strain to the moorings, which support the entire boat through suspension. Similarly, pelvic floor laxity may place excessive strain on the connective tissue suspensions in the pelvis. So, it means that strengthening pelvic floor muscles can prevent to delay the damage, stretching, or breaking of the connective tissues of suspensory ligaments. Even The American College of Obstetrics and Gynecology's Patient Education Bulletin on pelvic floor recommends patients to strengthen their pelvic floor to improve their POP. Hypothetically, strength training of pelvic floor muscles would have a very positive effect on prolapse as stronger pelvic floor muscles could prevent unnecessary burden on the pelvic suspensory—connective tissue components. Many postnatal women can live completely asymptomatic life even after laxity of pelvic floor muscles because the unstrained suspensory ligaments compensate for a few years. It becomes symptomatic after suspensory ligaments begin to strain. Delayed training of these muscles, especially after prolapse has developed, will significantly reduce the effectiveness of pelvic floor muscles. It is strongly recommended to strengthen weak PFM for every mother as a preventive training.

Splinting for Prolapse

Placing one or more fingers in the vagina to manually push back the malpositioned organ will straighten the kink. It will help to facilitate emptying of bladder or bowel. In other words, pushing the prolapsed organs back into the position is known as splinting.

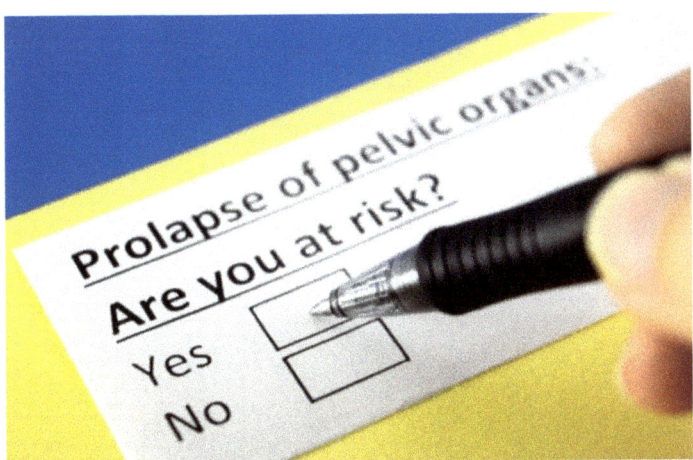

Types of pelvic organ prolapse (POP).

- Cystocele
- Rectocele
- Enterocele
- Uterine prolapse
- Vaginal vault prolapse

1. *Cystocele (Figs. 9A and B)*

Cystocele is prolapse of posterior wall of bladder out of vagina. It is an anterior compartment prolapse. Prolapse of urethra is urethrocele or both cystourethrocele.

- Vaginal penetration of the penis can displace the bladder into its normal anatomical position, which relives the obstruction. As a result, it leads to urinary leakage during sexual activities.
- A central cystocele happens when the bladder wall falls into the roof of the vagina due to PFM weakness.

Clinical features:

- Bulge or lump into or outside the vagina
- Necessity of pushing cystocele back to position to urinate
- Obstructive urinary symptoms like weak stream and incomplete bladder emptying. It happens because of prolapsed bladder, which causes urethral kinking
- Frequent urination
- Urge to urinate
- Vaginal pain or dyspareunia.

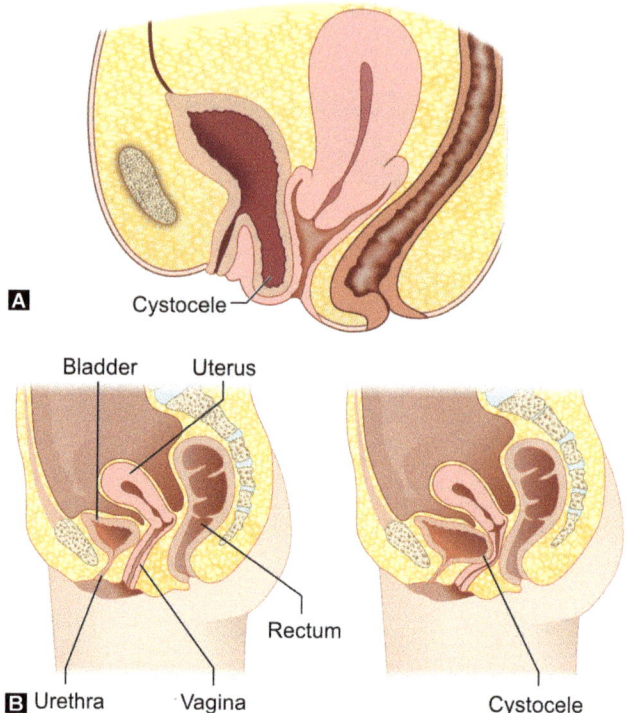

Figs. 9A and B: Cystocele.

Courtesy: DC Dutta's Textbook of Gynecology, Edited by Dr Hiralal Konar, New Delhi, Jaypee Brothers Medical Publishers, 2016; p171

2. Rectocele (Fig. 10)

Rectocele is a prolapse of wall of rectum. It is a prolapse of posterior compartment. The rectal wall pushes against posterior vaginal wall, creating bulge. The bulge becomes more obvious during bowel movements. Some patients might present with a history of habit of using their thumb to splint and push inside vaginal wall for defecation. Remember, supportive function of strong pelvic floor muscles can work as muscular net against rectocele.

- Normally, rectum should be anatomically straight without a kink to facilitate bowel movements.
- Rectal descent due to weak PFM.
- Protrusion of rectum through vagina due to weak PFM.

Clinical features:

- Bulge or lump in vagina, and it is more noticeable during bowel movements
- Kink of rectum causes difficult bowel movement
- Need of vaginal splinting by fingers to empty rectum
- Fecal incontinence
- Vaginal pain
- Dyspareunia.

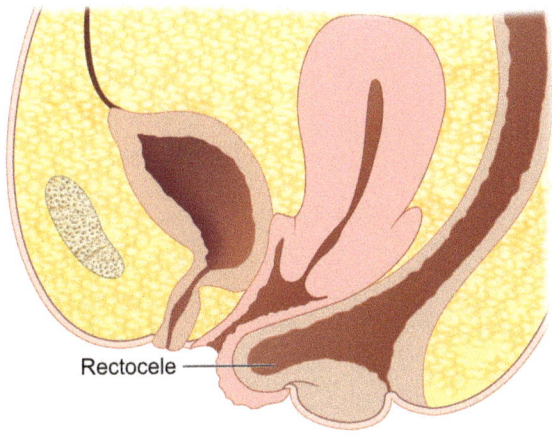

Fig. 10: Rectocele.
Courtesy: DC Dutta's Textbook of Gynecology, Edited by Dr Hiralal Konar, New Delhi, Jaypee Brothers Medical Publishers, 2016; p172

3. *Enterocele (Fig. 11)*

Enterocele is the prolapse of middle compartment. It is also known as herniation of small bowel. Enterocele can mainly occur posthysterectomy, as it leads to separation of anterior and posterior wall of vagina, which allows the intestines to push against the vagina.

Clinical features:
- Bulge or lump at vagina
- Cramping of intestine due to trapping of small intestine
- Vaginal pressure
- Dyspareunia.

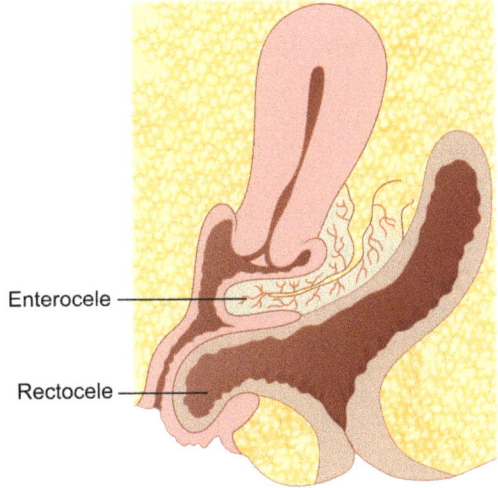

Fig. 11: Enterocele.
Courtesy: DC Dutta's Textbook of Gynecology, Edited by Dr Hiralal Konar, New Delhi, Jaypee Brothers Medical Publishers, 2016; p172

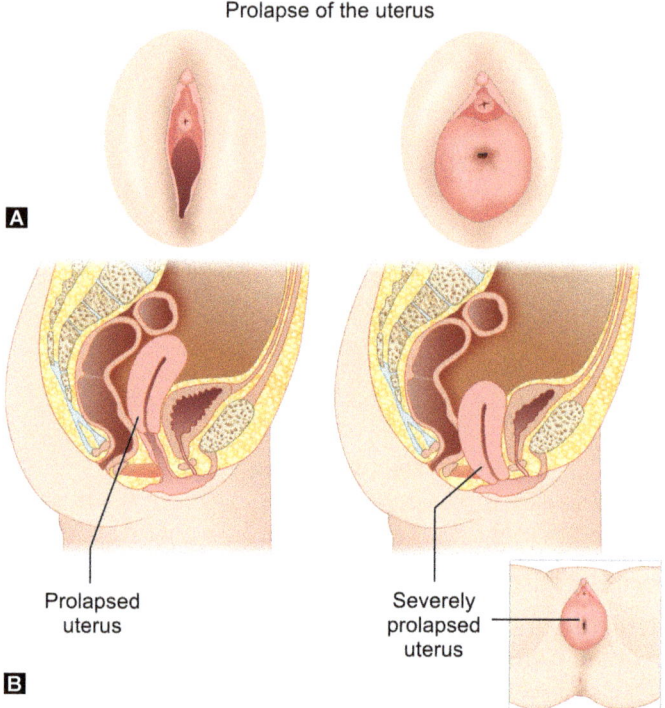

Figs. 12A and B: Uterine prolapse.

4. Uterine Prolapse (Figs. 12A and B)

Uterine prolapse is a type of middle compartment prolapse, which occurs due to lax pelvic floor and weakening of uterosacral ligaments at the top of vagina, which causes the uterus to fall.

Stages of uterine prolapse (Figs. 13A and B):
- *Normal*: External os at the level of ischial spines.
- *First-degree*: Drop of uterus into upper portion of the vagina. But the external os still remains above the introitus.
- *Second-degree*: The external os protrudes outside the vaginal introitus. However, the uterine body still remains inside the vagina.
- *Third-degree*: The uterine cervix, body, and the fundus drops to lie outside the introitus.
- *Fourth-degree*—procidentia: Prolapse of the uterus with the eversion of the entire vagina.

Clinical features:
- Bulge or lump
- Difficulty in urinating
- Increased urinary urgency and frequency
- Pelvic or vaginal pain during sitting and walking

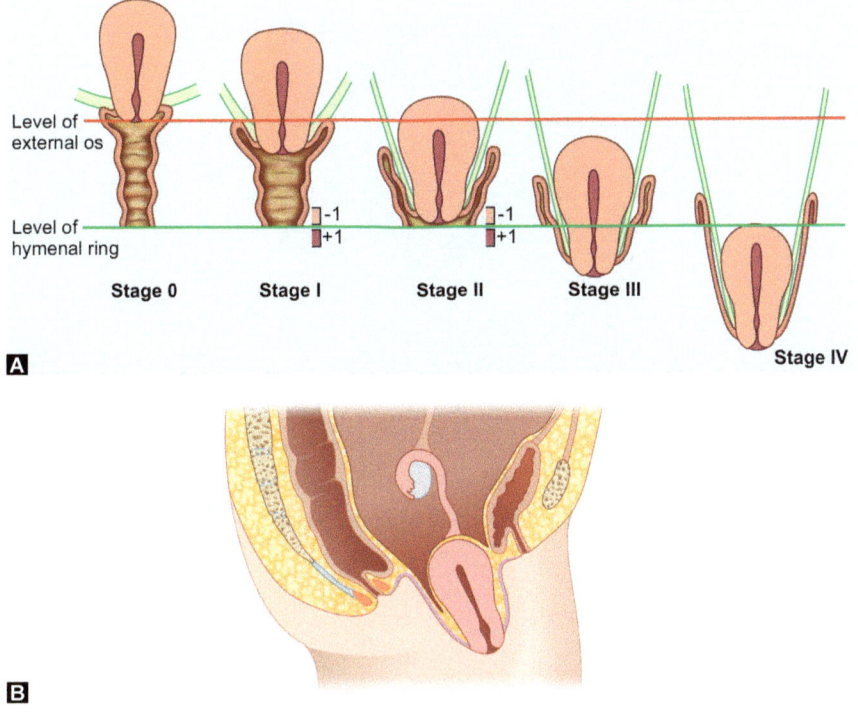

Figs. 13A and B: Stages of uterine prolapse.
Courtesy: DC Dutta's Textbook of Gynecology, Edited by Dr Hiralal Konar, New Delhi, Jaypee Brothers Medical Publishers, 2016; p169 and 170

- Dyspareunia
- Spotting or discharge due to the malpositioned uterus
- Procidentia—complete uterine prolapse—leads to ulceration and bleeding.

5. *Vaginal Vault Prolapse (Fig. 14)*

The top of the vagina gradually falls toward the vaginal opening. It can cause the walls of vagina to weaken. It occurs mainly posthysterectomy, as uterus provides support for the top of the vagina. Eventually, it can lead to protrusion of the top of the vagina out of the body through vaginal opening and turns the vagina inside out. Many times vaginal vault prolapse is associated with enterocele.

Key clinical features of pop or pelvic organ prolapse:
- Feeling of something coming down
- Vaginal heaviness
- Abdominal pressure or pain
- Lump at vaginal opening
- Reduction of symptoms of pain or pressure as women lie down with pillow under her hips

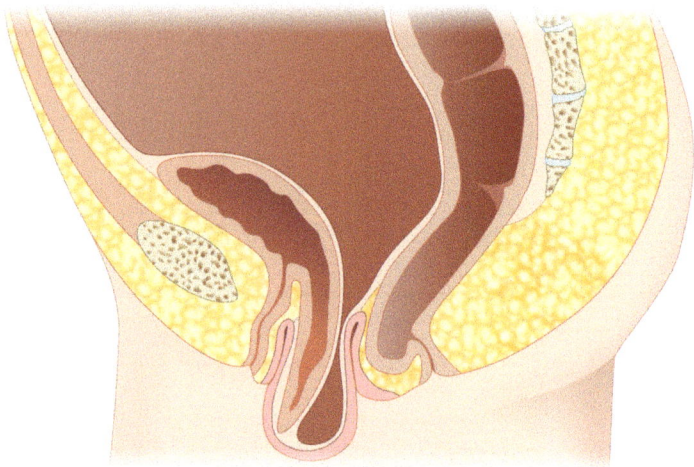

Fig. 14: Vaginal vault prolapse.

- Recurrent UTI
- Stress incontinence
- Diurnal and nocturnal frequency
- Urge incontinence
- Feeling of incomplete emptying
- Manual or thumb reduction or positional changes to start or complete emptying
- Difficulty in defecation
- Incontinence of flatus, liquid stool, or solid stool
- Urgency of defecation
- Digitation or splinting of vagina, perineum, or anus to complete
- Postdefecation rectal prolapse
- Lack of sensation or satisfaction during orgasm
- Incontinence during sex
- Unwillingness to have frequent intercourse
- Dyspareunia.

Remember, supportive function of fit pelvic floor muscles can work as muscular net against prolapse.

HEMORRHOIDS AND PELVIC FLOOR MUSCLES

Hemorrhoids or piles are enlarged, swollen, and inflamed veins in your lower rectum and anus. It is most common in pregnant women and people who suffer from constipation. ABC News from USA in December, 2012 reported that "hemorrhoids" were Google's biggest health search. Overweight, prolonged

Hypotonus Pelvic Floor Dysfunction (Vaginal Laxity and Health Issues)

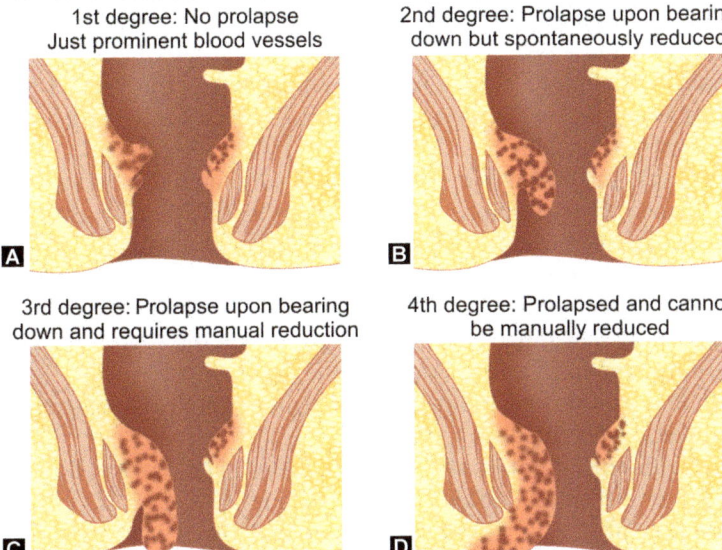

Figs. 15A to D: Grading of hemorrhoids.

constipation, pregnancy, heavy lifting, and prolonged diarrhea can cause piles (Figs. 15A to D).

Pelvic floor muscles can help to prevent hemorrhoids by increasing blood flow to the anal region while flushing out waste products and poor blood flow, which develops hemorrhoids. Strengthening PFM works as a strong support system for internal hemorrhoids and prevents protrusion, which leads to external hemorrhoids. Also, it helps to control leaking around the hemorrhoid problem areas.

MEDICAL RESEARCH: VAGINAL LOOSENESS AND BULGING OF ORGANS (PELVIC ORGAN PROLAPSE)

- Studies show that "4-10% of all women have severe enough prolapse where they experience symptoms."
- Very important information—"43-76% of all women do not even know they have prolapse; they know about it during their regular gynecological examination." That means you might have beginning of organ bulge/organ prolapse and you might not be even aware of it.
- Research shows that "strengthening pelvic floor muscles with pelvic floor muscle exercise can help delay or even prevent pelvic organ prolapse symptoms" which means tight vaginal muscle will keep your organs well supported.
- "Women from families with a genetic predisposition for hernias are 1.4 times as likely to experience pelvic organ prolapse", which means, if your mother or grandmother had a problem, you are likely to have it.

- "About 7% of women will have surgery for the prolapse by the age of 80." That means it is smart to be preventive in early and try to avoid surgery.
- "About 3-6% of women have organ prolapse below the vaginal opening, they generally feel as if they are sitting on a ball and may see actual bulge outside of their vagina."
- Gravity, age, and effects of childbirth, especially vaginal delivery, can easily cause pelvic organ prolapse. No scientific evidence that elective cesarean sections can decrease the risk of developing a prolapse.
- Sooner you find out if you have a pelvic organ prolapse, more likely you can delay or even prevent prolapse with pelvic floor exercises.
- Studies show that muscle retraining can reduce the severity of prolapse symptoms and can delay the onset of the prolapse.
- Pelvic floor muscle retraining has been demonstrated to help women with various urinary and pelvic symptoms.
- 50% of women can not locate correct muscles to do a pelvic floor muscle contraction based on written directions alone.
- On average of 13% of women who have prolapse surgery will require a repeat procedure within 5 years.

MULTIPLE CHOICE QUESTIONS

Q1. Which factors can cause vaginal laxity?
(a) Increased abdominal pressure
(b) Decreased abdominal pressure
(c) Hormonal imbalance
(d) Both (a) and (c)

Q2. The hormone which is responsible for increasing laxity of the connective tissues like ligaments and muscles is _____.
(a) Relaxin
(b) Prolactin
(c) Oxytocin
(d) Follicular-stimulating hormone (FSH)

Q3. How many degrees of perineal tear can occur during labor?
(a) 5 degrees
(b) 4 degrees
(c) 6 degrees
(d) None of these

Q4. Which muscle is incised in midline episiotomy?
(a) Bulbocavernosus and central tendon portion of perineal body
(b) Only through ischiocavernosus muscle
(c) Deep transverse perineal muscle
(d) All muscles of pelvic floor are involved

Q5. What type of incontinence can occur due to obstetric fistula?
(a) Only urinary incontinence
(b) Only fecal incontinence
(c) No incontinence
(d) Urinary and fecal incontinence

Q6. Which muscle bears the largest stretching of almost 3.26 times of its original length during delivery?
(a) Pubococcygeus
(b) Iliococcygeus
(c) Pubovaginalis
(d) Coccygeus

Q7. What is the main cause of vaginal laxity?
   (a) Tight pelvic floor muscles
   (b) Loose pelvic floor muscles
   (c) In coordinated pelvic floor muscles
   (d) It is due to the weakness of smooth muscles of vagina

Q8. All the symptoms listed below are the consequences of vaginal laxity, except:
   (a) Prolapse of pelvic organ
   (b) Urinary incontinence
   (c) Female sexual health problems
   (d) Pelvic pain and trigger points

Q9. What will be the grade of genuine stress incontinence, if the person gets incontinence while changing posture?
   (a) Grade 1
   (b) Grade 2
   (c) Grade 3
   (d) Grade 4

Q10. What is the cause of urge urinary incontinence?
   (a) Weak pelvic floor muscles
   (b) Involuntary contraction of detrusor
   (c) Weak support to urethra
   (d) All of the above

Q11. Which type of urinary incontinence has typical symptoms like "key in the lock" or "garage door syndrome"?
   (a) Stress urinary incontinence
   (b) Genuine stress incontinence
   (c) Urge urinary incontinence
   (d) Overflow incontinence

Q12. Which type of urinary incontinence can be caused by cystocele?
   (a) Stress urinary incontinence
   (b) Urge urinary incontinence
   (c) Overflow incontinence
   (d) Genuine stress incontinence

Q13. Prolapse of which organ is known as cystocele?
   (a) Urinary bladder
   (b) Vaginal vault
   (c) Rectum
   (d) Uterus

Q14. The most common type of pelvic organ prolapse posthysterectomy is:
   (a) Uterus prolapse
   (b) Rectal prolapse
   (c) Prolapse of some part of small intestine
   (d) Urinary bladder prolapse

Q15. What is the other name of fourth degree prolapse of uterus?
   (a) Rectocele
   (b) Enterocele
   (c) Procidentia
   (d) Cystocele

Q16. Vaginal vault prolapse is many a time associated with which other type of pelvic organ prolapse?
   (a) Enterocele
   (b) Cystocele
   (c) Prolapse of uterus
   (d) None of these

Q17. Which hormone deficiency postnatally can cause genuine stress incontinence?
   (a) Progesterone
   (b) Estrogen
   (c) Relaxin
   (d) Luteinizing hormone (LH)

Section 1: Female: Pelvic Floor Dysfunction

Q18. According to Q-tip test, if the cotton swab inserted up to the level of bladder shows a marking more than 30° when the patient is asked to cough, indicates:
    (a) Urethral hypermobility
    (b) Vaginal laxity
    (c) Urethral hypomobility
    (d) Tight pelvic floor muscles

Q19. Which type of urinary incontinence is more predictable?
    (a) Urge urinary incontinence
    (b) Stress urinary incontinence
    (c) Overflow incontinence
    (d) Mixed

Q20. Hypotonus detrusor muscle can result in:
    (a) Urge urinary incontinence
    (b) Overflow incontinence
    (c) Stress urinary incontinence
    (d) Mixes

ANSWERS

1: (d) Both (a) and (c)
2: (a) Relaxin
3: (b) 4 degrees
4: (a) Bulbocavernous and central tendon portion of perineal body
5: (d) Urinary and fecal incontinence
6: (a) Pubococcygeus
7: (b) Loose pelvic floor muscles
8: (d) Pelvic pain and trigger points
9: (c) Grade 3
10: (b) Involuntary contraction of detrusor
11: (c) Urge urinary incontinence
12: (c) Overflow incontinence
13: (a) Urinary bladder
14: (c) Prolapse of some part of small intestine
15: (c) Procedentia
16: (a) Enterocele
17: (b) Estrogen
18: (a) Urethral hypermobility
19: (b) Stress urinary incontinence
20: (b) Overflow incontinence

Chapter 7
Female Sexual Dysfunction (Pelvic Floor and Female Sexual Dysfunction)

FEMALE SEXUAL HEALTH DISORDER

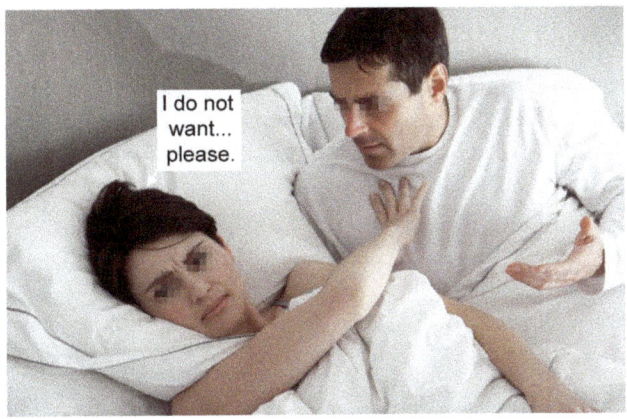

Pelvic floor muscles (PFMs) are responsible for sexual health of women. If the PFMs are too tight or too loose, they can lead to female sexual dysfunction (FSD). It is important to understand some of the key points of women's reproductive system to clearly understand pelvic floor and its relation to FSD.

- Female sexuality is a psychosomatic event involving dynamic process of psychological, physiological, hormonal, emotional, and cultural factors, which affect desire, arousal, lubrication, and orgasm.
- Sexual arousal is a combination of hormonal state, psychological, and emotional factors. However, it requires erotic physical stimulus which causes increased pelvic blood flow, genital engorgement, vaginal lubrication, and physiological changes in vagina, which prepare vagina for penetration.
- Master and Johnson demonstrated in their research that vasocongestion or increased blood flow is the primary reaction to sexual stimulation and increased muscle tension is a secondary reaction.
- Pelvic floor muscles are responsible to firmly grip the penis. Stronger PFM can give a tighter hug to the penis and weaker PFM gives a lazy low energy hug to the penis.

- The strength and duration of PFM contractions are directly proportional to orgasmic potential.
- The FSD is a very common problem which affects up to 55% of women.
- Too weak or loose PFM and too tight PFM can lead to FSD.
- Pelvic organ prolapse (POP) can also lead to FSD due to vaginal laxity and painful intercourse. Body image issues with vaginal appearance also contribute negatively.
- *Urinary incontinence (UI)*: Anticipation of urine leakage during intercourse can cause emotional distress which contributes negatively to sex life. Concerns about odor, hygiene, and embracement also negatively affect sex drive, excitement, and ability to orgasm.
- Upon stimulation, pelvic blood congestion and lubrication happens due to increased blood flow, and from Bartholin's and Skene's glands. Vagina expands. The cervix and uterus pull back and up.

FUNCTIONAL ANATOMY

The female genitalia can be divided into two categories: (1) external genitalia vulva which includes the mons pubis, clitoris, labia majora and minora; and (2) internal genitalia which includes organs like vagina, cervix, uterus, fallopian tubes, and ovaries (Figs. 1 to 3).

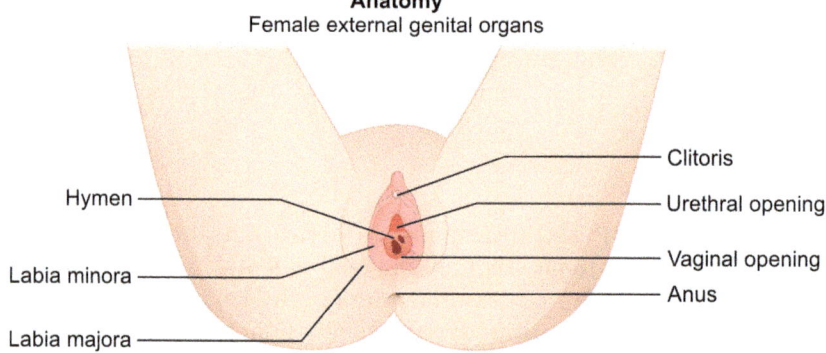

Fig. 1: Anatomy of female external genital organs.

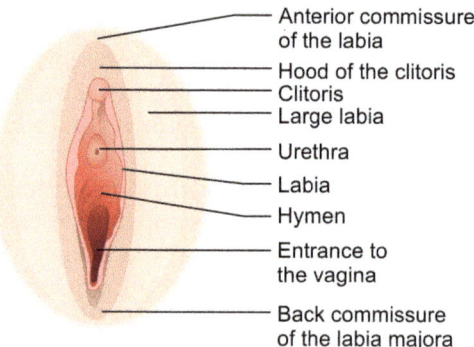

Fig. 2: Anatomy of female genital organs.

Female Sexual Dysfunction (Pelvic Floor and Female Sexual Dysfunction)

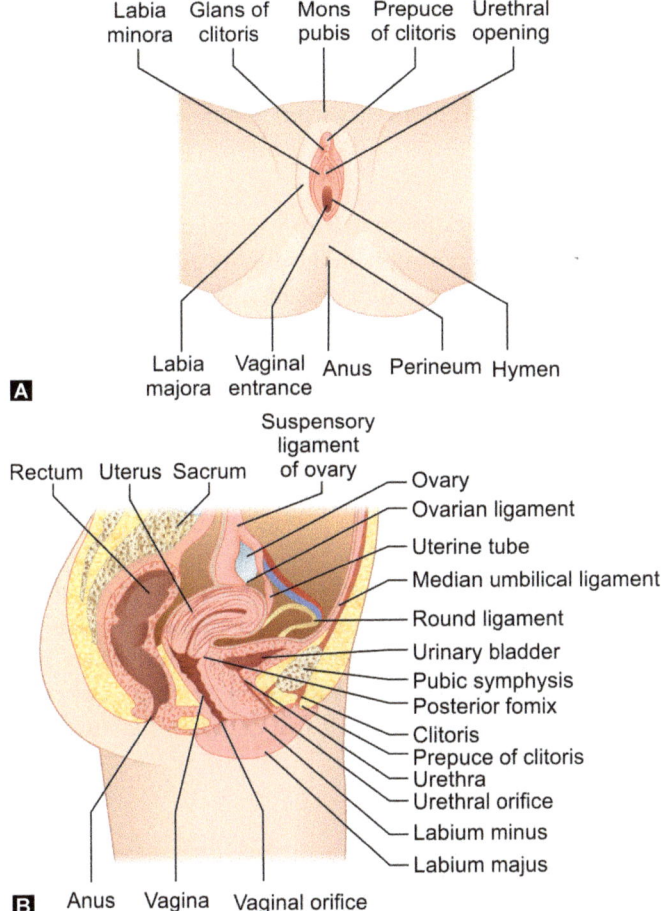

Figs. 3A and B: (A) Female external genitalia and (B) urogenital system.

Mons Pubis

Mons pubis is also known as mons veneris. It is the fatty layer of skin covering the pubic bone. It covers pubis hair at the age of puberty. The pubic hair grow on the mons pubis and between the labia majora and minora which helps to protect the vagina from the bacteria and pathogens. Also provides cushion to the pubic bones and mons.

Labia Majora

The two outer folds of the fatty layers of skin on the exterior of the vulva which serve as a physical barrier to protect the sensitive parts of the inner vulva. Pubic hair on labia majora helps to protect the vulva. Labia majora swells and becomes darker during sexual arousal as a result of vasocongestion.

Labia Minora

They are folds located between the labia majora, smaller in size and hairless. They help to protect vaginal opening. They contain more nerve endings and therefore they are erotically sensitive. Labia minora have blood vessels throughout the tissues which help to increase blood flow during arousal. As a result of vasocongestion, the tissue increases in the size and helps with sexual arousal. Sizes, shapes, and colors vary from female to female.

Vaginal Opening

Vaginal opening is vaginal entrance into vaginal canal. It is also known as "introitus". The vaginal opening is located between the labia minora into vestibular area. The opening is in a closed status, however, it opens when penetrated.

Vestibule

Vestibule is an intralabial smooth surface area. The vaginal and urethral openings are inside the vestibule.

Hymen

The hymen is a thin flap of mucosal tissue which covers opening of vagina. Hymen can be different from female to female. Some are completely stretched out, some are fully intact, and others are perforated. Penetrative sexual activities, any other penetrative activities like inserting finger or nonsexual activities like horseback riding, exercises, or activities like inserting tampons can also stretch hymen.

Uterus

Please review functional anatomy of uterus from Chapter 1. During sexual arousal, the uterus lifts up, which creates more space. It lowers and returns to its original position upon end of stimulation or orgasm is accomplished.

Urethral Opening

The location of the urethra is between the clitoris and vaginal orifice, which allows urine to exit from the body. Main purpose of urethra is urination. Some females report the experience of "squirting" at orgasm when fluid is released through urethral opening.

Clitoral Structures (Fig. 4)

The clitoral structures are the group of organs that make up the clitoris.

Clitoris is made up of (Fig. 5):
- Clitoral glans
- Clitoral hood
- Clitoral shaft
- Corpus cavernosa
- Crura.

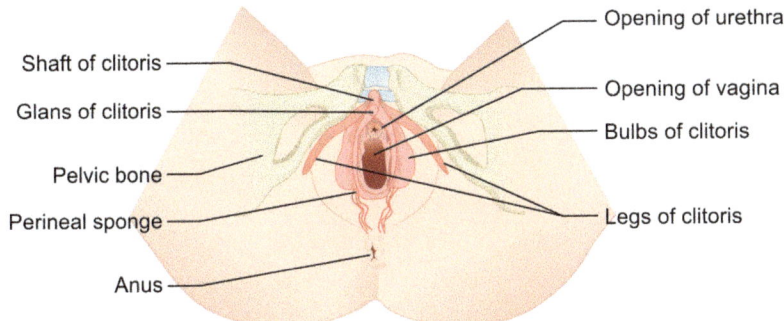

Fig. 4: Group of organs that make clitoris.

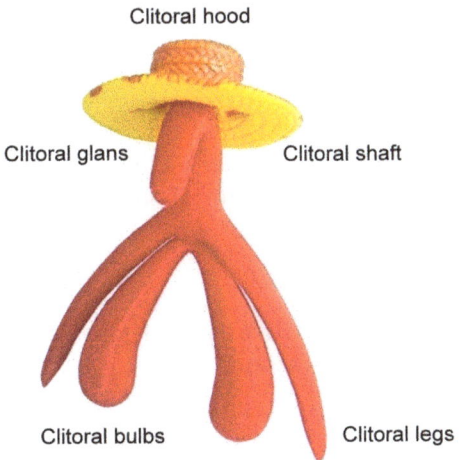

Fig. 5: Structures of clitoral.

Clitoral Glans

Clitoral glans is located close to the top of the vulva, it is the visible portion of the clitoris. It is covered by the clitoral hood, which can retract and expose more of the clitoris during arousal. Clitoral glans contains many nerve endings like the glans of the penis. It is sensitive part of the clitoris which is sexually pleasurable. The clitoral glans gets stiff and turns red due to increased blood flow into the erectile tissues during arousal (Fig. 6).

Clitoral Hood

Clitoral hood is made up of connective tissue located between the two labia minora that covers a portion of the clitoris. Clitoral hood helps to protect clitoral glans. Clitoral hood retracts during arousal like a foreskin of a penis.

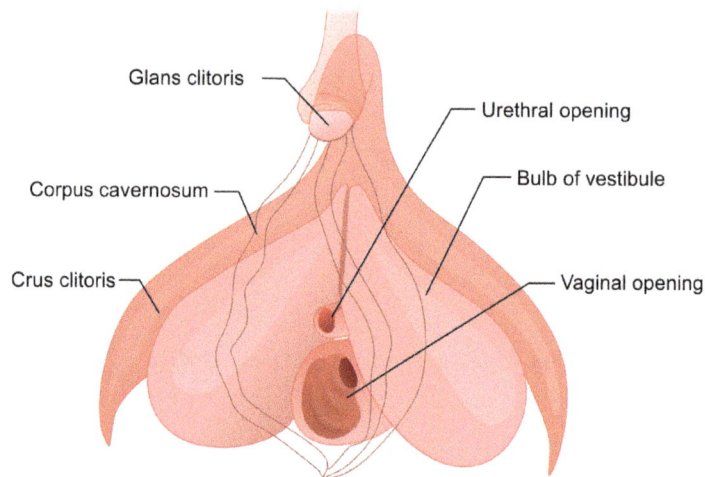

Fig. 6: Clitoral details.

Clitoral Shaft

Clitoral shaft is a small size, approximately 1 inch, structure that is attached to the clitoral glans. It is located under clitoral hood. It is a very sensitive structure, just like the shaft of the penis.

Corpus Cavernosa

The corpus cavernosa are tissues like corpus spongiosum in males which fills up with blood during clitoral erection.

Crura

It is the internal part of the clitoris. It is located near the vestibular bulbs. It contains two corpus cavernosa and erectile tissue. During sexual arousal, the crus gets rise in the blood flow and it becomes firm. Both crus are stretched back toward the pubis on either side of the clitoral glans and wrap around a portion of the urethral opening.

Pelvic Floor Muscle and Clitoris

- The clitoris engorges and erects during sexual stimulation.
- Contraction of bulbocavernosus (BC) and ischiocavernosus (IC) muscles compresses the deep internal portions of the clitoris.
- Contraction of BC and IC muscles maintains blood pressure within the erectile chambers of clitoris. It leads to higher pressure in erectile chambers of clitoris than systemic blood pressure.

Bulbocavernosus reflex (BCR)

- The clitoris stimulation leads to contraction of the BC and IC muscles along with anal wink.
- In other words, the PFM reflexively contract upon clitoral stimulation.

- Each contraction of BC and IC muscles increases blood flow to the clitoris, which helps to clitoral engorgement and they help to maintain clitoral rigidity.

Vagina

Vagina is the part from the vaginal introitus to the cervix. It is the muscular canal that is approximately around 3–4 inches deep when not aroused.
- Many people are confused between identification of vulva and vagina. If you put your hand on your private part—that is vulva. If you enter your finger internally within the vaginal opening—that is vagina.

During sexual arousal, it is approximately from 5 inches to 7 inches deep. During sexual arousal, blood flows to the vagina while the pelvic floor muscles relax and the vagina is expanded to allow the insertion. It includes:
- Vaginal opening
- Hymen
- Vaginal canal
- Vestibular bulbs
- G-spot
- Paraurethral gland
- Bartholin's gland.

The vaginal opening, hymen, and the vagina are discussed before.

Vestibular Bulbs

Vestibular bulbs are situated underneath the labia minora. During sexual arousal, the blood flow increases at the bulbs, which helps the vagina to lengthen and the vulva expands outward.

G-spot

- *G-spot*: Dr Ernst Grafenberg described it in 1950. It is a hypersensitive, erogenous zone located on the wall between vagina and the urethra. Some studies are showing that the G-spot is a small cluster of numerous nerve endings. Proper stimulation of G-spot can promote arousal and vaginal orgasm.

  It is named as Grafenberg spot. G-spot is located approximately 2 inches into the vagina on upper side in the direction of the bladder. There are many point of views about the G-spot. Some researches suggest that appropriate stimulation of G-spot not only increases the pleasure, it can also lead to female ejaculations in many women.
- *Female ejaculation: Squirting*—some women ejaculate fluid during climax. Some researches think that it is due to lubrication, other research thinks it is the secretion from Bartholin's and Skene's glands. Many researches think it is due to urine release because of an involuntary contraction of bladder that can happen during orgasm (Fig. 7).

Skene's Gland—Paraurethral Gland

The Skene's glands, also known as paraurethral glands, are located on the vaginal wall next to urethra. It could also be considered as a part of G-spot

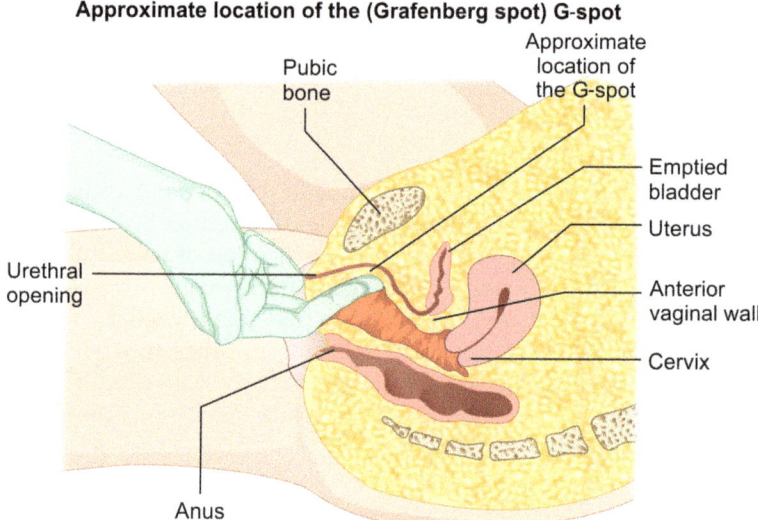

Fig. 7: Location of the G-spot.

and includes clitoris. They are highly sensitive. During sexual arousal, paraurethral glands swell up with blood and female ejaculations may occur in the paraurethral glands. Proper stimulation of paraurethral gland can also produce an orgasm in many women.

Bartholin's Glands

They are located in both sides of the vaginal opening. Their main function is lubrication. They secrete mucus onto the vulva and into the vagina upon sexual arousal.

Perineum

The perineum is located between the vaginal opening and anus. It is hairless and can be sexually sensitive.

Pelvic Floor Muscle and Arousal and Lubrication

- Pelvic floor muscles help to increase pelvic blood flow during arousal. PFMs also contribute to vaginal lubrication.
- Pelvic floor muscle helps with genital engorgement and clitoral rigidity from flaccid state of clitoris.
- Pelvic floor muscle helps to compress the roots of the clitoris and help to elevate blood pressure within the clitoris to maintain clitoris erections.

Pelvic Floor Muscle and Orgasm

- Master and Johnson's described the "Orgasmic Platform" where the outer third of the vagina with engorged inner lips is considered as a base of pelvic congestion.

- The arousal and sensations gradually builds and it is followed by rhythmic contractions of PFM, the uterus, and anus. It is followed by complete release and PFM relaxation.
- A total of 10–15 PFM contractions occur.
- First 3–5 contractions occur at 0.8 seconds intervals during orgasm. After that, the interval between the contractions increases and the intensity of contraction reduces.
- Without PFM, women might not even able to have real orgasms.
- It is generally associated with increased heart rate, respiratory rate, and blood pressure.
- As a woman develops better muscle memory and reflexive high-intensity contractions of PFM, it becomes easier to achieve orgasms and even multiple orgasms.

FEMALE SEXUAL DYSFUNCTION

Occurrence

Laumann et al., 1999 studies reported that up to 50% of general female population have some form of sexual dysfunction with postpartum aging women and those who have undergone gynecological surgery experiencing an even higher prevalence of this condition.

Definition

Sexual dysfunction is defined by World Health Organization (WHO 2010, Chapter V, F52) as "the various ways in which an individual is unable to participate in a sexual relationship he or she would wish"—WHO, 2006 defines sexual health as a state of well-being.

Causes of Female Sexual Dysfunction

- *Physical*: Medical conditions like cancer, kidney problems, multiple sclerosis, cardiac disease, and bladder dysfunctions can lead to sexual dysfunction. Medications like antidepressants, blood pressure medications, chemotherapy drugs, etc. can also decrease sexual desire and lead to orgasmic dysfunction.
- *Hormonal*: Hormonal imbalance or postmenopause lower estrogen level may lead to changes in genital tissues and sexual responsiveness. Also, reduced estrogen leads to decreased blood flow to the pelvic region which can lead to difficulty with arousal, genital sensations, and orgasms.
- The vaginal lining also becomes thinner and can loose elasticity particularly in sexually inactive or hypoactive patients, which can lead to painful intercourse (dyspareunia). Sexual desire also decreases when hormonal levels decrease. Hormone levels also shift after giving birth and during breastfeeding, which can lead to vaginal dryness and can lead to sex health issues.
- *Psychological and social*: Psychological conditions like anxiety and depression can cause sexual dysfunction. Low self-esteem, low self-

confidence, cultural and religious issues, long-term stress, history of sexual abuse, stress about pregnancy, and being a new mother may have similar effects. Couple issues about sex or any other aspects of relation can reduce sexual responsiveness.
- *Pelvic floor dysfunctions*: Above mentioned causes can lead to hypotonus, hypertonus, or incoordinated pelvic floor muscles. As a result, it leads to sexual health issues with desire, arousal, sensation, and orgasms.

Sexual Problems due to Pelvic Floor Dysfunction

- Lack of use
- Weakness of core muscles
- Poor body mechanics/poor posture
- *Chronic inflammatory conditions*: Prostatitis, cystitis, endometriosis, pelvic inflammatory disease (PID), colitis, irritable bowel syndrome (IBS)
- Urinary tract infections (UTIs)
- Habitual holding patterns
- History of sexual abuse
- Direct trauma like a fall on to tail bone
- Referred pain from pelvic organs pathology
- Positions hold for prolong period of time
- Surgical trauma like C-section
- Hysterectomy
- Episiotomy
- Laparoscopy.

APA Classification

According to the diagnostic and statistic manual of mental disorders of the American Psychiatric Association (APA) female sexual dysfunction (FSD) could be classified in three groups:
1. Orgasm disorders
2. Sexual interest or arousal disorders
3. Genito-pelvic pain and penetration disorders.

Basson Classification of Female Sexual Dysfunction (Box 1)

(Adapted from Basson et al., 2000)

BOX 1: Basson classification of female sexual dysfunctions (FSD).

According to Basson et al., 2000, FSD can be classified in to following categories:
- *Sexual desire disorders:*
  - Hypoactive sexual desire disorder (HSDD)
  - Sexual aversion disorder
- Sexual arousal disorder
- Sexual pain disorder
  - Dyspareunia
  - Vaginismus
  - Other sexual pain disorder
- Female orgasmic disorder

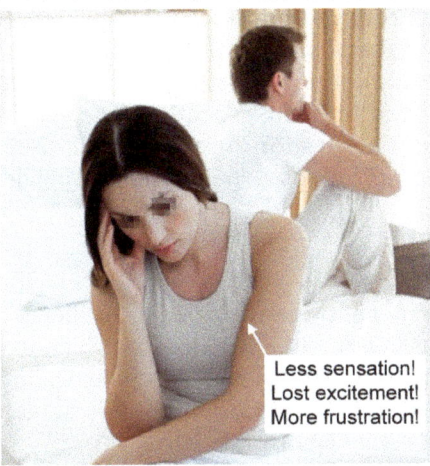

Sexual Desire Disorder

1. **Hypoactive sexual desire disorder**
   It is persistent or recurring deficiency of sexual fantasies/thoughts, and/or receptivity to sexual activity that causes personal distress. However, it is usually associated with other psychological, medical, emotional, or endocrine disorders. Hypotonus pelvic floor muscles create vaginal laxity which causes reduction of the friction during intercourse. It decreases neural and muscular stretching during sex. It also leads to reduced blood flow and ultimately reduced sexual sensation. It compromises on overall pleasure which results in reduced libido and hypoactive sexual desire disorder (HSDD). Hypotonus pelvic floor muscles can cause pain and spasm which leads to HSDD.
2. **Sexual aversion disorder**
   It is persistent or recurrent phobic aversion to and avoidance of sexual contact with a sexual partner that causes personal distress.

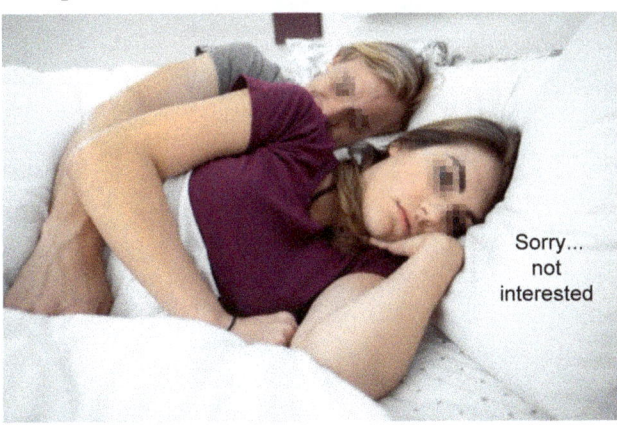

Sexual Arousal Disorder

It is persistent or recurring inability to attain or maintain sufficient sexual excitement that causes personal distress. Sexual arousal disorder is presented by the lack or absence of desire for sexual activity with sexual stimulations that normally induce sexual arousal. It could also be reduced ability to maintain sexual responses during sexual arousal. Hypotonic or hypertonic pelvic floor muscles cause reduced intimate sensation, and reduced vaginal smooth muscle relaxation and lubrication. Sexual arousal disorder can be because of the side effect of medications or pelvic, neural, pelvic floor, or peripheral vascular problems.

Sexual Pain Disorder

Sexual pain disorder means presence of pain in the pelvis or vagina during any stage of normal sexual intercourse including desire, arousal, or orgasm. Sexual pain disorder is usually associated with psychological trauma, physiological pelvic diseases, and associated pelvic floor dysfunctions. Sexual pain disorder includes dyspareunia and vaginismus.

Dyspareunia

- Recurrent or persistent genital pain associated with sexual intercourse. Pain during penile, digital, or any other form of vaginal penetration can be considered as dyspareunia.
- Dyspareunia is painful intercourse where patients present with pain during initial or deep vaginal penetration. Pain may have a presentation of localized introital tenderness or diffused deep soreness.
- Sometimes, it can be sustained for a few hours or up to 3 days. Conditions like endometriosis, adhesions, inflammatory pathologies, vaginal atrophy, hormonal imbalance, trauma to urethral and bladder wall, and other pelvic organ pathologies can lead to dyspareunia.

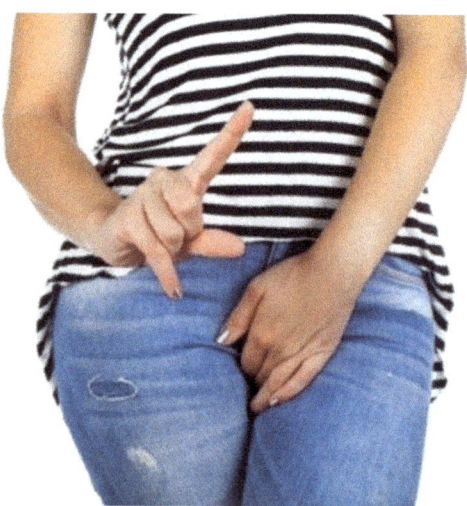

- According to research, 57% of patients with hypertonus pelvic floor muscles and 41% of patients with incontinence may have dyspareunia.
- Generally, it is due to dry stretching and microtrauma of tightened pelvic floor muscles or adhesions. Multiple trigger points can be present at pelvic

floor muscles. Spasms of obturator internus, coccygeus, iliopsoas, or levator ani can be found with deep penetration.

Pain or discomfort generally during initial penetration. However, she can tolerate and continue with penetration, thrusting, and the completion of intercourse.

Painful stages:

Stage 1: Woman experiences some level of pain during intercourse.

Stage 2: Vaginal penetration, thrusting along with completion of intercourse happens with continuous pain.

Stage 3: Penetration is tolerable, however, cannot tolerate thrusting. She cannot complete intercourse. Generally, women avoid sex at this stage.

Stage 4: Vaginal penetration becomes intolerable. Generally, woman stops having intercourse.

Sexual abuse or other relationship issues needs to be addressed for efficient management. Research suggests that during high level of women arousal, the vaginal apex expands and uterus moves upward. We believe and advise patients to prevent deep thrusting during intercourse, especially if women are not highly aroused. Adoption of sexual positions like being side to side, vaginal entry from behind, and women on top are helpful. Any position where it gives more control to women for depth, force, and speed of penetration can give them opportunity to relax better. Devices like pelvic floor 360 can provide great help.

Vaginismus

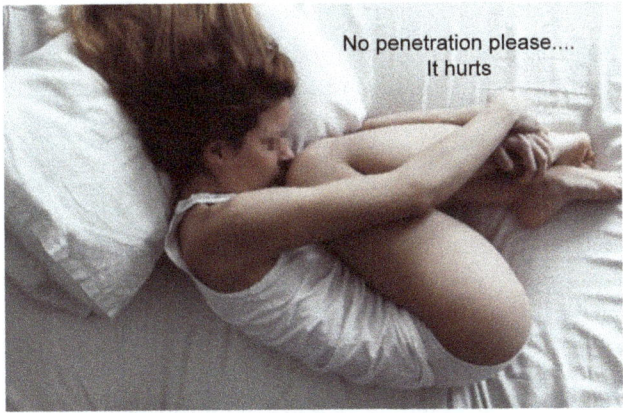

- Recurrent or persistent involuntary spasms of the muscles of the outer third of the vagina. Spasmodic muscles interfere with vaginal penetration and cause personal distress.
- Vaginismus is a condition that limits or prevents vaginal penetration due to unwanted, unintentional, and involuntary contraction of PFM. Primary vaginismus can be congenital and secondary vaginismus can be due to muscle spasms with history of trauma, sexual abuse, psychological conflicts, pelvic pain, intrapelvic pathology, etc. Vaginal examination may

not completely diagnose pelvic floor spasm, as sometimes vaginismus can be stimulus-based.
- However, majority of time, palpation of pelvic floor can reproduce the pain. Patients with pathologies like urethral syndrome or vulvar vestibulitis can improve vasodilation which can lead to deficient arousal response and ultimately dyspareunia.

> *"Some old wounds never truly heal, and bleed again at the slightest sword."*
> —*George RR Martin*

Pelvic floor spasms are the wounds that could keep getting worse at the slightest penetration. Pelvic floor rehabilitation (PFR) is extremely essential.

Female Orgasmic Disorder

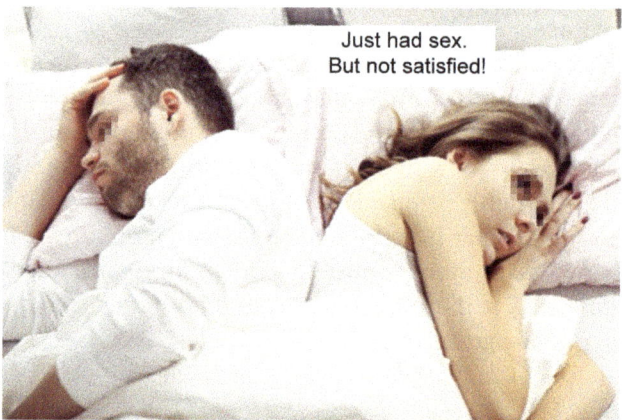

It can be defined as persistent or frequent difficulty with delay in or absence of orgasm after appropriate sexual stimulation and arousal that causes personal distress. It could be associated with neural or spinal cord disorders. Proper sensory stimulation can lead to female orgasm and creates repeated 1-s motor contraction of the pelvic floor muscles, and it is also associated with contractions of smooth muscles of vagina and uterus. Intensity of orgasms is directly related with pelvic floor positioning, endurance, strength, and tone of the muscles. Patients with pelvic pain have inhibitory response of pelvic floor muscles which leads to lack or reduced intensity of orgasm. Nonorgasmic women who cannot achieve orgasm are mainly due to reduced pelvic floor action, inadequate stimulation, anxiety, vaginismus, and psychological factors. Loose, stretched, or damaged pelvic floor muscles can lead to reduced amount of sensation that a woman feels during sex. Most of the sensation during sex comes from the pelvic floor muscles because vagina alone has a very few sensory nerves. Pubococcygeus muscles, also known as the "love muscle", are the muscles that wrap around the vaginal and anal opening as well as clitoris. According to research, strength and squeeze pressure of pubococcygeus muscle is significantly related to woman's ability to orgasm. PFR can significantly improve the sexual sensation, ability to reach orgasms, and intensity of orgasms which leads to increased libido.

FEMALE SEXUAL FUNCTION INDEX

The questionnaire like female sexual function index (FSFI) and WOW IIPRE Group questionnaire can subjectively measure sexual functioning in women and pelvic floor functioning.

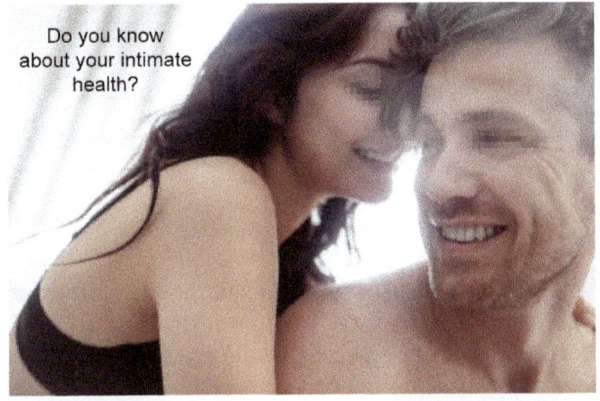

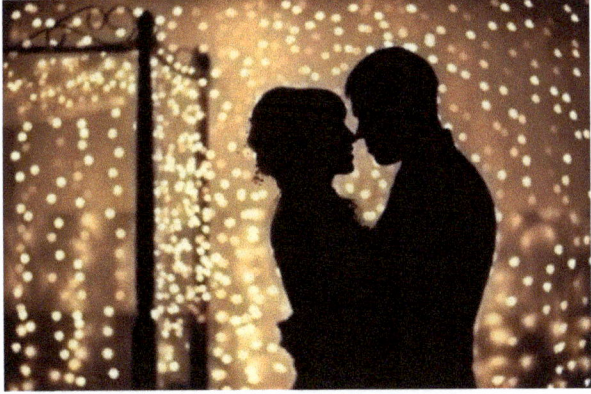

SIGNIFICANCE OF PELVIC FLOOR MUSCLE IN FEMALE SEX HEALTH

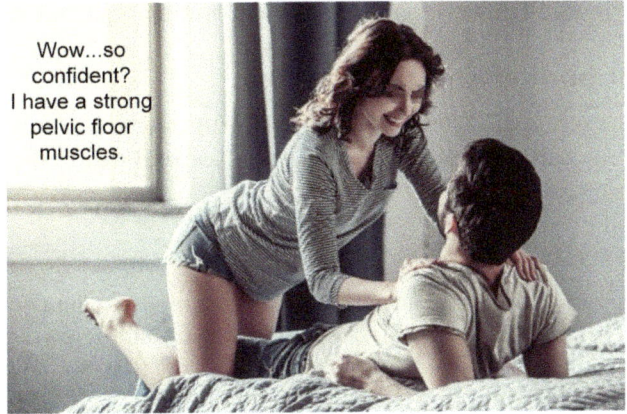

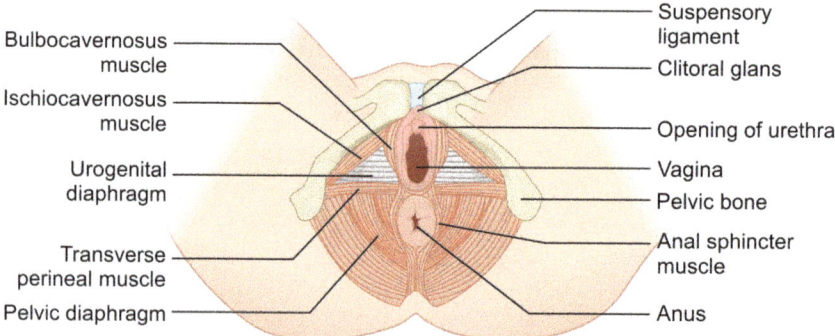

Fig. 8: Perineal muscle.

The perineal membrane consists of ischiocavernosus, bulbospongiosus, and superficial perineal muscles which are anatomically close to the vestibular bulbs and clitoris, and these all muscles enhance sexual responses (Fig. 8).
- The ischiocavernosus muscle is attached with clitoral hood, which helps to raise clitoral blood flow together with bulbocavernosus muscle.
- Contractions of these muscles place pressure on the deep dorsal vein of the clitoris. Ultimately, it prevents venous escape from clitoris. IC muscle is extremely important for arousal and attainment of orgasm.
- The bulbocavernosus and puborectalis muscles also assist in vaginal closure which facilitates more vaginal friction during intercourse. The activation of the LA including pubococcygeus and iliococcygeus muscles facilitates vaginal ballooning.
- Pathophysiological reasoning suggests that increased blood flow following pelvic floor activation encourages microvascular blood flow and ultimately lubrication, efferent sensations, and autonomic responses.
- During sexual activity, sexual pleasure can be improved for both partners by genital responses provided by contraction of levator ani including pubococcygeus and iliococcygeus muscles.
- Weak or lax muscles provide insufficient activity necessary for vaginal friction or blood flow which can ultimately inhibit orgasmic potential.

Persistent Genital Arousal Disorder

Rare sexual dysfunction generally presents with unwanted, arousal, genital engorgement, and multiple orgasms without sexual desire or stimulus. It resolves after orgasm.

Penis Captivus

Condition where male penis can get stuck within female's vagina due to intense contractions of PFM. Most of the time, it resolves after female orgasm or male ejaculation. Withdrawal of penis can happen only after that. Sometimes, couple has to call for emergency and get medical attention.

Female Sexual Dysfunction (Pelvic Floor and Female Sexual Dysfunction)

VAGINAL SPASMS AND FEMALE SEX HEALTH

"Turn your wounds into wisdom."

—Oprah Winfrey

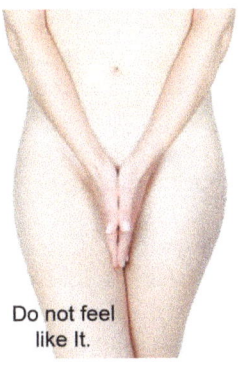

Do not feel like It.

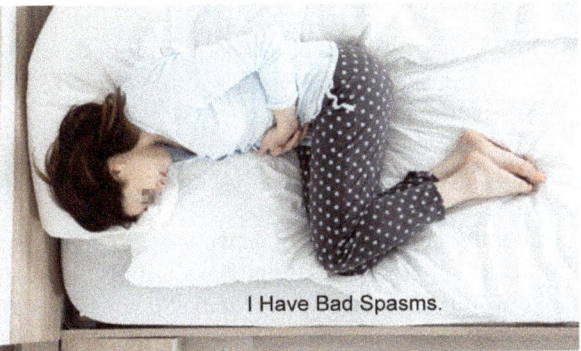

I Have Bad Spasms.

Any disorder related to female sexual desire, arousal, orgasm, and/or sexual pain is known as FSD. Sexual arousal is associated with vaginal lubrication, depends on integrity of sympathetic nervous system, and can be significantly reduced by anticipation of pain. The anticipation of pain or discomfort leads to anxiety which ultimately leads to reduced libido, arousal response, and can prevent vaginal lubrication. Vaginal lubrication can also be decreased by estrogen deficiency, pain medication, anticholinergic, antidepressant, and antihistamine medications. Poor lubrication causes vaginal dryness and causes microtrauma to vaginal tissue and pain. Conditions like dyspareunia and vaginismus create pain with sexual activity. It is important to treat sexual pain at earliest possible as it can cause low self-confidence, low self-esteem, personal distress, negative experience, relationship disputes, husband's or partner's disappointment and can negatively affect on quality of life concerns for the couple.

ONCOLOGY AND FEMALE SEXUAL DYSFUNCTION

Sexual dysfunction in oncological patients regardless of the origin of neoplasia is huge quality of life concern for most of the patients. Gynecologic and breast cancers have negative impact on woman's sexual health due to reduced body image especially postsurgical anatomical damages. It causes them to perceive their body as sexually substandard which creates changes in the response to the sexual stimuli. It ultimately influences desire, inadequate vaginal lubrication, and reduced pleasure and sexual well-being.

Surgical procedures like salpingo-oophorectomy lead to the physical and hormonal changes like early menopause.

Studies also suggest that cancers like head and neck can also hurt self-esteem which leads to distress in interpersonal and couple relationships.

Patients with breast tumors may lead to FSD due to multiple reasons. Mastectomy, conservative survey, endocrinological manipulations, and estrogen deprivation may create premature menopausal state. It leads to vaginal dryness, dyspareunia, reduced libido, and orgasmic disorders. Poor body image and anxiety about relations with partner make it worst.

Surgical procedures of gynecological cancer may include removal of sexual organs (uterus, tubes, ovaries, cervix, and vulva), which can lead to severe level of FSD.

MENOPAUSAL CHANGES

- Lower estrogen level leads to vaginal dryness, thinning, fragile tissue, reduced vaginal length and width, reduced expansive ability, and reduced lubrication.
- Physical changes of menopause can lead to reduced sexual desire, arousal, and orgasmic ability. Pain, burning, itching, and irritation during or after intercourse are common.
- If patient is sexually not well active, it can increase the symptoms. Regular sexual activity is very helpful as vaginal penetration increases vaginal blood flow, lubrication, and elasticity. Strong PFM can support all above.
- Vaginal lubrication and vaginal estrogen application can help to mange postmenopausal changes by restoring suppleness in vaginal tissues.

RADIOTHERAPY, CHEMOTHERAPY AND FEMALE SEXUAL DYSFUNCTION

Radiotherapy has a key role in the treatment of rectal, anal, bladder, cervix, and vulvar carcinomas along with breast cancers. Damage caused by radiation therapy may include bleeding, reduced elasticity of vaginal walls and vulva, vaginal dryness, thin and fragile genitalia, subsequent scarring, narrower and shorter vagina along with psychological repercussions. Chemotherapy may also lead to weakening of immune system, general tiredness, nausea, hair loss, and poor body image can lead to FSD.

VAGINAL LAXITY AND FEMALE SEX HEALTH

"If opportunity doesn't knock, build the door!"

—**Milton Berle**

If your patient does not feel best sensation down there, build their pelvic floor.

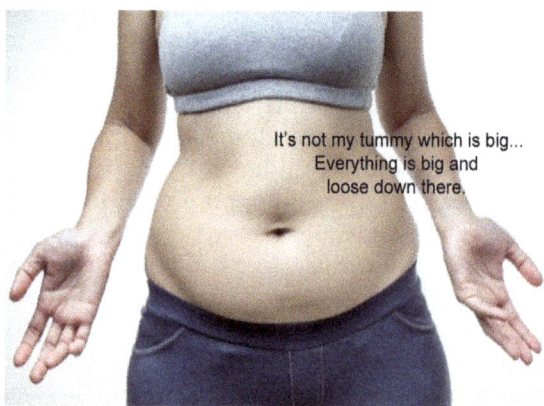

Many researches have confirmed that PFMs are responsible for intensity of pleasurable sensation during intercourse. Strong PFMs are tighter and thicker, which can increase the experience of stretch during intercourse. Also, fitter and tighter PFMs have more nerve endings and better blood circulation which help to engorge the clitoris and increase sexual sensations. Weaker and flabby PFM might not provide good neural stretch and leads to reduced blood circulation. As a result, it may lead to decreased vaginal sensation and reduced intensity of orgasms which negatively affects intimate life of a woman.

URINARY INCONTINENCE AND FEMALE SEX HEALTH

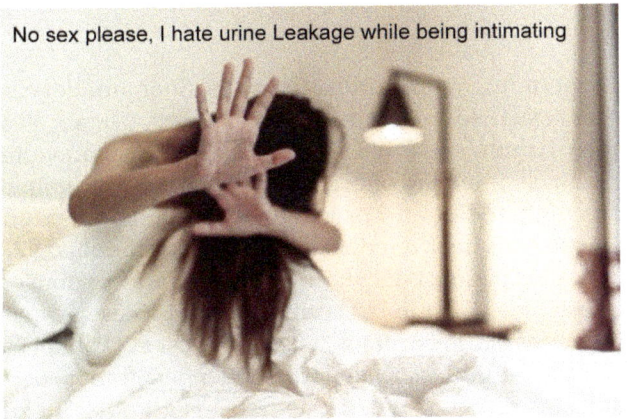

Women present with urinary incontinence (UI) especially mixed type report more of the sexual dysfunction. Anticipation of UI during sexual intercourse reduces the libido. According to research, incontinence during sexual intercourse can happen in up to 56% of women with lower urinary tract dysfunction. This problems are more visible after age of 50 years. Factors like frequent UI during sex, wetness during night, and compulsiveness to wear pads reduce the sexual desire of a woman. Conditions like overactive bladder lead to significantly higher level of pain and UI during sexual activities compare to stress urinary incontinence (SUI). The UI can happen during penetration, orgasm, or both. Involuntary detrusor contractions can lead to urine leakage during orgasm. Urodynamic studies during orgasm have demonstrated simultaneous bladder contraction and urethral relaxation.

POSTSURGICAL SEXUAL PROBLEMS

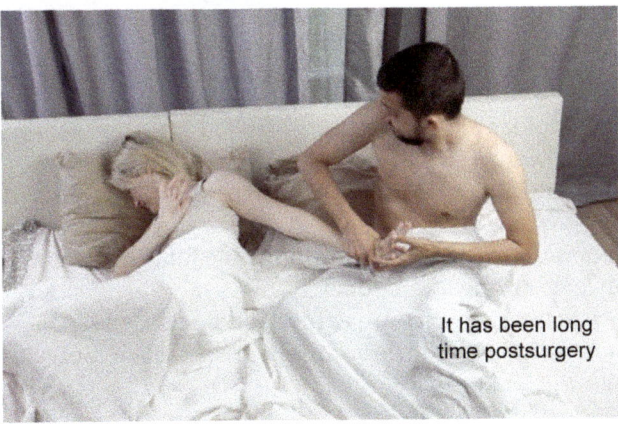

Poor sexual outcomes are very common issues after urological surgeries. Postsurgical sexual dysfunctions may include diminished or altered orgasmic response, postoperative reduced or loss of or reduced libido, and postoperative dyspareunia. Operative damage to the dorsal nerve of the clitoris may lead to orgasmic dysfunction. Vaginal shortening following excessive vaginal excision may lead to dyspareunia. Pain due to postsurgical scarring, reduced mobility, and decreased sensation are common postsurgical side effects.

SUMMARY

Hypotonus, hypertonus, or incoordinated pelvic floor muscles can negatively affect women's sexual desire, arousal, orgasms, and, overall, all sexual well-being of women. Healthy and fit pelvic floor muscles can improve libido, vaginal sensations, arousal, intensity of orgasm, and sexual well-being of women. PFR should be directed toward psychological evaluation, finding physical causes, and neuromuscular re-education to sexual stimulus. PFR should be started with detailed patient education, spouse or partner counseling, muscle awareness, muscle identification, relaxation training, Glazer's protocol. Tactile biofeedback devices like pelvic floor 360 are very useful. Patient can start self-relaxation, deep breathing associated with finger penetration, partner's finger penetration, tampon, dilator, etc. We believe it is very helpful for women to have complete control of penetration in women and educate her to progress with penetration when she feels comfortable.

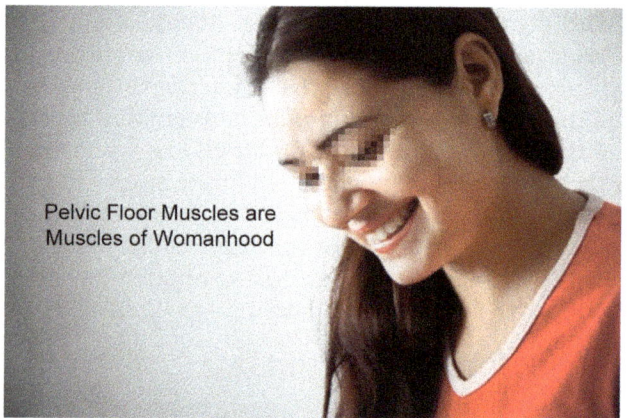

RESEARCH FINDINGS ABOUT FEMALE SEX HEALTH

- Orgasm difficulties affect 24% of women.
- About 10% of women have never experienced an orgasm.
- Between 33 and 50% of women are unhappy with how often they achieve orgasm.
- Pelvic floor muscles are directly responsible for the intensity of sensation a woman feels during intercourse.
- Toned pelvic floor muscles are tighter and thicker.
- Tighter and thicker pelvic floor muscles experience more stretch during intercourse.

- Firm pelvic floor muscles create more pleasurable sensation from stretch because they have more nerve endings.
- Well-toned vaginal pelvic floor muscles also have more blood circulation which helps to engorge the clitoris and increases sensation even more.

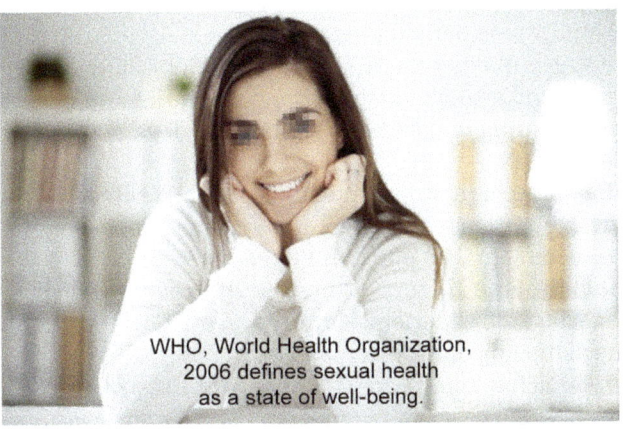

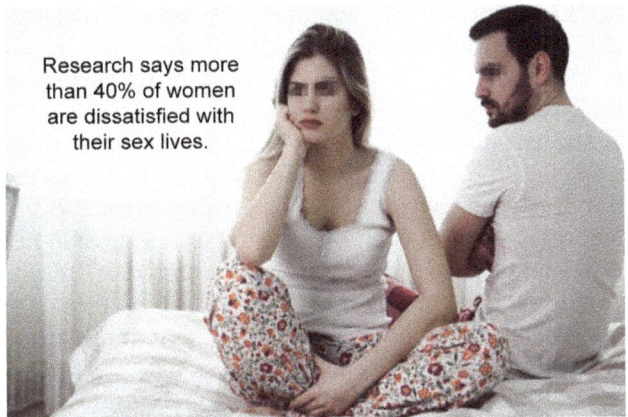

Women with higher reported level of sexual satisfaction also report a higher sense of purpose in life.
- Women who explore ways to have a better sex life, with expectations for improvement, can experience better sexual well-being.
- According to a study published in American Journal of Obstetrics and Gynecology, sexual dysfunction affects 48% of women, and these same women had decreased sexual sensation specifically in their clitoris which increased the chances of sexual dysfunction.
- Some studies have found that more than 40% of women report sexual dissatisfaction.
- National Survey of Sexual Health and Behavior states an "orgasm gap" with only 64% of women report having an orgasm at their most recent sexual event.
- Loose, stretched or damaged pelvic floor muscles can lead to reduced amount of sensation that a woman feels during sex. Most of the sensation

- during sex comes from the pelvic floor muscles because vagina alone has a very few sensory nerves.
- Pelvic floor muscles weaken and sag with age due to reduced tone. Also, less estrogen hormone after menopause causes the vaginal tissues to become thin and weaker. As a result, it decreases sexual sensation and leads to reduced ability to experience orgasms.
- Research shows that nerves within the pelvic floor muscles can stretch only 15% before damage occurs, which happens during the stretch and tear of the muscles during childbirth. It has a clear negative effect on women's sexual sensation.
- According to research, improvement in sexual desire and ability to reach more powerful orgasms with greater ease are great benefits shown by postpartum women who perform PFM exercises.
- Women who had a history of inability to reach orgasm due to poor pelvic muscle, tone experience improved sexual desire and performance including achieving orgasms.
- With age, we all lose muscle mass. After age of 40, women lose half a pound of muscle mass every year; after menopause, women lose one pound every year. Muscle loss is combined internal and external. As a result, women also lose PFMs with age which can lead to diminished sexual satisfaction. However, fit and healthy PFMs kept in good shape with exercises contribute to sexual pleasure and satisfaction.
- According to research, even women with the history of urinary leakage during sexual activities demonstrate positive difference with sexual satisfaction (including desire, arousal, lubrication, and orgasm)
- Studies show significantly better score on sexual satisfaction survey for the women who perform PFM exercises compared to the women do not do vaginal muscles exercise.
- Studies show that women with weak PFMs must relearn natural and unconscious contractions.
- Pelvic floor muscles surround the internal parts of clitoris which is invisible. So contraction of these muscles increases blood flow and sensation of the clitoris.

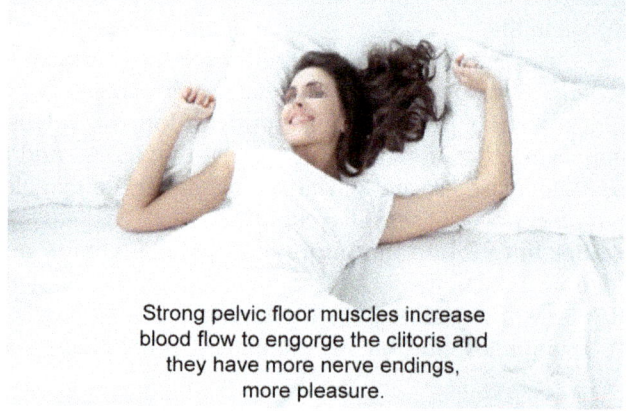

Strong pelvic floor muscles increase blood flow to engorge the clitoris and they have more nerve endings, more pleasure.

- Using pelvic floor muscles to stimulate clitoris can increase pleasure because clitoris has between 6,000 and 8,000 sensory nerve endings.

- Exercising pelvic floor muscles during foreplay increases blood flow to genitals, promotes lubrication, improves arousal, and improves over all intimate health of the women.

ORGASM AND PELVIC FLOOR

A research by Graber and Klin-Graber found a positive correlation between the strength of pelvic floor muscles and intensity of woman's orgasm.

Chambless et al. suggested that strong pelvic floor muscles are crucial for the attainment of orgasm, which means PFM training can help to prevent and treat arousal and orgasmic disorders.

Desire Enhancement by Pelvic Floor

In a Turkish study, improvement in sexual desire, "performance during coitus", and achievement of orgasm were reported in women who received pelvic floor rehabilitation, which means PFM training can help to prevent or treat sexual desire disorders.

> Female sexual dysfunctions (FSD) due to hypotonus, hypertonus, or incoordinated pelvic floor muscles.
> - *Hypertonus PFM:* Too tight or spasms mainly associated with pain, vaginismus, dyspareunia, etc.
> - *Hypotonus PFM:* Too loose or weak; mainly associated with reduced sensations, orgasmic dysfunctions, etc.
> - *Incoordinated PFM:* Inability to coordinated PFM action during penetration and thrusting movements.
>
> For example, patient might hold PFM tight during penetration or it might go for reflexive spams. Even if patient is able to relax PFM voluntarily.

(PFM: pelvic floor muscle)

MULTIPLE CHOICE QUESTIONS

Q1. What is the approximate length of the vagina during sexual activity?
- (a) 5–7 cm
- (b) 5–7 inches
- (c) 3–5 cm
- (d) 3–5 inches

Q2. What is the full form of HSDD?
- (a) Hyperactive sexual desire disorder
- (b) Hypoactive sexual desire disorder
- (c) Hyperactive sleep disturbance disorder
- (d) Hypoactive sleep disturbance disorder

Q3. Which term can be used to describe painful vaginal insertion?
- (a) Vaginismus
- (b) Dyspareunia
- (c) None of the above
- (d) Both of the above

Section 1: Female: Pelvic Floor Dysfunction

Q4. Which among the levator ani group of muscle is related to female orgasm?
 (a) Puborectalis (b) Pubococcygeus
 (c) Iliococcygeus (d) Coccygeus

Q5. Which term can be used to describe the condition in which due to very intense and sudden contraction of pelvic floor muscle the penis gets stuck in the vagina during sexual intercourse?
 (a) Vaginismus (b) Penis captivus
 (c) Dyspareunia (d) Vaginal lock

Q6. Which hormone is responsible for vaginal lubrication and its expandability?
 (a) Progesterone (b) Oxytocin
 (c) Estrogen (d) FSH

Q7. Vaginismus and dyspareunia are commonly related to which type of pelvic floor muscle dysfunction?
 (a) Hypotonus muscle dysfunction
 (b) Hypertonus muscle dysfunction
 (c) Incoordinated dysfunction
 (d) Visceral dysfunction

Q8. Orgasmic dysfunction generally results due to:
 (a) Hypertonus muscle dysfunction (b) Hypotonus muscle dysfunction
 (c) Incoordinated dysfunction (d) Visceral dysfunction

Q9. What is the other name of female ejaculation?
 (a) Squirting (b) Leaking
 (c) Overflow (d) Squeezing

Q10. Which bulbs are located underneath labia minora?
 (a) Bartholin's gland (b) Vestibular bulbs
 (c) Paraurethral glands (d) Bulbourethral glands

ANSWERS

1: (b) 5-7 inches
2: (b) Hypoactive sexual desire disorder
3: (b) Dyspareunia
4: (b) Pubococcygeus
5: (b) Penis captivus
6: (c) Estrogen
7: (b) Hypertonus muscle dysfunction
8: (b) Hypotonus muscle dysfunction
9: (a) Squirting
10: (b) Vestibular bulbs

Section 2

Male: Pelvic Floor Dysfunction

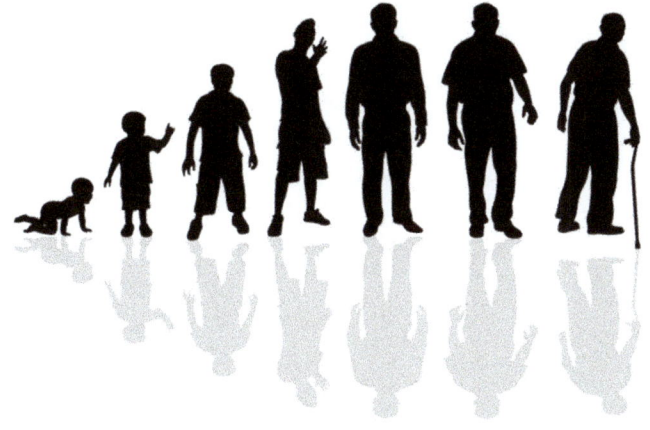

Men's Lifecycle,

It is harder to stand straight as you grow Older.....

I'm not a relationship expert. I'm an expert on manhood.
—Steve Harvey

....Be an expert on manhood

Chapter 8

Quick Reminder: Functional Anatomy

▎INTRODUCTION

The male pelvis contains the lower urinary tract, ureter, bladder, urethra, prostate gland, and pelvic floor muscles (PFMs). Following is a quick reminder of what you already know about male reproductive (Fig. 1) and urinary system (Fig. 2).

▎BLADDER AND VOIDING

- Urine from kidneys is propelled along the ureters into the bladder.
- It happens by peristaltic activity of the ureters.
- The elasticity of the bladder helps to maintain the pressure at zero.
- The intravesical stretch receptors are stimulated via S2-S4.
- It happens after filling of the bladder at 350–500 mL.
- It triggers detrusor muscle activity.
- Person feels a strong desire to void.

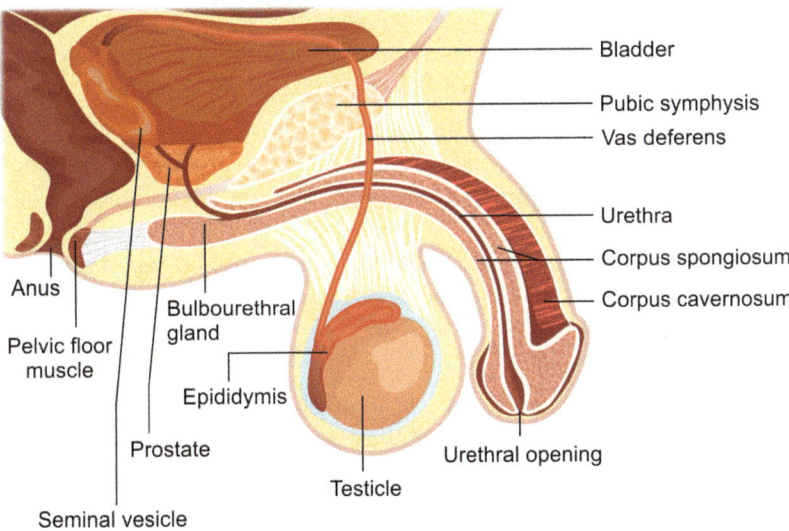

Fig. 1: Male reproductive system.

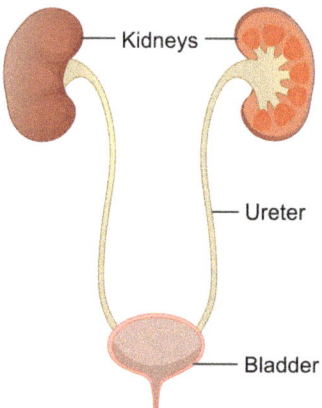

Fig. 2: Urinary system.

- The first sensation to void is usually at 200 mL.
- The relaxation of the striated PFM under voluntary control and completed by reflex action helps to void.
- After voiding is completed, bulbocavernosus (BC) muscle helps to eject the last few drops of urine and other PFM contracts while detrusor relaxes and bladder refills.

URETHRA

- Urethra is approximately 8 inches long. It passes through the prostate gland and opens through the tip of the penis. Urethra has two sphincter muscles—internal (involuntarily) and external (voluntarily). External sphincter muscle is thicker in male than female. Internal sphincter can get damaged during prostate cancer surgery.
- Urethra helps to pass urine outside the body. Urethra also helps to pass semen from the ejaculatory duct to the outside of the body.

The urethra in men has three portions:
1. *External portion*: The portion of urethra within the penis is external portion
2. *Internal portion*: The portion of the urethra within the perineum is internal portion
3. *Inner portion*: The portion of the urethra that travels through prostate and enters the bladder is the inner most portion.

PROSTATE (FIG. 3)

- Prostate gland is located at the base of the bladder. It is walnut-shaped fibromuscular gland. It is pierced through proximal urethra.
- The young adult prostate gland weighs about 20 g. The size of the prostate gland is about 4 cm × 3 cm × 2 cm. The size of the prostate gland increases

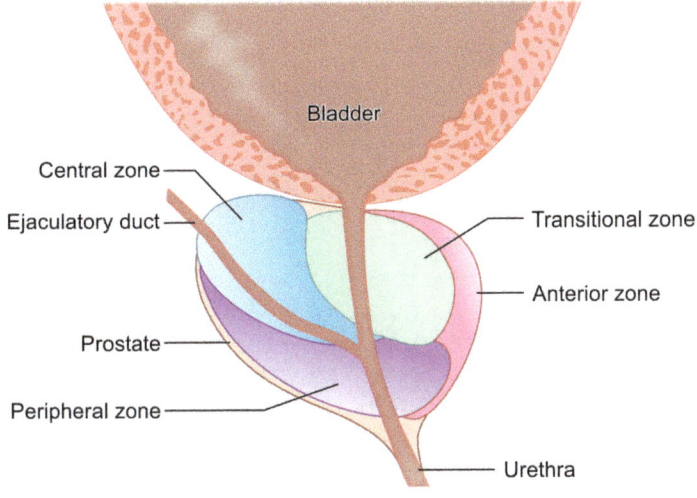

Fig. 3: Prostate gland.

with age. The prostate gland has three lobes: Anterior, right, and left. Left lobe is intraurethral.
- Main function of prostate is the manufacture of secretions, which become components of semen. Also it helps with entry of semen. The contractions of smooth muscle tissue of prostate help to control the flow of urine or semen.
- Milky white fluid of the prostate gland contains antibacterial nutrients, citrate for sperm transport and protein like prostate-specific antigen. Contraction of smooth muscles of the bladder neck during ejaculation helps to prevent urine leakage.
- Healthy pelvic floor muscles improve overall blood circulation to the pelvis and improve the support to overall health of the pelvis.

SCROTUM (FIG. 4)

- The scrotum is made of skin and muscles.
- It helps to hold the testis. It is anatomically situated inferior and posterior to the penis in the pubic region.
- It is made up of two testis located in two pouches. The smooth muscles of the scrotum are responsible for maintaining ideal distance between the testis and the rest of the body.
- The scrotum goes down for relaxation to move the testis away from the body's heat, while body heat goes up.
- As a result, it helps with thermoregulation and to support spermatogenesis. The scrotum contracts to move the testes closer to the body's heat when temperatures drop down. It indirectly helps to maintain the ideal range for spermatogenesis.

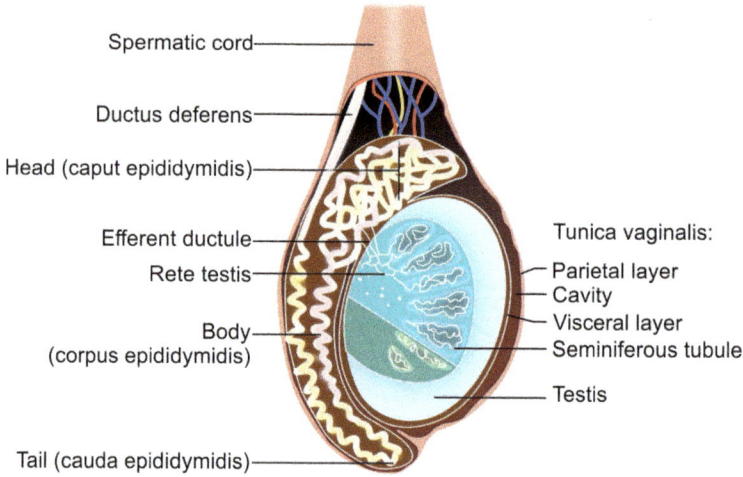

Fig. 4: Scrotum.

TESTICLES

- There are two testicles. They help the production of sperm and testosterone.
- The testes are ellipsoid glandular organs.
- The size of the testes is approximately 1.5–2 inch long. The diameter of testes is approximately an inch.
- Each testicle is located inside its own pouch on one side of the scrotum.
- The spermatic cord and cremaster muscle connect them with abdomen. The contraction and relaxation of cremaster muscles with the scrotum help to regulate the temperature of the testicles. Small compartments inside of the testicles are known as lobules.

EPIDIDYMIS

- The epididymis is an area where sperm is stored. It is around the superior and posterior edge of the testicles. The epididymis is made up of thin tubules.
- They are a few feet long. Sperm is produced inside the testes, which move into the epididymis to mature. Sperm gets time to mature because of the length of the epididymis.

SPERMATIC CORDS AND DUCTUS DEFERENS (FIG. 5)

- Spermatic cords are located within the scrotum. They contain the ductus deferens, nerves, veins, arteries, and lymphatic vessels.
- They help to connect testicles to the abdominal cavity and support the function of the testicles.

Ductus Deferens

- Vas deferens is another name of ductus deferens. It is a muscular tube. It is responsible to carry the sperm from the epididymis into the abdominal

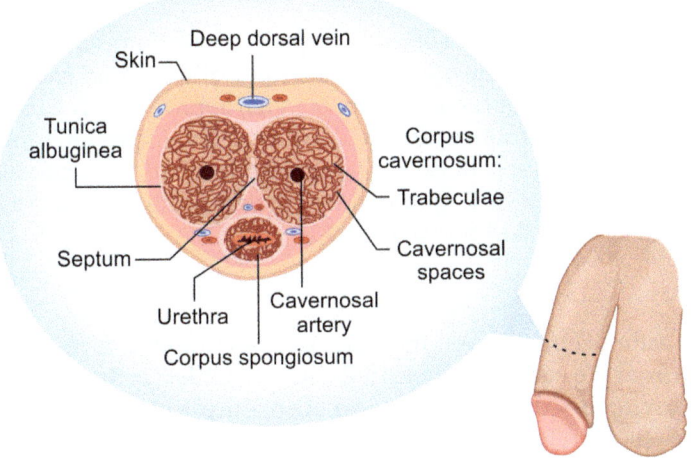

Fig. 5: Medical anatomy of penis.

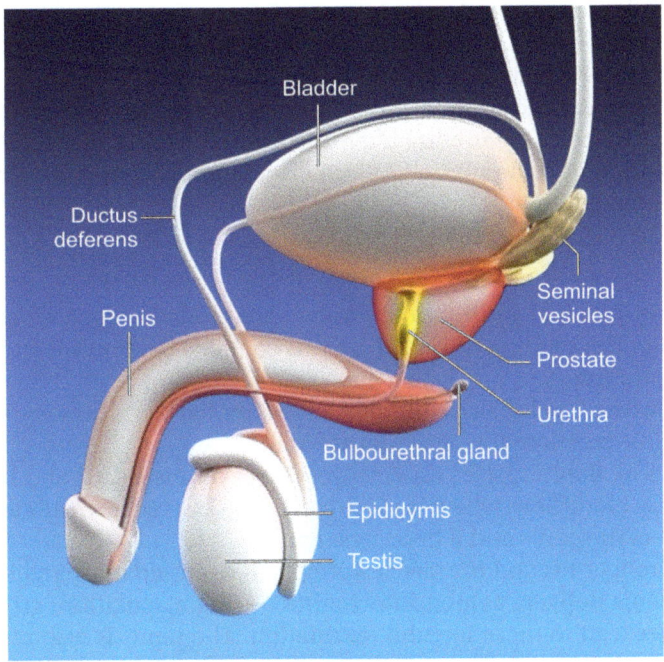

Fig. 6: Male urogenital anatomy.

cavity and to the ejaculatory duct. It has wider diameter than the diameter of epididymis.
- The storage of mature sperm happens in the internal space of ductus deferens. The ductus deferens mobilizes the sperm toward the ejaculatory duct.

SEMINAL VESICLES

- Some of the liquid portion of semen is produced and stored by the seminal vesicles, exocrine glands. They are anatomically situated anterior to the rectum and posterior to the urinary bladder, approximately 2 inches long. Seminal vesicles produce the liquid, which is rich in proteins and mucus.
- Alkaline pH helps sperm to survive against the acidic environment of the vagina. The fructose of the liquid feeds sperm cells. It helps to increase duration of survival of the sperm cell.

EJACULATORY DUCT

- The ductus deferens passes through the prostate and joins the urethra. The ducts from the seminal vesicles are within ejaculatory duct.
- The ejaculatory duct expels sperm. Also, during ejaculation, expels the secretions from the seminal vesicles into the urethra.

COWPER'S GLANDS

- The bulbourethral glands are another name of Cowper's glands. They are a pair of exocrine glands.
- They are pea-sized. They are located anterior to the anus and inferior to the prostate. It secretes a thin fluid into the urethra.
- This alkaline fluid lubricates the urethra. It also neutralizes acid from residual urine in the urethra after urination. During sexual arousal, entry of this fluid into the urethra before ejaculation prepares the urethra for the semen flow.

PENIS

- Penis is the male genitourinary organ, anatomically situated externally, and superior to the scrotum. The penis contains the urethra and opening of the urethra.
- Erectile tissue, pelvic floor muscles, and increased blood flow work together for penile erection during sexual arousal.
- The pelvic floor muscles especially ischiocavernosus (IC) and BC lead to increase blood flow, which leads to erection. The erection leads to increase in size of the penis and it becomes rigid.
- The stronger BC and IC muscles provide longer and more rigid erection. The penis delivers semen into vagina during ejaculation; stronger BC muscles lead to more forceful ejaculation. The penis is also responsible for excretion of urine through the urethra.

SEMEN

- Semen is generated by male sexual organs and expelled out of the body through ejaculation during sexual intercourse. Semen contains sperm. It is thick and sticky. It also helps sperm to remain within the vagina after intercourse due to its consistency.

- It has slightly alkaline pH, which helps to counterbalance and neutralize the acidic environment of the vagina. Semen contains approximately of 100 million sperm cells per milliliter in healthy adult male.

NERVE SUPPLY (FIG. 7)

Pudendal nerves.

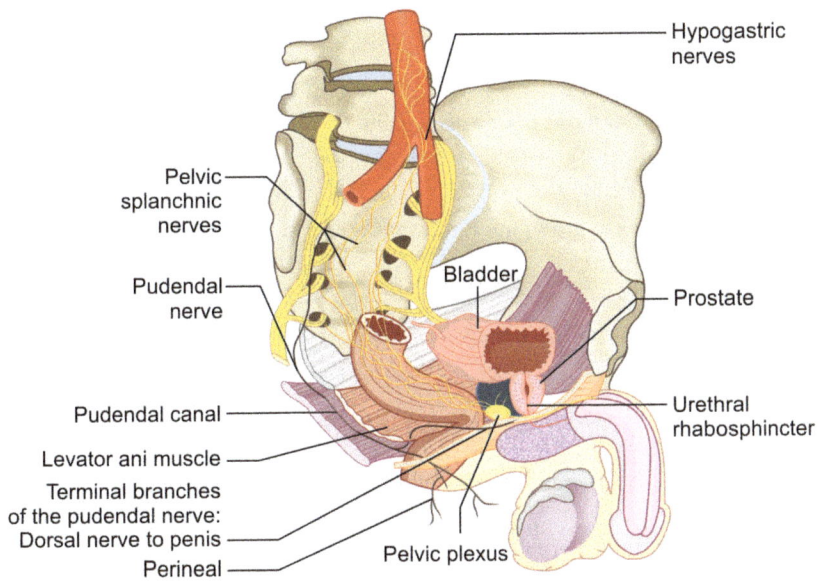

Fig. 7: Pelvic plexus.

MULTIPLE CHOICE QUESTIONS

Q1. Which nerve roots stimulate intravesical stretch receptors of urinary bladder?
- (a) L2-L4
- (b) S2-S3
- (c) S2-S5
- (d) S2-S4

Q2. Which muscle helps to eject last a few drops of urine out of urethra?
- (a) Ischiocavernosus
- (b) Bulbocavernosus
- (c) Levator ani
- (d) Sphincter urethra

Q3. What is the approximate length of male urethra?
- (a) 8 cm
- (b) 8 inches
- (c) 7 cm
- (d) 7 inches

Q4. What is the weight of prostate gland?
- (a) 40 g
- (b) 20 g
- (c) 50 g
- (d) 25 g

Q5. The contraction of which smooth muscle during ejaculations prevents urine leak?
- (a) Urinary bladder
- (b) Prostate
- (c) Seminal vesicle
- (d) Bulbourethral gland

Section 2: Male: Pelvic Floor Dysfunction

Q6. What is the main role of scrotum?
(a) Thermoregulation for spermatogenesis
(b) Thermoregulation for homeostasis
(c) Both of the above
(d) None of the above

Q7. Which structure connects the testicles to the abdomen?
(a) Spermatic cord and cremaster muscle
(b) Only spermatic cord
(c) Only cremaster
(d) Scrotum

Q8. What is the other name of Cowper's gland?
(a) Bulbourethral gland
(b) Seminal vesicle
(c) Bartholin's gland
(d) Vas deferens

Q9. Semen contains approximately how many sperms per milliliter?
(a) 10 million/mL
(b) 100 million/mL
(c) 10 million/dL
(d) 100 million/dL

Q10. What is the nerve supply of pelvic organs?
(a) Pelvic nerve
(b) Pudendal nerve
(c) Sciatic nerve
(d) Iliac nerve

ANSWERS

1: (d) S2-S4
2: (b) Bulbocavernous
3: (b) 8 inches
4: (b) 20 g
5: (b) Prostate
6: (a) Thermoregulation for spermatogenesis
7: (a) Spermatic cord and cremaster muscle
8: (a) Bulbourethral gland
9: (b) 100 million/mL
10: (b) Pudendal nerve

Chapter 9

Pelvic Floor Muscles and Functions

"A man must stand erect, not be kept erect by others."
—Marcus Aurelius

Proper functioning of PFM is extremely essential for your patients to stand erect. Otherwise, age-induced atrophy will slouch them forever!

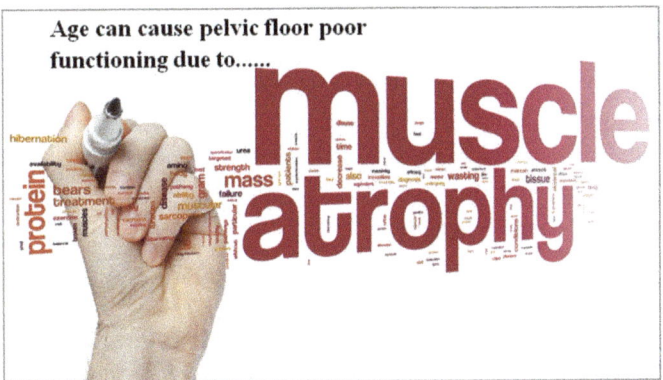

■ PELVIC FLOOR MUSCLE LAYERS (FIG. 1)

- The pelvic floor is hammock-shaped and group of muscles extending from the base of the spine to the pubic bone. PFMs are interconnected and work together as a unit. They collectively help with solidity, longevity, and quality of erection along with ejaculation. Pelvic floor dysfunction (PFD) can lead to conditions like erectile dysfunction (ED), urinary incontinence, pelvic pain, or poor prostate health.
- Just like women, pelvic floor muscles (PFMs) are extremely important part of men's urinary, prostate, and sexual health. PFM provides basic platform for prostate gland.
- There are three different layers of PFMs in men. They provide base of very important functions of men's health.
    1. Superficial layer—urogenital and anal triangle
    2. Middle layer—urogenital diaphragm
    3. Third layer—pelvic diaphragm.

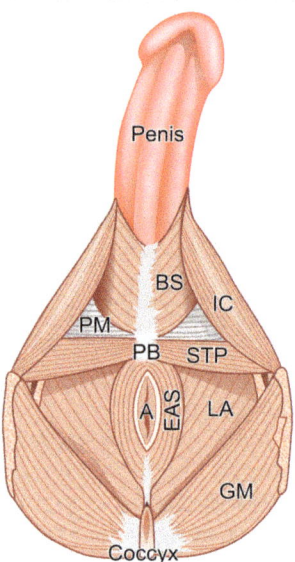

Fig. 1: Pelvic floor muscle layer.
(IC: ischiocavernosus; BS: bulbospongiosus; PM: perineal membrane; PB: perineal body; STP: superficial transverse perineal; EAS: external anal sphincter; GM: gluteus maximus)

Superficial Layer

Urogenital and Anal Triangle

It is mainly responsible for continence and sexual functions. It helps levator ani, but is not directly responsible for support.
- *Superficial transverse perineal muscle (STP)*: It is from ischial tuberosity to perineal body. It helps action of deep transverse perineal muscles to stabilize perineal body.
- *Bulbocavernosus (BC) muscle/bulbospongiosus*:
  - It is from perineal body to corpus cavernosum. It connects and compresses with the bulb of the penis to the urogenital diaphragm.
  - It contracts during ejaculation. It also surrounds deeper portion of the urethra and compresses urethra.
  - Stronger BC muscles compress the urethra to expel last few drops of urine that sit in the deep urethra. It also helps to support corpus spongiosum and the glans. It helps to move blood from the penis into glans.
  - It maximizes engorgement of the corpus spongiosum and glans. BC muscles in female are split around the vagina.
  - Bulbocavernosus muscles contraction compresses venous return by compressing the dorsal vein of the penis. At the climax, BC muscle is responsible for the expulsion of the semen through rhythmic contractions. Rhythmic contraction of stronger BC muscles helps with more powerful ejaculations.

- *Ischiocavernosus (IC) muscle*: It is from ischial tuberosity to corpus cavernosum on each side of the penis. It covers and compresses each corpus cavernosum of the penis.
  - It is a compressor muscle. IC muscle compresses the corpora and stabilizes the erect penis.
  - It helps to move blood from body of crura into the body of penis.
  - It erects the penis by increasing the intracavernous pressure.
  - It is mainly responsible for the solidity or rigidity of erection. It decreases the return of the blood flow to help and maintain the rigidity of the penis.
  - At climax, IC contracts in rhythmic fashion and provides maximum erectile rigidity at the time of ejaculation.
- *External anal sphincter*: From anal canal, it is anchored to perineal body and anococcygeal body, and loops around the anus to provide continence. It is always contracted to a baseline, which is known as tonic contraction. It can also vigorously contract along with PFM. It should be relaxed for bowel movement and expelling gas.
(Credit to Dr Henry Gray, Gray's Anatomy of the Human Body, 20th edition, Original Publication 1918, Public Domain)

Middle Layer/Urogenital Diaphragm

- *Deep transverse perineal muscle (DTP):* It is from ischial ramus to perineal body. It stabilizes position of perineal body. It consists of additional fibers like sphincter urethra which loops around urethra and helps with continence. It is under voluntary control and can be activated and trained. It contracts to help PFMs to expel semen and urine.
- *External urethral sphincter:* External uretheral sphincter also called sphincter urethera are circular fibers which originates from inferior pubic arch from both the sides and loops around the urethra.

Deep/Innermost Layer: Pelvic Diaphragm

Pelvic diaphragm is made up of levator ani, which is the most important supportive muscle. It is a hammock-like muscle between the pubic bones in front and coccyx. The difference between levator ani and other skeletal muscle is higher resting tone. Main function of levator ani is to provide support to pelvic organs and to provide continence at night. It is innervated by pudendal nerve. Advanced contractions are required to maintain continence during coughing, sneezing, laughing, jumping, etc. This muscle has approximately 70% slow twitch and 30% fast twitch muscle fibers. This muscle has different parts as per direction.
- *Pubococcygeus (PC) muscle*: It is from the pubic bones to coccyx. In male, you can feel the muscle between coccyx and anus by putting index finger on the coccyx and track it down to a soft tissue groove where the bone ends, at insertion of coccyx, especially during contraction. Contraction can be felt at tip of the coccyx. It supports pelvic viscera.

- *Puborectalis (PR) muscle*: It is from pubic bone to anococcygeal body, slings around the junction of rectum and anal canal, and loops around rectum. It pulls the rectum forward during contraction, toward pubic symphysis to assist fecal continence.
- *Levator prostate (LP)*: It is present only in men. It supports prostate gland and contributes to prostate health.
- *Iliococcygeus*: It is from coccyx to each of the ischial tuberosity. Mainly supportive work, not much contribution on lifting anus.
- *Coccygeus muscle*: It is from ischial spine to coccyx. It contributes with stability of sacroiliac joint. It lies close to iliococcygeus muscles. Supports pelvic viscera and pulls coccyx forward after defecation.

Other Key Muscles

- *Obturator internus*: From pelvis to greater trochanter of femur. Lateral rotation of extended hip and abduction of flexed hip L5-S1.
- *Piriformis*: From sacrum to greater trochanter of femur. Lateral rotation of extended hip and abduction of flexed hip.
- *Nerve supply*: The pudendal nerve.
- *Blood supply*: The pudendal arteries.

FUNCTIONS OF PELVIC FLOOR MUSCLES

The PFM has functional differences between men and women. Followings are key functions of PFM when it comes to men's health:
- Improves sexual health
- Prevents muscle loss and helps to treat erectile dysfunction
- Prevents and helps to treat premature ejaculation
- Helps to improve urinary health
- Helps to improve prostate health
- Helps in bowel control
- Prevents pelvic pain.

PFM Improves Sexual Fitness

Strong pelvic floor muscles increase sexual fitness. Men with weak pelvic floor muscles report some sort of sexual dysfunctions.

PFM Prevents Muscle Loss and help to treat Erectile Dysfunction

More than 50% of men over 40 years experience some form of erectile dysfunction. Fitter pelvic floor muscles can help to prevent age-related muscle loss and right treatment can even treat erectile dysfunction.

PFM prevent and treat Premature Ejaculations

A weak pelvic floor generally leads to premature ejaculation, the most common male sexual disorder.

PFM Helps to Improve Urinary Health

Conditions like postvoid dribbling, urinary incontinence, and an overactive bladder can affect men's lifestyle and confidence.

PFM Helps to Improve Prostate Health

Pelvic muscle exercises can increase pelvic blood flow, which is very helpful for prostate health.

PFM Helps in Bowel Control

Strong pelvic muscles can improve the tightness and ultimately closure of the sphincter muscles to alleviate bowel urgency and leakage.

PFM Prevents Pelvic Pain

Strong pelvic floor should also be capable enough to create complete relaxation. Proper relaxation ability of pelvic floor muscles can prevent pelvic pain.

MULTIPLE CHOICE QUESTIONS

Q1. What is the collective function of pelvic floor muscles during ejaculation?

(a) To provide solidity, longevity, and quality of erection
(b) To provide only solidity
(c) To provide only longevity
(d) None of the above

Q2. What is the attachment of deep transverse perineal muscles?

(a) Ischial spine to perineal body
(b) Ischial ramus to perineal body
(c) Ischial tuberosity to perineal body
(d) Ischial tuberosity to sphincter urethrae

Q3. What is the attachment of superficial transverse perineal muscle?

(a) Ischial tuberosity to perineal body
(b) Ischial ramus to perineal body
(c) Ischial tuberosity to sphincter urethrae
(d) Ischial spine to the fibers of deep transverse perineal muscles

Q4. What is the role of bulbocavernosus muscle during urination?

(a) It contracts to expel last a few drops of urine
(b) It relaxes to expel last a few drops of urine
(c) It contracts and gives signal to detrusor to relax
(d) It relaxes and gives signals to detrusor to contract

Section 2: Male: Pelvic Floor Dysfunction

Q5. Which muscle helps for powerful ejaculation?
- (a) Ischiocavernosus
- (b) Bulbocavernosus
- (c) Smooth muscles of penis
- (d) Deep transverse perineal muscle

Q6. Which one of the below muscles is present only in males?
- (a) Levator ani
- (b) Bulbocavernosus
- (c) Ischiocavernosus
- (d) Levator prostate

Q7. Which one of the following is false for pelvic floor muscle function?
- (a) It is not playing any active role in sexual health
- (b) It helps to maintain urinary hygiene
- (c) It helps for maintaining closure of anal canal
- (d) None of the above

Q8. How does age affect the pelvic floor muscle function?
- (a) Aging causes muscle weakness
- (b) Aging causes hypertrophy of pelvic floor muscles thereby increasing their strength
- (c) Age causes hypotrophy of prostate
- (d) All of the above

Q9. What is the shape of pelvic floor muscles?
- (a) Square
- (b) Oval
- (c) Hammock shaped
- (d) Circular

Q10. The structure can be trained by exercise, except for:
- (a) Endopelvic fascia
- (b) Levator ani muscle
- (c) Bulbocavernosus
- (d) Piriformis

ANSWERS

1: (a) To provide solidity, longevity and quality of erection
2: (b) Ischial ramus to perineal body
3: (a) Ischial tuberosity to perineal body
4: (a) It contracts to expel last a few drops of urine
5: (b) Bulbocavernosus
6: (d) Levator prostate
7: (a) It is not playing any active role in sexual health
8: (a) Aging causes muscle weakness
9: (c) Hammock shaped
10: (a) Endopelvic fascia

Chapter 10

Pelvic Floor Muscles Dysfunction (Types of PFD)

"The defining function of the artist is to cherish consciousness."
—Max Eastman

Defining function of the men's pelvic floor is to cherish manhood.

PFD can be depressive for any man

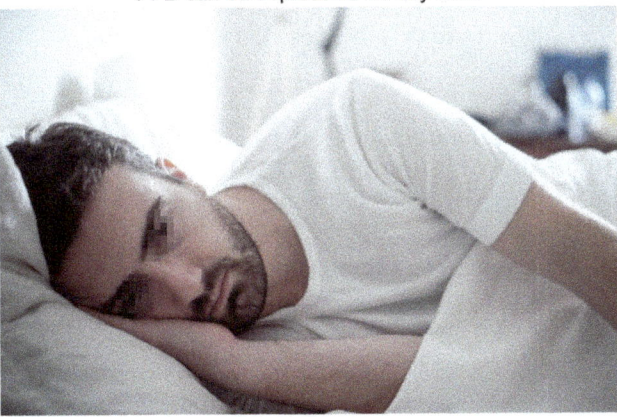

PELVIC FLOOR DYSFUNCTION

We all understand pelvic floor muscle (PFM) functions. We understand how they can help with men's sexual, prostate, and urinary health. PFM can become too loose, too tight, or incoordinated. They can fail to continue with their normal function which is known as pelvic floor dysfunction (PFD) (Figs. 1A to C).

Causes of Pelvic Floor Dysfunction

- Age
- Overweight or obesity
- Prostatitis
- Prostatectomy
- Pelvic trauma
- Perineal trauma
- Pelvic organ pathologies, etc.

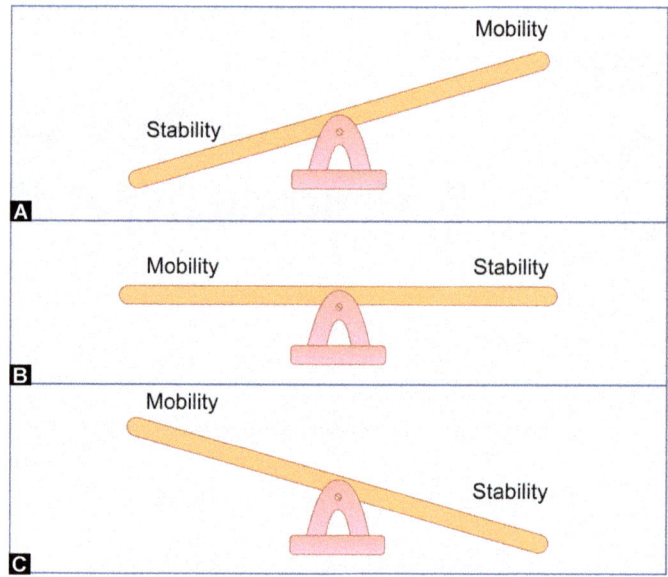

Figs. 1A to C: Types of pelvic floor dysfunction.

TYPES OF PELVIC FLOOR DYSFUNCTION

It is very important to maintain delicate balance between stability, mobility, and usability for best functioning of PFM. Too much stability leads to tightness, spasm or hypertonus PFM, too much mobility and looseness leads to hypotonus PFM.

Key function is a balance with stability, mobility, and usability.

Pelvic floor dysfunction is divided into mainly two categories:
1. Hypertonus
2. Hypotonus.

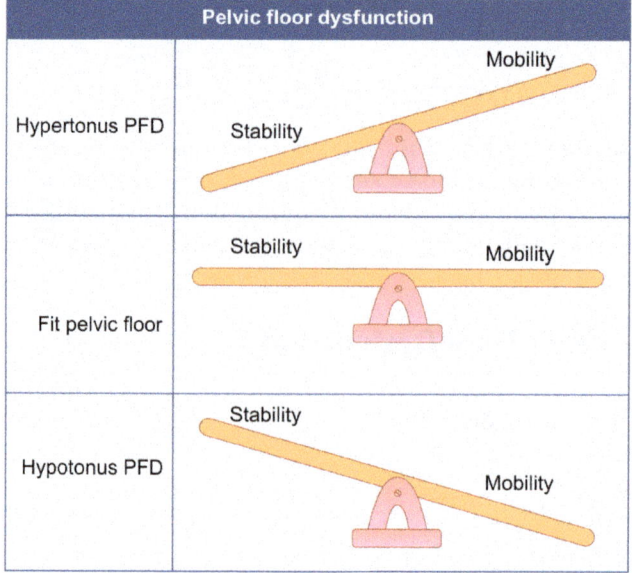

1. **Hypertonus dysfunction or PFM pain:** Hypertonus means overactive pelvic floor muscles. They do not let the organs fully expand due to adhesions, surgery, or trauma. Hypertonus pelvic floor muscles cannot relax properly. Symptoms are pressure, pain, constipation, and urinary frequency. Hypertonus or spasmodic pelvic floor muscles create impairment of muscle isolation, contraction, and relaxation. Pain can be localized to the suprapubic area, coccyx, lower sacrum, rectal pain, and pelvic discomfort. PF do not know that how to relax completely. Also, they contract or spasm when full relaxation is necessary, e.g. pelvic pain conditions.
2. **Hypotonus dysfunction or erectile dysfunction:** Pelvic floor muscles fail to maintain normal tone or create a strong contraction when it is necessary. It means too weak or lax pelvic floor muscles. It generally happens with age, atrophy, or lack of use, e.g. erectile dysfunction, premature ejaculations, postvoidal dribbling, etc. (Fig. 2).

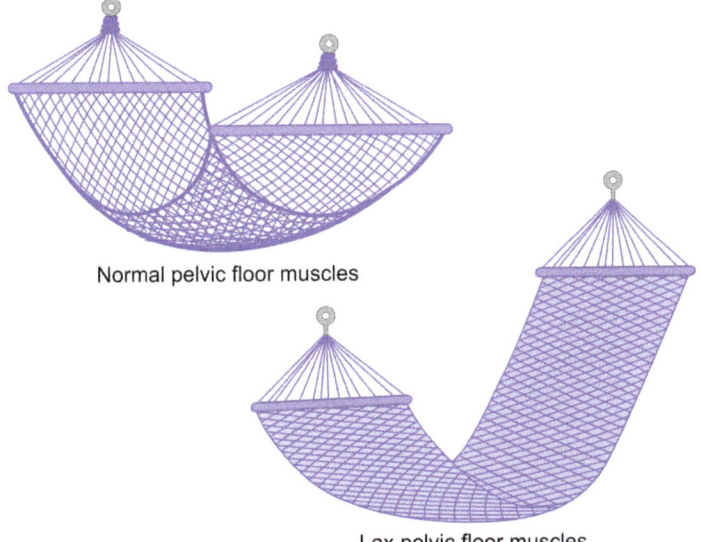

Fig. 2: Hammock shaped: Pelvic floor laxity.

OTHER CLASSIFICATIONS OF PELVIC FLOOR DYSFUNCTION

Incoordination Dysfunction/Combined Dysfunction

It can be defined as difficulty to create proper or complete sequencing of pelvic floor or abdominal muscles contractions and relaxations. It can be due to neurological, functional, or habitual incoordination. Difficulty in the contraction or relaxation sequencing of pelvic floor (PF). Neurological incoordination, functional incoordination, and habitual incoordination are different types of incoordination dysfunction.

Visceral Dysfunction

It is dysfunction of pelvic floor muscles due to visceral pathology like irritable bowel syndrome (IBS), etc.

Nonfunctional Dysfunction

Nonpalpable pelvic floor muscle contraction and relaxation for example paralytic muscles.

MULTIPLE CHOICE QUESTIONS

Q1. A proper pelvic floor function means balance between:
- (a) Stability and mobility
- (b) Stability and flexibility
- (c) Mobility and flexibility
- (d) Flexibility and fixation

Q2. Impairment in muscle isolation, contraction, and relaxation leads to which type of pelvic floor muscle dysfunction?
- (a) Hypotonus
- (b) Hypertonus
- (c) Incoordination
- (d) Any type of dysfunction

Q3. Erectile dysfunction and postvoidal dribbling fall in which type of pelvic floor dysfunction?
- (a) Hypotonus
- (b) Hypertonus
- (c) Incoordination
- (d) Any type of dysfunction

Q4. Irritable bowel syndrome leads to which type of pelvic floor dysfunction?
- (a) Visceral
- (b) Hypertonus
- (c) Hypotonus
- (d) Incoordinated

Q5. When there is abnormal contraction and relaxation of pelvic floor muscles, it is called as:
- (a) Visceral
- (b) Hypertonus
- (c) Hypotonus
- (d) Incoordinated

ANSWERS

1: (a) Stability and mobility
2: (d) Any type of dysfunction
3: (a) Hypotonus
4: (b) Hypertonus
5: (d) Incoordinated

Chapter 11

Assessment of Pelvic Floor Muscle

"Being male is a matter of birth. Being a man is a matter of age. But being a gentleman is a matter of choice."
—**Vin Diesel**

Proactive pelvic floor assessment and fitness is a matter of choice. Choose to educate "muscles of manhood."

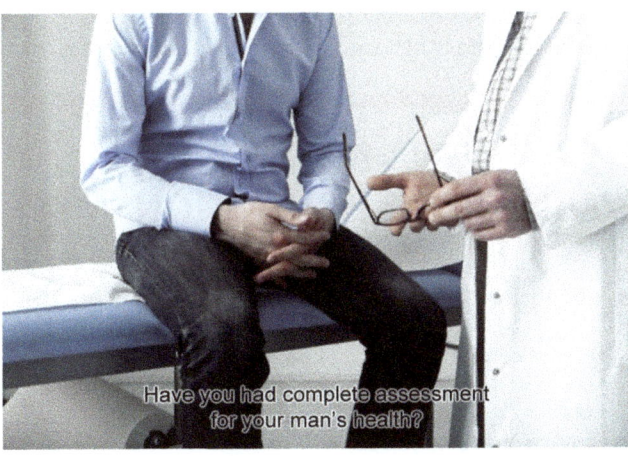

Surprisingly, when it comes to pelvic floor muscle (PFM), most of the attention is commonly given to women PFM as its connection to vaginal laxity, urinary incontinence, pelvic organ prolapse, and pelvic pain is well understood and well discussed in many literatures. Dr Kegel has put a lot of attention by developing Kegel exercises which are commonly used by educated mothers especially during prenatal, perinatal, and postnatal phases.

When it comes to PFMs in men, it commonly becomes the issue of muscles of manhood. It is commonly observed in our practice that many men have chosen a silent suffering as it is the muscles about man-ego. However, the truth is that the PFM of men has the same meaningful potential of examination and treatment effectiveness like female. However, it is commonly ignored or neglected.

Female PFMs can be palpated transvaginally or transrectally. However, male PFMs need to be assessed transrectally or externally.

Section 2: Male: Pelvic Floor Dysfunction

SUBJECTIVE

Subjective History

- When it comes to pelvic floor dysfunction (PFD), each patient is a teacher. It is very important to take detailed subjective history. Following parts of history taking are essential to understand type of PFD.
- Chief complaints—exact complaint in patient's own words would be easily able to provide signal toward type of PFD.
- Take detailed history of surgery, pelvic trauma, pelvic pain, prostate health, urinary incontinence and erectile dysfunction (ED), etc.
- Urinary leakage: Detailed history about types of activities that creates leakage, number of times of leakage, ability to hold urine for prolonged time, e.g. while travelling, amount of leakage, need to wear or change pads, postvoidal dribbling, etc.
- Prostate health: Detailed history about pelvic pain, prostate health, and prostatectomy.
- Sexual health or pelvic pain: Detailed history about pain, discomfort. History about ED like solidity of erection, longevity of erection, difficulty with erection, premature ejaculation, etc. *IIEF*
    - *International Index of Erectile Function Questionnaire*
- Other associated history like undiagnosed low back pain, etc.

Het's MSF SCALE
MALE SEXUAL FUNCTION (MSF)

WOW IIPRE

- Are you sexually active?
  a. Yes ☐   b. No ☐
- If yes, what is your current frequency of sexual intercourse?
  _____/week
  _____/month
- What was your past frequency of sexual intercourse?
  _____/week
  _____/month
- Do you have any other medical condition which might be affecting your sexual health?
  a. Yes ☐   b. No ☐
  Specify_____
- Are you apprehensive of urine leakage during intercourse?
  a. Yes ☐   b. No ☐   c Sometimes ☐
- Do you have any problems with prostate health?
  a. Yes ☐   b No ☐
  Specify_____
- Do you suffer from any type of urine problems?
  a. Yes ☐   b No ☐

- Do you have history of any surgery like prostatectomy or any other?
  a. Yes ☐   b. No ☐
  Specify_____

Pain and Discomfort

- Do you have pain in your private area (penis, scrotum, perineal body, anus or any other pain).
  a. Yes ☐   b. No ☐   c. Sometimes ☐
  Specify_____
- Are you able to have pain free sexual activity?
  a. Yes ☐   b. No ☐
- If no, what is your level of pain or discomfort during sexual activity?
  a. Intense ☐   b. Moderate ☐   c. Mild ☐
- How frequently do you feel pain or discomfort during intercourse?
  a. Always ☐   b. Sometimes ☐   c. Rarely ☐
- Are you able to complete intercourse even with pain?
  a. Yes ☐   b. Most of the time ☐   c. Have to stop ☐
- If there is pain, does it lasts even after intercourse?
  a. Yes ☐   b. No ☐   c. Sometimes ☐
  For how long_____
1. Please rate level of pain free and comfortable experience during sexual intercourse.

0	1	2	3	4	5	6	7	8	9	10

Uncomfortable and painful   Comfortable and pain free

Sexual Desire

- What is the level of your sexual desire or interest?
  a. High ☐   b. Moderate ☐   c. Low ☐
- How will you rate your desire to have sex compared to past or before?
  a. More intense ☐   b. Same ☐   c. Less intense ☐
- Do you always feel receptive towards your partner's initiation?
  a. Yes ☐   b. No ☐
- If no, how often do you feel receptive towards your partner's initiation.
  _____/10
2. Please rate your overall desire to have sex.

0	1	2	3	4	5	6	7	8	9	10

No desire   High desire

Sexual arousal (erectile functioning)

- Can you get penile erection during sexual activity?
  a. Yes ☐   b. No ☐
- If yes, how often can you get penile erection during sexual activity?
  a. All the time ☐   b. Sometimes ☐   c. Rarely ☐
- Do you feel that you have hard enough erection for successful vaginal penetration?
  a. Yes ☐   b. No ☐

Section 2: Male: Pelvic Floor Dysfunction

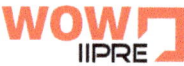

- If yes, how often can you have hard (enough penile erection for successful vaginal penetration?)
  a. All the time ☐   b. Sometimes ☐   c. Rarely ☐
- Are you able to maintain penile erection throughout sexual intercourse?
  a. Yes ☐   b. No ☐
- If you cannot maintain erection, how frequently do you lose erection during intercourse?
  a Always ☐   b. Sometimes ☐   c. Rarely ☐
- If you lose erection, can you regain erection by manual stimulation or any other way to complete intercourse?
  a. Always ☐   b. Sometimes ☐   c. Rarely ☐
- How satisfied you are with your erection throughout sexual intercourse?
  a. Very satisfied ☐   b. Somewhat satisfied ☐   c. Dissatisfied ☐
- How many times did you get satisfactory erection in your last 10 sexual intercourse? _____/10
- How would you rate your erection compared to past?
  a. Better ☐   b. Same ☐   c. Worst ☐
- How would you rate your confidence level for maintaining erection throughout intercourse?
  a. High ☐   b. Average ☐   c. Low ☐

3. Please rate your overall erectile ability during sexual intercourse.

0	1	2	3	4	5	6	7	8	9	10

Inability   Best ability

Orgasm (ejaculations)

- Do you feel that you find difficulty/delay in reaching orgasm?
  a. Yes ☐   b. No ☐   c. Sometimes ☐
- Do you feel that you are able to last long enough in sexual intercourse?
  a. Yes ☐   b. No ☐
- If no, how frequently you experience premature ejaculations?
  a. Always ☐   b. Sometimes ☐   c. Never ☐
- How intense is your ejaculation force?
  a. Very intense ☐   b. Moderate   c Mild ☐
- Are you satisfied with the intensity of ejaculation you reach during sexual intercourse?
  a. Yes ☐   b. No ☐   c. Sometimes ☐

4. Please rate your overall ejaculation experience?

0	1	2	3	4	5	6	7	8	9	10

Bad   Very good

Satisfaction

- Do you feel like you are completely satisfied with sexual intercourse?
  a. Yes ☐   b. No ☐
- If no, how frequent are you satisfied with sexual intercourse?
  a. Always ☐   b. Sometimes ☐   c. Never ☐

- How is your level of satisfaction compared to past?
  a. Same ☐   b. Less ☐   c. More ☐
5. Please rate your overall satisfaction with your sexual life.

| 0 | 1 | 2 | 3 | 4 | 5 |

Dissatisfied   Completely satisfied

Confidence

- Do you feel any nervousness or performance anxiety with sexual intercourse?
  a. Yes ☐   b. No ☐
- If yes, how often do you feel any nervousness or performance anxiety with sexual intercourse?
  a. All the time ☐   b. Sometimes ☐   c. Rarely ☐
- Does nervousness or performance anxiety negatively affects your sexual desire or sexual performance?
  a. Yes ☐   b. No ☐   c. Sometimes ☐
6. Please rate your level of confidence about overall sex life.

| 0 | 1 | 2 | 3 | 4 | 5 |

No confidence   Best confidence

Other Questions

- How well is your emotional bonding with your partner?
  a. Good ☐   b. Average ☐   c. Bad ☐
- How well is your intimate bonding with your partner?
  a. Good ☐   b. Average ☐   c. Bad ☐
- Do you feel that emotional distress negatively affects your sexual life?
  a. Yes ☐   b. No ☐   c. Sometimes ☐
- Do you feel that you get distracted due to some negative thoughts during sexual intercourse?
  a. Yes ☐   b. No ☐   c. Sometimes ☐
- Does your sexual well-being negatively affects other aspect of your life?
  a. Yes ☐   b. No ☐

Please answer these questions:
1. Since when are you suffering from this problem? _____
2. Have you ever had any treatment for this problem?
   a Yes ☐   b. No ☐
3. If the answer to the above question is yes (specify), what was your success rate?
   _____
4. Please describe your problem in your own words.
   _____

Interpretation of Het's MSF Scale

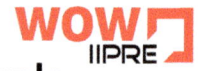

The Het's MSF scale is designed to find the sexual score of a patient suffering from male sexual dysfunction. The scale has 5 components, desire, arousal (erectile functioning), orgasm (ejaculation) and satisfaction.

The last question in all the component except for psychological factors has a score from 0-10, so the maximum score of the whole scale will be 50.

The initial questions in all the component are not used to find the score they are designed mainly for clinical understanding and to check the progress.

Only the last questions score will give the value. 0-25 is poor sexual health
25-40 is average sexual health 40-50 is good sexual health.
(0 is worst and 50 is best male sexual health).
The accurate cause of MSD can be diagnosed by seeing the individual score of the 5 components.

Component	Minimum score	Maximum score	Patient score
Pain, discomfort	0	10	
Desire	0	10	
Arousal (erectile functioning)	0	10	
Orgasm (ejaculation)	0	10	
Satisfaction	0	10	
Total score	_____	50	

Too tight or spasmodic pelvic floor muscles may lead to pain during sexual activity, which can negatively affect desire, arousal (erectile functioning), intensity and longevity of orgasm and over all satisfaction.

Too weak pelvic floor muscles especially the ischiocavernousus may lead to reduced blood flow into the penile arteries and the bulbocavernosus may fail to prevent the venous return.

Over all weak pelvic floor muscles may lead to conditions like softer erection, inability to sustain erection, premature ejaculation, reduced intensity and force of ejaculation, performance anxiety, nervousness, lack of confidence, poor self-esteem and compromised male sexual health.

Psychological Factors:
Any psychological factors like performance anxiety, relationship issues, low self-esteem, emotional distress other health issues, partners sexual health issues etc. can also greatly lead to compromised sexual well-being. Treating sexual dysfunction is not only about pelvic floor rehab specialists, the role of pelvic floor experts is to make sure that pelvic floor functioning is normal.

Simultaneously patient should also be referred to other medical specialists like psychiatrists, psychologists, sexologists, urologists, etc.

In this scale the unrelated questions to pelvic floor are kept with a purpose of better clinical understanding so the patients can be referred to appropriate medical specialist for the complete treatment.

Important note: On the scale of Het's MMT (-3/-3) that is complete relaxation and (+3/+3) that is complete contraction can greatly enhance overall sexual well-being of the patient, provided psychological and other medical factors are simultaneously addressed.

Please visit www.visionwowgroup.com" to download the forms.

OBJECTIVE

Chronic Pelvic Pain Posture

- Increased lumbar lordosis
- Anterior pelvic tilt
- Lordosis kyphosis
- Reduced spinal range of motion (ROM)
- Positive thomas test
- Typical pelvic pain posture.

Prolonged sitting can lead to overflexion of the coccyx.
And any other form of changes in the frequent static and dynamic biomechanics of lumbopelvic junction can lead to overstretched or over compressed PFMs dysfunctions. It fails to maintain normal tone of PFMs which can lead to trigger point formation and hypertonus dysfunction as per Lukban, 2002. Even the presence of any kind of sacroiliac joint dysfunction at any stage can lead to trigger points development of PFMs.

Perineum Observation

- Identify structures
- Positions
- Scar
- Skin condition
- Symmetry of tissues
- How perineum reacts to increase in intra-abdominal pressure?
- Visual–biofeedback
- Verbal cues
- Biofeedback tools.

Internal examination of PFMs is a valid way for physical therapists to access and treat PFD. American Physical Therapy Association "examination of the pelvic floor muscles is consistent with physical therapy practice. It complies with national physical therapy policies requiring the performance of tests and measurements of neuromuscular function as an aid to the evaluation and treatment of a specific medical condition".
Adopted February 1993, revised August 2000.
Guide to Physical Therapy Practice Musculoskeletal pattern—impaired muscle performance includes dysfunction of the PFMs. Initial publication 1997 physical therapy 77:11, pages 1,252.

DISCLAIMER

Professional Responsibility

- Check with state, national, and international practice act
- Use of correct terminology like internal examination of pelvic floor muscles
- Should have undergone specific training
- Respect patient privacy, comfort
- Patient always has a choice to opt in or out for internal examination

- Patient always has a choice to proceed or terminate during any phase of examination
- Chaperone by regional standards and business policy is very important
- Verbal and written consent is must
- Very important to identify yourself and support staff with their name tags.

SELF TEST

For bulbocavernosus muscle (BC) and ischiocavernosus muscle (IC) muscle test or self test:

Check for change in erection angle and the duration of maximum time during contraction and relaxation of PFM. For this test, patient needs to obtain full erection for test to be more reliable and valid.

Patient could be instructed in detail and can do following test at his own convenience:
- Patient in standing 0° = flaccid penis; 90°= horizontal or parallel to ground; 180°= abdominal or almost vertical level.
- Three measurements are recorded in standing:
  1. Erection angle with PFM relaxation
  2. Erection angle with PFM contraction
  3. Time until PFM fatigue.

External Palpation

- *PC—pubococcygeus muscles*: Place your finger at soft tissue groove where the coccyx ends at the insertion. You can feel PC muscles between the coccyx and anus. Ask your patient to contract PFM.
- *BC—bulbocavernosus muscles*: Place your finger in the midline between the scrotum and the perineal body and ask your patient to contract PFM strong contraction of BC will be palpable.
- *IC—ischiocavernosus muscles*: Place your fingers between the scrotum and perineal body. From there, run your finger on either side of the BC muscles, over the course of inner corpus cavernosum. Get to the side at the deep limbs of the IC muscles. Ask patient to contract PFM and it is hardly palpable.
- *STP— superficial transverse perineal muscles*: Place your fingers between the ischial tuberosities can be palpated from ischial tuberosity above the anus. Ask the patient to contract PFM.

During Procedure

- Patient should be in left-lateral position and relaxed for transrectal examination
- Place the nonexamining hand on patients knees or legs
- Therapist should be seated on the side
- Maintain eye contact and check body language of the patient
- Verbally explain the examination procedure before you initiate, verbalize how you will insert your finger rectally

Assessment of Pelvic Floor Muscle

- What you will expect when you ask for PFC, how you will palpate, how you will turn your fingers inside to access different areas?
- Educate patients about trigger points, sweet-spot and how you will need patient's feedback.
- Suggest them how much pressure you intend to put and what level of discomfort patient may experience.
- Let them know in advance if you plan to apply quick stretch or ischemic pressure technique.
- Tell them if you want them to squeeze finger.

Modified Oxford Grading System

0: Complete lack of contraction

1: Minor flicker

2: Weak activity without a circular contraction or inner and upward movement

3: Moderate with inner and upward movement

4: Good—significant inner and upward movement

5: Strong—strong contraction with significant inward and upward movement.

Anteriorly, you can palpate prostate gland, and explain the patient that palpation of prostate gland might make him feel like urinating. Normal prostate is walnut shaped with distinct palpable lobes.

Het's—MANUAL MUSCLE TESTING (MMT) GRADING— PELVIC FLOOR MUSCLE

CONTRACTION	Grade 3	Strong upward and inward pull against resistance
	Grade 2	Grip with complete circumference
	Grade 1	Mild contraction (from any side)
0	Grade 0	Baseline tone
RELAXATION	Grade -1	Inability to penetrate
	Grade -2	Symptomatic penetration (pain, tightness, discomfort or any other symptom)
	Grade -3	Asymptomatic penetration (easy penetration)

Anal Wink Test

Light stroking the anus while the provider observes for anal contraction—the anus wink. Stimulated S2-S4 nerve root results in reflex contraction of anal sphincter.

Bulbocavernosus Reflex

Gentle squeeze the glans penis in men (the clitoris in women) and observe for anal contraction. Muscle is innervated by S2-S4 nerve root.

Transrectal Examination of Pelvic Floor Muscle

- Patient should be in left lateral position at the edge of examination table.
- Properly inspect anus, or perineal areas for lumps, ulcers, inflammation, or rashes, from outside, noting for any fecal staining.
- Suggest the patient to bear down or cough and inspect for any lesion or discharge.
- Suggest patient to relax and the therapist will insert lubricated index finger into the anal canal in a direction pointing toward the umbilicus.
- Note for the resting tone of muscles of the anal sphincter.
- Normally, it is expected that the muscles of the anal sphincter close around the circumference of the examiner's finger (Figs. 1 to 3).
- The distal external sphincter is felt just inside the anal canal.
- Puborectalis (PR)—portion of the levator ani muscle can be palpated approximate 3.5-4 cm inside. Ask the patient to tighten their anus and examiner should feel a ring pulling in and around entire circumference of the finger.

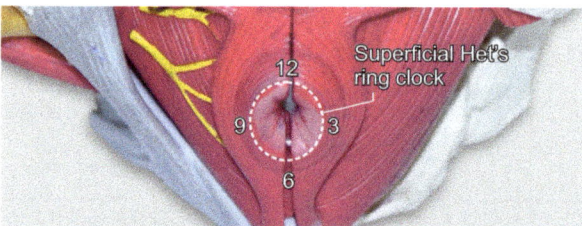

Fig. 1: Showing the orifice of superficial Het's ring clock, transrectal opening only in male.

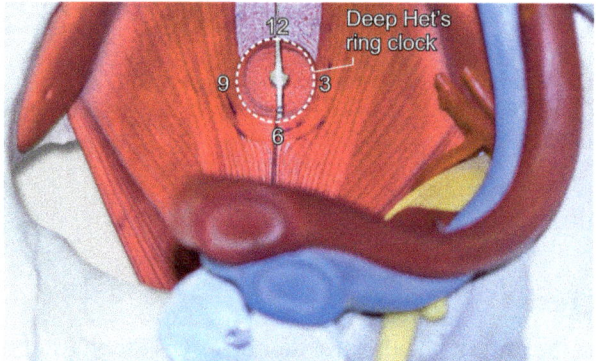

Fig. 2: Showing the orifice of deep Het's ring clock, at transrectal opening only in male.

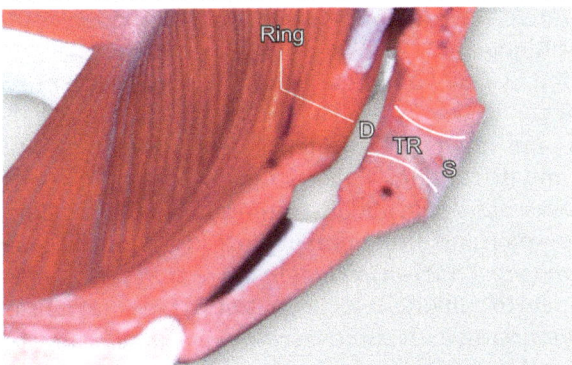

Fig. 3: Side section of Het's ring (skeletal muscle ring).

Optional Transrectal Examination in Supine

The optional transrectal examination has been shown in Figure 4.

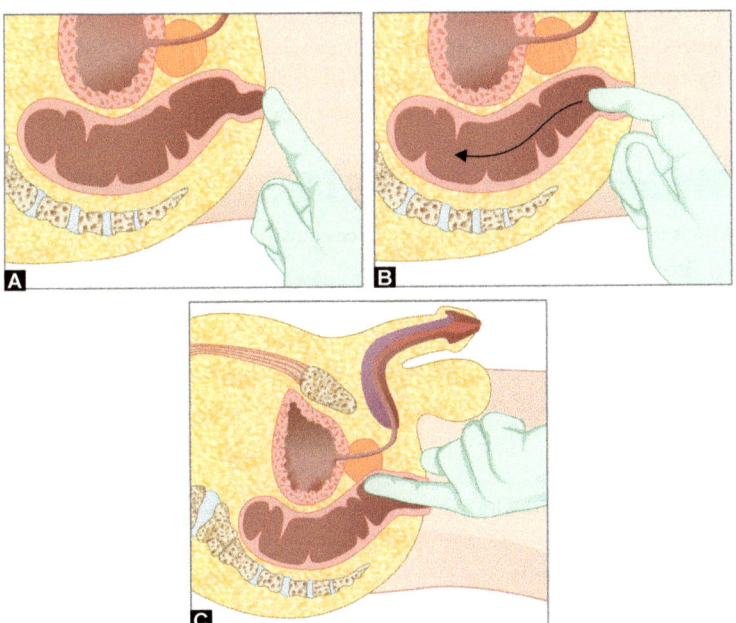

Figs. 4A to C: Transrectal examination in supine: (A) Insert the lip of the gloved index finger into the anus; (B) Introduce your finger to follow the curve of the sacrum; (C) Rotate the finger anteriorly to palpate the anterolateral and lateral walls of the prostate.

MALE PELVIC FLOOR HYPERTONUS DYSFUNCTION AND TRIGGER POINT SYMPTOMS

Adapted from Stanford Protocol

- *PC muscles*—referred pain to perineum and base of penis. Urethral pain, urgency, and frequency.

Section 2: Male: Pelvic Floor Dysfunction

- *IC muscle*—referred to anterior levator, prostate, lateral wall, and perineal and anal sphincter.
- *LA*—referred as *Golf ball in the rectum,* presents with urinary frequency and urgency.
- *Coccygeus*—pre- and post-bowel movement pain associated with full bowel sensation and discomfort.
- *Anterior lower abs*—pain and discomfort in bladder and lower abs.
- *Lateral abs*—pain and discomfort in the testis, stomach, coccyx, and groin.
- *Adductor magnus (AM)—Golf ball in the rectum*
- *Gluteals*—pain in tailbone, testicles, buttocks, hips, sacrum, and hamstrings
- *Laycock quantitative assessment scale*—please refer to women's assessment and follow the same technique for intrarectal examination and rehabilitation plan.
- *Electromyography (EMG) and ultrasound assessment*:
  - You can also use electromyography assessment of PFM by using surface electrodes at perianal junction or rectal electrodes.
  - Provider can use EMG display to differentiate between too much or too less tone. However, it could be misguided due to sensitivity of EMG especially from use of accessory muscles.
  - Specialized sonography with full bladder can display the activation of PFM. (Refer to assessment of female section for more details).

MULTIPLE CHOICE QUESTIONS

Q1. Which muscle is palpated between coccyx and anus?
  (a) Pubococcygeus muscle
  (b) External anal sphincter
  (c) Iliococcygeus
  (d) Coccygeus

Q2. Which nerve root is stimulated during anal wink test?
  (a) S1-S3
  (b) S2-S4
  (c) L5-S1
  (d) L4-S1

Q3. Which reflex is elicited by gently squeezing the glans of penis?
  (a) Anal reflex
  (b) Cremasteric reflex
  (c) Bulbocavernosus reflex
  (d) None of these

Q4. During transrectal examination which muscle is palpated approximately 3.5-4 cm inside the anal opening?
  (a) Levator ani muscle
  (b) Pubococcygeus
  (c) Puborectalis
  (d) Coccygeus

Q5. Overflexion of coccyx is caused by:
  (a) Prolonged sitting
  (b) Prolonged standing
  (c) Bending forward and working for long time
  (d) None of these

Q6. Which superficial pelvic floor muscle is palpated in the midline from scrotum to the anus?
- (a) Bulbocavernosus
- (b) Ischiocavernosus
- (c) Superficial transverse perineal muscle
- (d) Perineal body

Q7. Which muscle runs on the either side of bulbocavernosus muscle?
- (a) Bulbospongiosus
- (b) Ischiocavernosus
- (c) Perineal body
- (d) Superficial transverse perineal muscle

Q8. In the self-test of bulbocavernosus and ischiocavernosus muscle which things are checked?
- (a) Erection angle of penis with pelvic floor muscle contraction
- (b) Erection angle of penis with pelvic floor muscle relaxation
- (c) Time till the erection is maintained
- (d) All of the above

Q9. EMG study of pelvic floor muscles is done by placing the surface electrode at?
- (a) Perianal area
- (b) Perineal area
- (c) At external anal sphincter
- (d) None of these

ANSWERS

1: (a) Pubococcygeus muscle
2: (b) S2-S4
3: (c) Bulbocavernosus reflex
4: (c) Puborectalis
5: (a) Prolonged sitting
6: (d) Perineal body
7: (b) Ischiocavernosus
8: (d) All of the above
9: (a) Perianal area

Chapter 12

Hypertonus Pelvic Floor Dysfunction (Pelvic Pain and Health Issues)

No one can hurt me without my permission.

—Mahatma Gandhi

But pelvic floor hypertonus can.

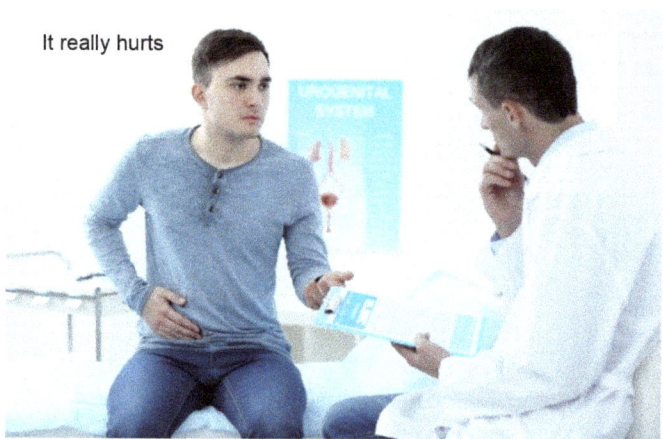

Too much tension of the pelvic floor muscles (PFMs) can be triggered by stress. PFM spasms can also be due to sexual, urinary, and bowel pathologies. Inability to relax PFM leads to chronic spasms of PFM.

PELVIC PAIN

Pelvic pain in men may include penile pain, pudendal nerve neuralgia, pudendal canal syndrome (PCS), prostate pain, perineal pain, proctalgia fugax, prostatodynia, or orchialgia.

Penile Pain

Intracavernosal injections, circumcision, or penile prosthesis surgery can cause penile pain. Conditions like Peyronie's disease, priapism, paraphimosis or herpes genitalis can also cause penile pain which can be relieved as underlying cause is treated. Patients with penile pain may develop secondary pelvic floor spasms due to pain.

Pudendal Nerve Neuralgia

Patients with pudendal neuralgia experiences severe pain on the side of the perineum. Pain is relieved on a toilet seat and gets worst by sitting.

Pudendal Canal Syndrome

It happens due to compression or overstretching of pudendal nerve in the Alcock's canal or clamp between the sacrospinal and the sacrotuberous ligaments. (Professor Ahmed Shafik, 1991). Patients present with perineal pain, hypo- or hypersensitivity, fecal incontinence, urinary incontinence or impotence. Pudendal neuropathy can be caused by cycling, trauma, and fall on buttocks. On examination, pressure on the nerve at the pudendal canal and medial to the ischial spine may reproduce symptoms. Patients with pudendal neuropathy present with tightness or spasmodic muscles.

Prostatitis

- It is inflammation of prostate gland (Figs. 1A and B). Patient presents with fever, chills, lower back pain (LBP), genital pain, body aches, urinary frequency, nocturia, painful urination, and penile discharge in case of acute prostatitis (Figs. 2, 3 and 4).

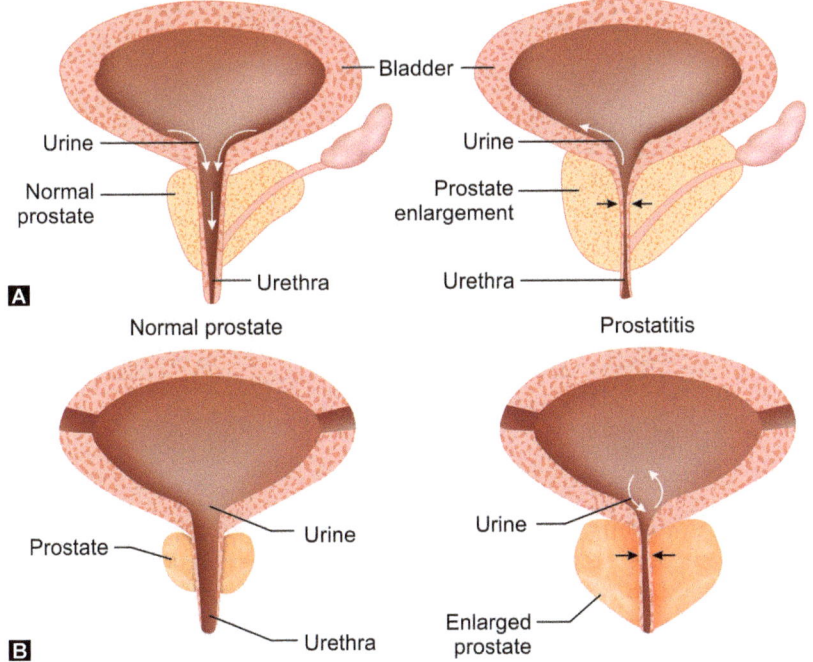

Figs. 1A and B: Prostatitis.

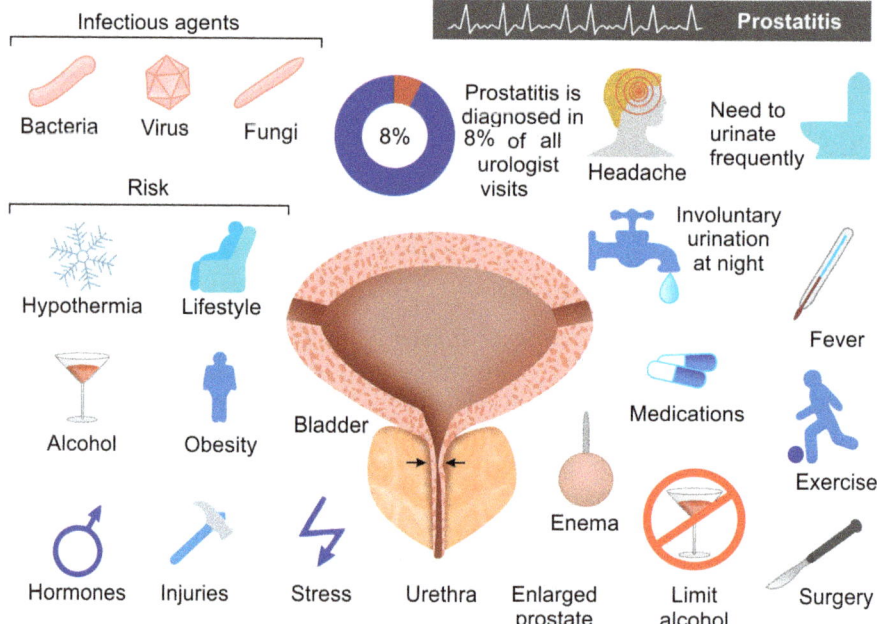

Fig. 2: Prostatitis: Causes, symptoms and treatment.

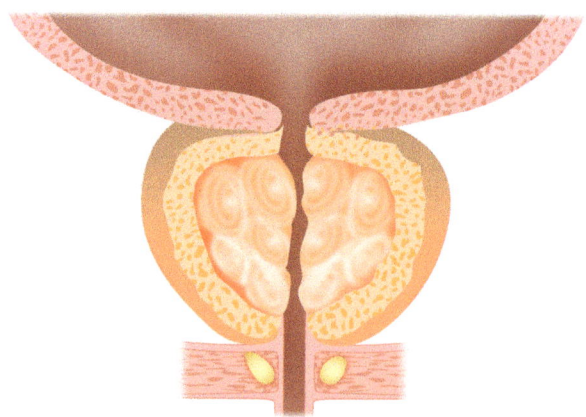

Fig. 3: Obstructed urethra.

- Men with prostatitis present with reduction in sexual interest, problems with sexual performance, and reduced strength of erections.
- Anticipation of pain can significantly reduce sexual interest. Any type of forceful sexual activity with already tighten PFMs can be very counterproductive. Some urologists advice the patients to increase the

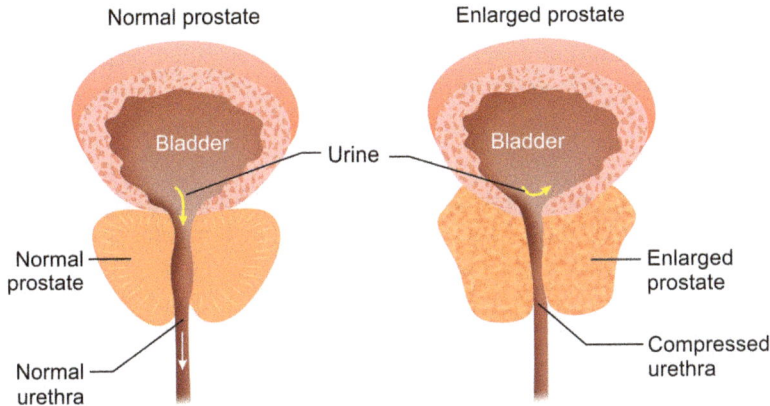

Fig. 4: Benign prostatic hyperplasia.

frequency of ejaculation. However, our experience suggests that it is more beneficial to wait and reduce the frequency of ejaculation and only increase the frequency once PFM has learned to relax. Even practice of relaxation during sexual activity can also help to reduce pelvic pain during sexual intercourse.
- Patients complain of rectal or suprapubic pain. The semen may be yellow or blood strained. Prostatitis can be acute or chronic bacterial (can be caused by ascending bacteria via urethra), prostatosis means nonbacterial inflammation of prostate.
- Bacterial prostatitis may be treated with antibiotics. According to Singh et al. 1997, nonbacterial prostatitis may be treated with pulse shortwave therapy.

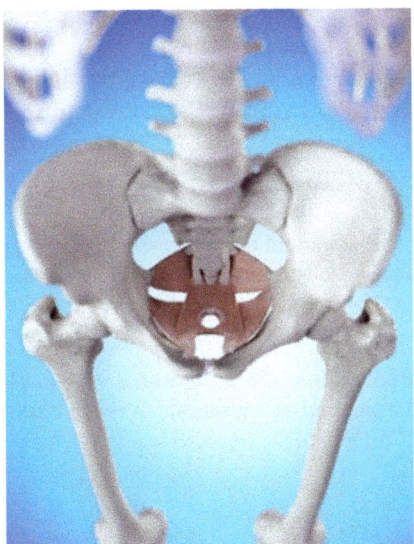

Prostatodynia

Nonbacterial inflammation of prostate and urethra is known as prostatodynia. PFM spasm might happen as result of pain.

Perineal Pain

Patient with testicular pain or prostatodynia can lead to perineal pain and ultimately perineal spasm which might present with myofascial restrictions in many cases.

Proctalgia Fugax

Patient of proctalgia fugax presents with pain due to spasm of the puborectalis/anal sphincter. Patient may experience relief by sitting on the toilet and bearing down as if voiding feces. This type of bearing down can trigger the relaxation of PFM which can relax the anal sphincter.

Tension Myalgia

- Any painful condition of pelvis or intrapelvic painful pathologies can lead to protective spasm of levator muscles or PFMs. State of hypercontraction of PFM can lead to tightness, pain, and inflammation. It is a spasmodic state of muscles which is often painful and tender.
- Patients lose their ability to relax PFMs. It can lead to genital, urinary or rectal pain. It has negative effects on urinary, bowel, and sexual functions.
- It can also be known as chronic postatitis or chronic pelvic pain syndrome (CPPS). CPPS may or may not go with inflammation.
- Patient presents with the pelvic pain or discomfort, pain in groin, genitalia, or perineum. Difficulty in sitting, pain radiating to rectum and to the tip of the penis with voiding and sexual dysfunction.

Any type of trauma or pathologies that creates pelvic pain could result in multiple trigger points, myofascial tightness, repeated spasms, and hypertonus dysfunction. Ultimately, PFM muscles go for chronic tension and inability for relaxation which is known as hypertonus dysfunction.

MULTIPLE CHOICE QUESTIONS

Q1. What will be the Het's manual muscle testing (MMT) grade of the pelvic floor muscle, if it is able to partially relax or partially contract due to the presence of pain?
(a) -1 (b) 1
(c) -2 (d) 2

Q2. Assume that your pelvic floor are like elevator and this elevator is stuck between ground floor and basement and is unable to reach basement, what grade will it be on Het's MMT?
(a) 0 (b) -1
(c) 1 (d) -2

Q3. The grade of MMT according to Het's protocol ranges from_____.
   (a) 0 to 5
   (b) -3 to 0
   (c) 0 to 3
   (d) -3 to 3

Q4. What is the full form of SERF?
   (a) Strength and relaxation, endurance, repetition, fast twitch
   (b) Strength, endurance, relaxation, fast twitch
   (c) Slow twitch, endurance, repetition, fatigue
   (d) Strength and relaxation, endurance, resting, fast twitch

Q5. When you are checking the endurance of the pelvic floor muscle by using Het's assessment scale, how much second hold will you expect to term it as a good endurance?
   (a) 1 second
   (b) 5 seconds
   (c) 8 seconds
   (d) 10 seconds

Q6. What is the *final goal* for pelvic floor rehab according to Het's assessment level?
   (a) Patient should be intentionally able to do activation of pelvic floor muscle
   (b) Patient is able to do reflexive activation of pelvic floor muscle
   (c) Both (a) and (b)
   (d) None of the above

ANSWERS

1: (c) -2
2: (b) -1
3: (d) -3 to 3
4: (a) Strength and relaxation, endurance, repetition, fast twitch
5: (d) 10 seconds
6: (b) Patient is able to do reflexive activation of pelvic floor muscle

Chapter 13

Hypotonus Pelvic Floor Dysfunction (Erectile Dysfunction and Other Health Issues)

*When I fight someone, I want to break his will. I want to take his manhood.
I want to rip out his heart and show it to him.*

—**Mike Tyson**

*Erectile dysfunction does the same thing to your patients.
"The only unnatural sex act is that which you cannot perform."*

—**Alfred Kinsey**

Help your patient now.

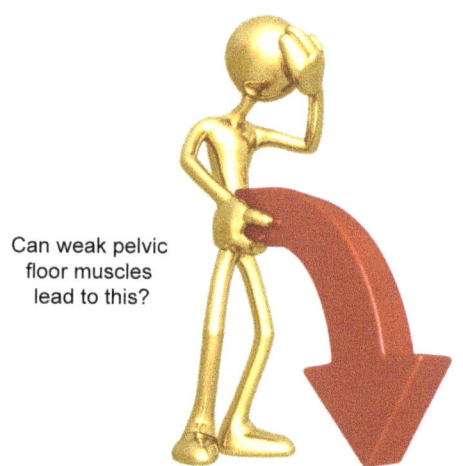

Can weak pelvic floor muscles lead to this?

▌INTRODUCTION

Men are generally busy building up their biceps and pecs. Pelvic floor muscles (PFMs) are most commonly ignored muscles.

It is important to understand basic anatomy of men's pelvis and private parts. Their anatomical attachment makes them most important muscle for their urinary, sexual, and prostate health. Fitness of PFM especially bulbocavernosus (BC) and ischiocavernosus (IC) muscles is extremely essential for erection, penile rigidity, and ejaculation. A weakness of the

PFMs may cause or worsen a number of problems like difficulty in gaining or maintaining erection, softer erections, etc. *Hypotonus dysfunction leads to weakness of PFM with age or under use. It can lead to conditions like*:
- Erectile dysfunction (ED)
- Premature ejaculation
- Postvoid dribbling
- Poor prostate health
- Urinary incontinence.

CAUSES

Many factors can weaken your PFMs, including:
- *Inadequate*: Under use of these muscles
- Age
- Prostate surgery
- Trauma, etc.

HYPOTONUS DYSFUNCTION

Following are some of the harmful effects of weak private muscles:
- Reduced perineal or intimate power, stamina, and performance.
- *Erectile dysfunction*: More than 20% of men under 40 years old and 50% of men over 40 years old experience some form of ED (this problem is getting worse even for younger population because of anxiety and stress of different phases of life).

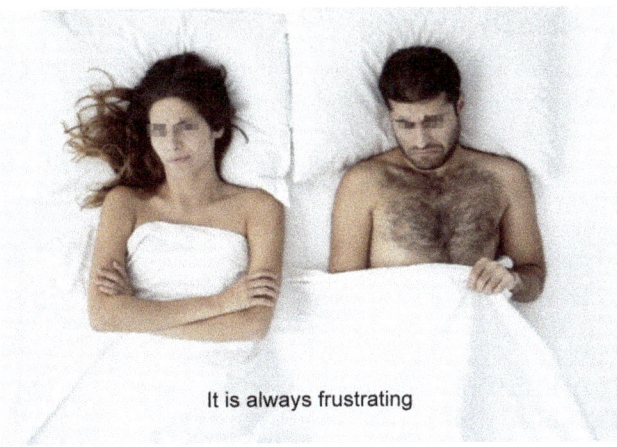

It is always frustrating

- *Premature ejaculation*: Weak pelvic floor can contribute to premature ejaculation (PE), one of the major concerned problems for most men.
- *Postvoid dribbling*: Urine drops after urination is also a sign of weak private muscles, urinary leakage and overactive bladder.
- *Weak prostate health*: Weak PFMs reduce pelvic blood flow which compromise on pelvic health.
- *Reduced bowel control*: Weak pelvic muscles can reduce the strength of the sphincter muscles.

Erectile Dysfunction

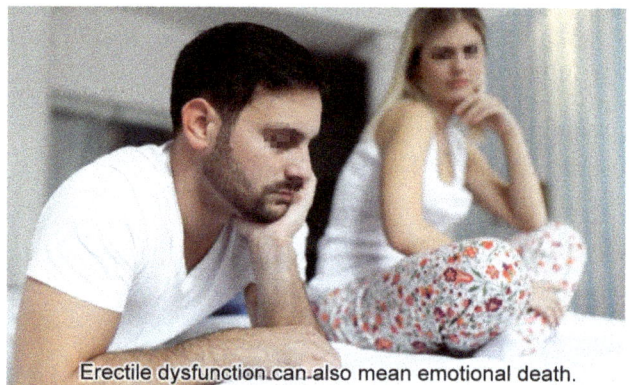
Erectile dysfunction can also mean emotional death.

Definition

According to National Institute of Health (NIH), ED is defined as "inability to achieve or maintain an erection sufficient for satisfactory sexual performance."

According to research by Aytac et al. 1999, approximately 152 million men worldwide suffered from ED in 1995, this number is projected to raise to 322 million men worldwide by 2015.

According to research by Feldman et al. 1994, found that 40% of all men at the age of 50 years old have ED, by 70 years 66% of men has ED. It gets worse with age.

Causes of Erectile Dysfunction

Most of the men are not aware of progressive weakness of PFMs due to:
- Inadequate—under use of BC and IC muscles
- Decreased PFM tone due to aging
- Overweight or obesity can cause high blood pressure which negatively affects erection
- Diseases like diabetes or surgery
- Prostate health problems
- Arteriogenic or venogenic
- Diabetic
- Drug-induced
- Trauma to pelvic floor or pudendal nerve
- Surgical trauma
- Lifestyle factors like cigarette smoking and alcohol abuse
- Chronic obstructive pulmonary disease (COPD)
- Long distance or prolonged bicycling or horse riding can restrict blood circulation to the PFM and penis and can also cause pudendal nerve compression or damage.

As mentioned, there may be many causes of ED. But it narrows down to two major reasons:
1. Insufficient blood flow to fill the erectile chambers of the penis
2. Poor venous trapping.

Biomechanics of Erection

- A penile erection is simple medical biomechanics where maximizing inflow of blood happens along with minimizing outflow. The penis has erection chambers that get filled with blood. These erection chambers are made of sinuses. An erection occurs when these sinuses become congested with blood.
- Smooth muscle relaxation in the penile arteries causes blood inflow to the penis and the sinuses of the erection chambers. Penile veins are compressed by filled sinuses to block the outflow of blood, which leads to expanded penis.
- The PFMs especially BC and IC helps transform an expanded penis to a rigid penis. They compress the deep and inner part of the penis, which leads to improving rigidity and elevating the blood pressure within the penis (it is above systolic blood pressure).
- In other words, an erect penis is a hypertensive penis (high blood pressure). Solid rigidity is maintained by this tremendous blood pressure.
- With age, the smooth muscle of arteries starts becoming stiff. The smooth muscle of the penile arteries and sinuses of the erection chambers also become stiff. As a result they reduce relaxation ability, which leads to ED.
- Additionally, PFMs weakens with age. Combined effect of the stiff smooth muscle and the weak PFMs leads to failure of the penis to fill with blood and to store blood. As a result, ED happens.

Step by Step Mechanism of Erection

- *Flaccid phase:* Low blood flow and low blood pressure exists in the penis.
- *Filling phase*: Stimulus initiates relaxation of smooth muscles of penile artery. This vasodilatation enables blood flow to lacunar space.
- *Corporal veno-occlusive mechanism*: Corporal veno-occlusive mechanism where the venous return is reduced by PFM and causes penis to expand and elongate.
- *Full erection and rigidity phase*: The intracavernous pressure rises higher than the diastolic pressure (Fig. 1).

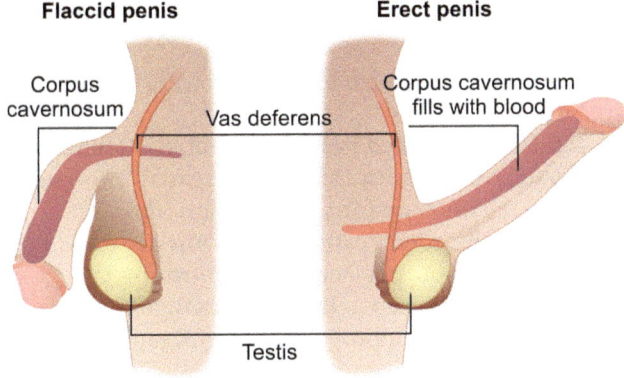

Fig. 1: Flaccid–erect penis.

- Systolic phase of the pulse creates more increase in the blood inflow leads to solid rigidity.
- Contractions or reflex contraction of IC and BC muscles creates more blood flow and more increase in the intracavernous pressure.
- That means weak IC and BC muscles fail to increase blood circulation and also fail to reduce venous return. It leads to lack of penile rigidity or ED. However, stronger IC and BC muscles increase the intracavernous pressure by increasing blood flow and reducing venous return. Stronger BC and IC muscles help with better, longer, and more solid erection.

Keypoints of Erectile Mechanism of Penis

- Bulbocavernosus and ischiocavernosus create penile erection by improving blood flow and preventing venous return.
- BC and IC helps to eject semen from the urethra.
- Sperm—produced in testis and stored in epididymis.
- Propelled up the vas deferens, 2 ducts that passes over the bladder.
- Seminal vesicles add fluids.

Classification

Severity-based classification of ED by Albaugh and Lewis, 1999:
- Mild ED—achieving satisfactory erection in 7–8/10 attempts
- Moderate ED—achieving satisfactory erection 4–6/10 attempts
- Sever ED—achieving satisfactory erection 0–3/10 attempts.

Reduced Intensity of Orgasm

- Genetics, hormonal changes, and age can lead to enlargement of the prostate gland. It may lead to less semen and reduced ejaculatory power.
- Bulbocavernosus muscle is like a source of power for ejaculatory force. Weaker BC muscles will result in dribbling of semen or orgasms with reduced intensity.
- Stronger BC muscles can intensify the pulse waves of ejaculations. Also, stronger BC muscles can engorge corpus spongiosum and pressurizes the urethra into much narrower space and maximizes the force of ejaculation.

Premature Ejaculations

- Over the age of 40 years, 50% of men experience PE. PE is the most common male sexual disorder.
- The cause of PE can be caused by hyperexcitable BC reflex, psychological factors, hypersensitive penis, infrequent sexual intercourse, extreme arousal, genetics, alcohol, performance anxiety, etc.
- Poor ejaculatory control can cause significant distress to the partners. Strength of PFM can improve ejaculatory control.
- Weak pelvic muscles may lead to PE. By strengthening the pelvic muscles, ejaculatory control can be improved along with longevity of erection.

- The strength of PFMs, especially BC, helps in ejaculation of semen from the penis. Most men loose PFM strength with age which leads to diminished force and reduced intensity of orgasm. It is important to proactively strengthen PFMs.

Postvoidal Dribbling

Weak PFMs leads to urinary health issues like postvoid dribbling, stress urinary incontinence, and overactive bladder. Postvoid dribbling occurs after completing urination. PVD is a leakage of urine immediately after completing urination. It is one of the key sign of the prostate enlargement. The urethra in men has 3 portions:
1. External portion: The portion of urethra within the penis is external portion
2. Internal portion: The portion of the urethra within the perineum is internal portion
3. Inner portion: The portion of the urethra that travels through prostate and enters the bladder is the innermost portion.

After urination, some of the urine stays in internal portion of urethra which drips out posturination. Mostly due to movement or gravity. PFM contractions, especially BC muscles help in expelling the residual urine.

Stress Urinary Incontinence (Fig. 2)

- It occurs mainly either following radical prostatectomy for prostate cancer or postprostectomy during activities like exercising, sneezing, coughing, bending, lifting. Increased intra-abdominal pressure in the presence of weak PFM leads to stress urinary incontinence (SUI).
- Stronger PFMs helps to prevent SUI.

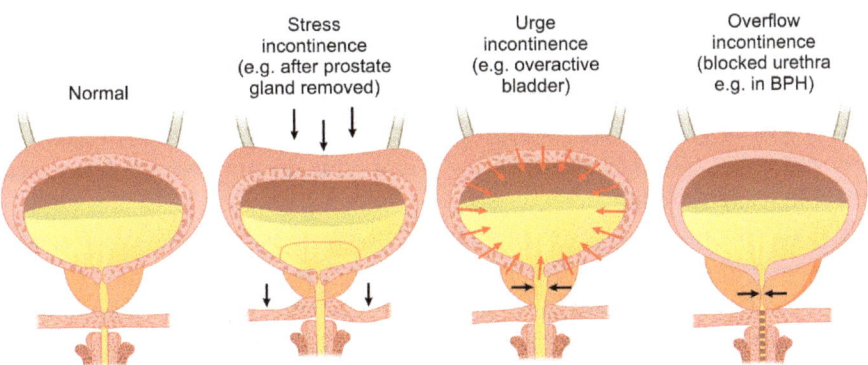

Fig. 2: Stress urinary incontinence in men.

Overactive Bladder

- Overactive bladder (OAB) happens because of involuntary contraction of bladder muscles. OAB can be due to reduced ability of brain to control the bladder.
- Patient presents with urinary urgency, frequency, and night-time urination with or without urine leakage.
- It can be triggered by positional changes, handwashing, exposure to running water, or when placing the key in the door. PFM play key role in inhibiting urgency.

Bowel Dysfunction

- Weak PFMs reduce strength of anal sphincter. Bowel urgency or fecal incontinence can happen due to abnormal rectal contractions, weakened PFMs, nerve damage, or conditions like diarrhea.
- The pelvic muscles support the anal sphincter. The stronger pelvic floor muscles gives better closure to the sphincter.

Poor Prostate Health

Pelvic muscle exercises do not prevent prostate enlargement, prostate cancer, and prostate infections. However, PFM strength will increase pelvic blood flow, which is beneficial for prostate health. Age-related prostate enlargement is associated with inflammation in which PFM strengthening can play a big role.

Benign Prostatic Hyperplasia

Multiplication of cells with age can lead to benign prostatic enlargement. The prevalence of Benign prostatic hyperplasia (BPH) increases with age.

There are two stages of BPH:
1. Microscopic stage
2. Macroscopic stage.

The microscopic nodular development can be seen in men between 30 years and 50 years of age. Symptoms include urinary hesitancy, straining, intermittency, weak stream, difficulty in emptying, incomplete emptying, and dribbling after voiding.

Benign hypertrophy of prostate, obstruction leads to overflow incontinence. transurethral resection of the prostate (TURP) procedure is common mode of intervention. Generally, the bladder neck is resected which can disturb complete closure. Postprostatectomy men also experience retrograde ejaculation. Some patients need to undergo suprapubic or retropubic prostatectomy (Fig. 3).

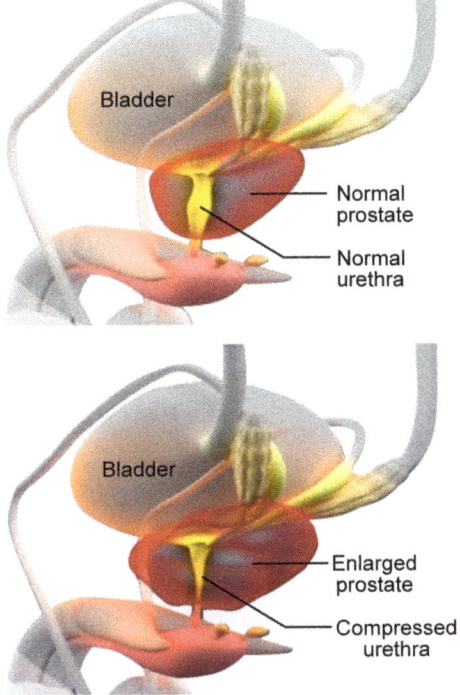

Fig. 3: Compressed urethra.

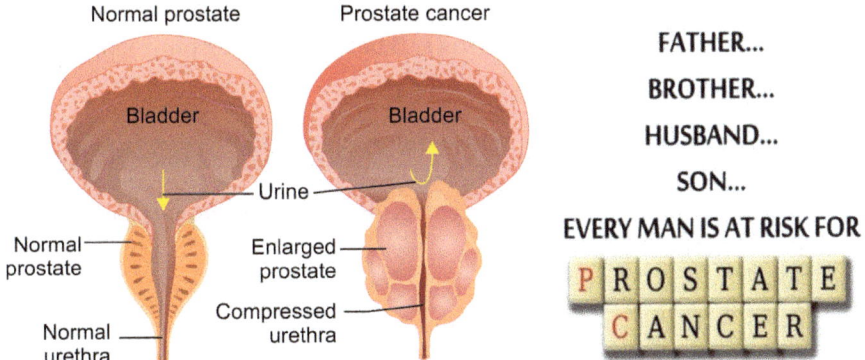

Figs. 4A and B: Prostate cancer.

Prostate Cancer (Figs. 4 and 5)

- According to National statistics of UK, lung cancer is most common cancer in men, after that prostate cancer is second most common cancer in men. And prostate cancer is different. They can coexist but generally does not lead to each other. Radiotherapy, radical prostatectomy can be a choice of treatment along with antiandrogen treatments.

Section 2: Male: Pelvic Floor Dysfunction

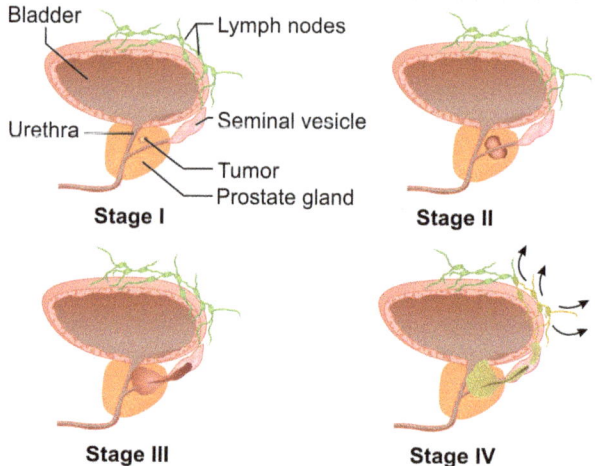

Fig. 5: Stages of prostate cancer.

- It can lead to erectile dysfunction or urinary incontinence like symptoms which can be greatly treated by PFM rehabilitation. Sometimes, pain can lead to PFM spasms or hypertonus or incoordination type of PFD.

Postprostatectomy incontinence:
- Prostatectomy may cause damage or disturbance of urinary sphincter which can lead to SUI, UI or mixed.
- The internal urethral sphincter which might be damaged, does not have any voluntary control. The continence depends exclusively on external urethral sphincter and PFMs. PREHAB before prostatectomy can be very beneficial.

MULTIPLE CHOICE QUESTIONS

Q1. According to statistics what percentage of men above 50 years suffers from erectile dysfunction?
- (a) 60%
- (b) 50%
- (c) 40%
- (d) 20%

Q2. Classification of erectile dysfunction was first given by:
- (a) Albaugh and Lewis
- (b) Albaugh and Edward
- (c) Edward and Lewis
- (d) Edward and Adams

Q3. If a person achieves satisfactory erection for 5 times out of 10 attempts it is which type of erectile dysfunction:
- (a) Mild ED
- (b) Moderate ED
- (c) Severe ED
- (d) Very severe ED

Q4. Which dysfunction can be caused by hyperexcitable bulbocavernosus reflex?
 (a) Erectile dysfunction
 (b) Premature ejaculation
 (c) Postvoidal dribbling
 (d) Incontinence

Q5. In which portion of urethra does the residual urine get stored after urination?
 (a) Inner portion
 (b) External portion
 (c) Internal portion
 (d) Throughout urethra

Q6. Overactivity of detrusor and weakness of PFMs lead to which type of incontinence?
 (a) Overactive bladder incontinence
 (b) Stress incontinence
 (c) Urge incontinence
 (d) Mixed incontinence

Q7. Which are the types of benign prostatic hyperplasia?
 (a) Microscopic and macroscopic
 (b) Microscopic and etiological
 (c) Macroscopic and etiological
 (d) None of these

Q8. Which type of ejaculation is common postprostate surgery?
 (a) Retrograde ejaculation
 (b) Premature ejaculation
 (c) Incomplete ejaculation
 (d) None of these

Q9. Which is the common treatment option for BPH?
 (a) Transurethral resection of prostate
 (b) Laparoscopic prostate removal
 (c) Medical management
 (d) All give same results

Q10. Prostate enlargement which leads to over pressure on PFMs can cause which type of pelvic floor dysfunction?
 (a) Hypotonus dysfunction
 (b) Hypertonus dysfunction
 (c) Incoordinated dysfunction
 (d) Visceral dysfunction

ANSWERS

1: (c) 40%
2: (a) Albaugh and Lewis
3: (b) Moderate ED
4: (b) Premature ejaculation
5: (c) Internal portion
6: (a) Overactive bladder incontinence
7: (a) Microscopic and macroscopic
8: (a) Retrograde ejaculation
9: (a) Transurethral resection of prostate
10: (a) Hypotonus dysfunction

Section 3

Pediatric Pelvic Floor

It is easier to build strong children than to repair broken men.
—**Frederick Douglass**

Easier to build strong pelvic floor than to repair them.
Diaper backward spells repaid. Think about it.
—**Marshall McLuhan**

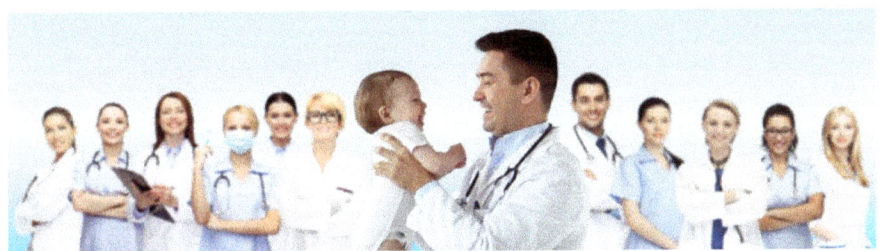

Chapter 14

Normal Continence Development, Enuresis and Encopresis

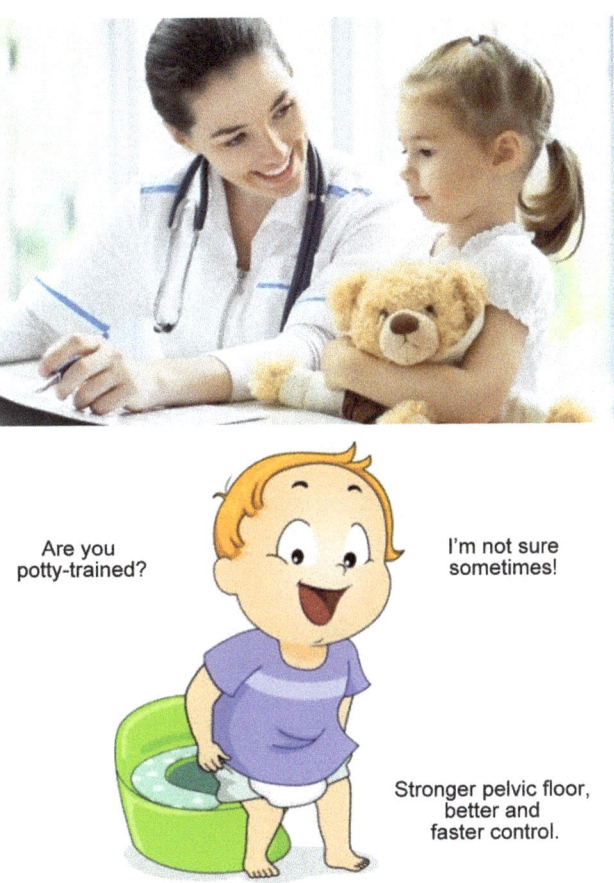

INTRODUCTION

Generally the children are accepted to be toilet-trained by the age of 3 in India and America. It is mostly because of the need of enrolment in daycare or preschool. In some cases, it takes more than 3 years for proper neuromuscular development of children's bladder and sphincters. Accepted age for a child to gain urinary continence could be 4 years.

Approximately by 18 months child is able to differ voiding. And toilet-training begins at 2–3 years of the age.

Age-wise toilet-training protocol approximately:
- Age 2–3—nocturnal bowel control
- Age 3–4—daytime bowel control
- Age 4 and above—daytime bladder control
- Age 5–6—nocturnal bladder control.

ENURESIS

According to Rushton (1995), enuresis is the persistence of involuntary voiding beyond the age of anticipated control.

According to the American Psychiatric Association (APA), enuresis is repeated voiding of urine during the day or at night into bed or clothes at least twice a week for at least 3 months.

Incidence of Enuresis

According to Statistics, enuresis occurs in 5–7 million children between the age of 6 years and 18 years (7% of boys and 3% of girls pediatric visits at the age of 5).

Up to 16–60% of pediatric visits are due to urinary incontinence.

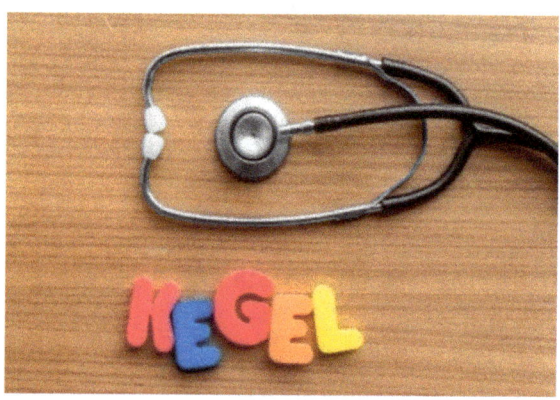

Enuresis affects child in so many ways:
- Low self-esteem
- Stress between parents and children
- Low self-confidence
- Depression
- Anxiety.

Het's ASSESSMENT LEVEL FOR PELVIC FLOOR MUSCLE

Het's assessment level for pelvic floor muscle has been described in Table 1.

Types of Enuresis

The different types of enuresis are described in Box 1.

Normal Continence Development, Enuresis and Encopresis

TABLE 1: Het's reflexive result scale (Het's RR scale).

Het levels/ stages	Diagnosis	Current status of patient
1	Unintentional—unable	• Patient is unaware of PFM • Patient is unable to do proper PFM contractions
2	Intentional—unable	• Patient is aware about PFM • Patient is trying to do correct PFM contractions or relaxation. But unable to do
3	Intentional—partially able	• Patient is aware about PFM • Patient is trying her best to perform PFM complete contraction or relaxation. But can only do partial contractions or relaxation of PFM
4	Intentional—completely able	• Patient is aware about PFM • Patient is completely able to do isolated complete PFM contractions and relaxations • But cannot use them properly during functional activities
5	Intentional—functionally able	• Patient is aware to use PFM in functional activities and patient intentionally uses PFM contraction and relaxation during functional movements • But still it is not automatic yet
6	Final goal—reflexive activation/ relaxation	• Patient automatically uses PFM contraction or relaxation during related functional activities • Patient does not to try to do PFM activity intentionally. • However, later on patient realizes that they did it. In other words, now it has become subconscious reflexive behavior to use PFM

BOX 1: Types of enuresis.

Types of enuresis:
- *Monosymptomatic/nocturnal enuresis:* Child presents with normal control and normal bladder function during the day. However, they wet their bed during sleep
- *Nonmonosymptomatic/diurnal enuresis:* Primary night-time bed-wetting with problems of voiding during the daytime
- Combined; child present with voiding and bed-wetting in day or night both

Enuresis also divided into two parts:
1. *Continues enuresis:* The child has completely failed to achieve dryness or complete continence
2. *Phasic enuresis:* The child is successfully continent for more than 3 months and then relapse

Symptoms
- Frequent cloth wetting
- Bed-wetting at least twice a week (Fig. 1).

Causes of Enuresis
- *Nonintentional or involuntarily:*
  - Small size of bladder
  - Frequent urinary tract infection (UTI)

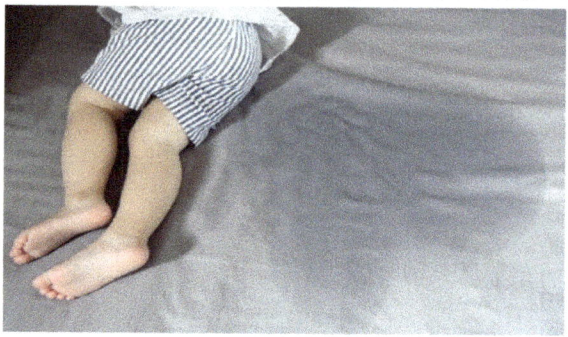

Fig. 1: Bed-wetting.

- Any pain which leads to enuresis
- Stress
- Frequent constipation causes pain leads to leakage
- Poor or delayed development of neuromuscular pattern of pelvic floor muscles.
- *Intentional or voluntarily mainly psychological:*
  - Another new baby
  - Relocation of house, loss of loved one
  - New school or teacher
  - Parental conflict
  - Problems with friends
  - Problems at school
  - Fear from parents
  - Physical or sexual abuse.

ENCOPRESIS

It is undesirable and involuntary loss of stool in day or night.

Incidence of Encopresis

- According to Sutphen et al. (1997), 25% of pediatric visits of gastroenterology are due to encopresis. These children are 10 times more affected with attention deficit hyperactivity disorder (ADHD). According to APA, encopresis is the repetitive leakage of feces in inappropriate places for at least once in a month for 3 months in children over 4 years of age.

KEYPOINTS FOR PEDIATRIC PELVIC FLOOR DYSFUNCTION

- Detailed subjective history to rule out and address causes
- Examination: Always with parent inside the room
- Pre-examination consent is very important

- Examine abdominal wall for muscle integrity, masses, symmetry, and pain
- Visual inspection of genitalia for scars, lesions, soiling or swelling, position of urethral and vaginal opening, only externally
- *No intravaginal examination should be done in premenstrual girls*
- Anal sphincter reflex: It can be tested by applying light stroking lateral to anus, resulting in anal wink or anal sphincter contraction.
- Bulbocavernosus reflex: It can be tested by squeezing glans or by applying stroking to the clitoral hood or clitoris that leads to pelvic floor contraction.
- Reflex arc is intact if above mentioned reflexes are present.
- Palpate perineum for tenderness or sensory awareness.

KEYPOINTS FOR PEDIATRIC PELVIC FLOOR REHABILITATION PRINCIPLES

- In children aged between 2 and 3, parental education is the key
- *Biofeedback* training can be initiated at age 2–3
- Biofeedback education may be given in nonmedical looking environment like not wearing doctors clothes
- Use the treatment on their toy or doll to create better acceptance
- Parental education in providing verbal, visual or tactile cues to inhibit hip adductors, gluteus, lower abs and other accessory muscles
- "If the child is not able to recruit pelvic floor muscles directly due to some pathology we can go for stronger contraction of the hip adductors or other associated accessory muscles which can irradiate the pelvic floor muscles" (Courtsey goes to "Dr Sunita Patel" CEO WOW IIPRE).
- Teach them to sit on the toilet seat and pelvic floor for reflex to work along with this any visual or auditory stimulus can be given.
- Teach them valsalva method and have them to avoid it
- Teach the children that they are teacher or boss of their bowel and bladder and they should control it (Figs. 2A and B).
- According to research published by National Institutes of Health (NIH), 1994, biofeedback is 60% more effective in the treatment of diurnal incontinence. The purpose of biofeedback is not only to strengthen the pelvic floor muscle but also to learn the coordination of pelvic floor with bladder and bowel.
- Use of biofeedback devices like pelvic floor 360 can be extremely efficient in providing proper treatments and desirable results.

Note: Please refer to following chapters about pelvic floor rehabilitation and rehabilitation devices, you can use similar techniques, rehabilitation protocols and rehabilitation devices including pelvic floor 360 for most efficient results. However, each rehabilitation plan should be customized by individual pediatric subjective and objective assessment.

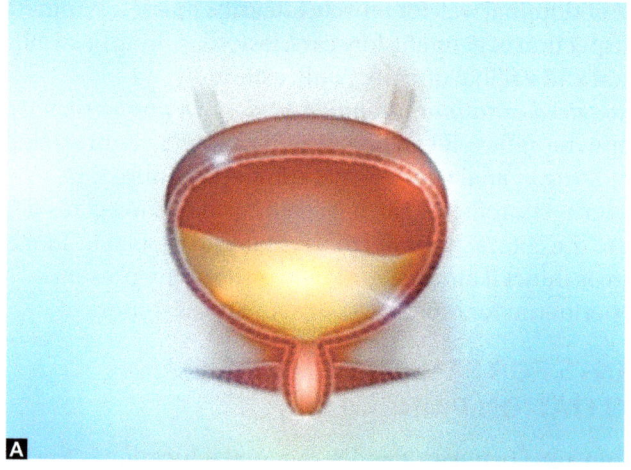

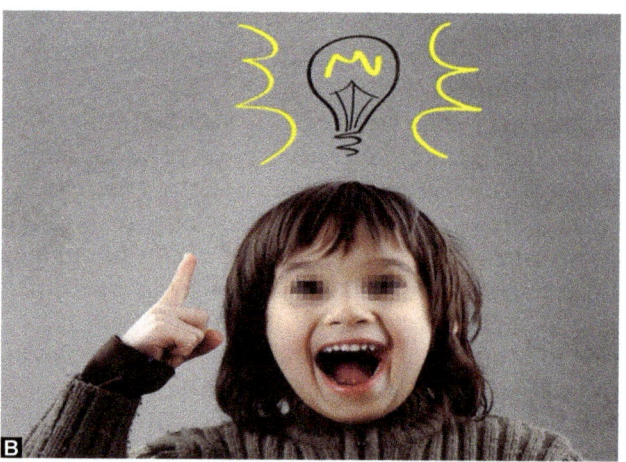

Figs. 2A and B: Continent, happy and confident chid.

MULTIPLE CHOICE QUESTIONS

Q1. Involuntary voiding of urine beyond the age of anticipated control is known as:
 (a) Enuresis
 (b) Encopresis
 (c) Incontinence
 (d) All of the above

Q2. If the child has a normal bladder control in the daytime but has problem of bed-wetting at night it is which type of enuresis?
 (a) Nocturnal enuresis
 (b) Diurnal enuresis
 (c) Continuous enuresis
 (d) Phasic enuresis

Q3. Which type of enuresis it will be if the child has normal continence for 3 months but there is relapse after 3 months?
 (a) Nocturnal enuresis
 (b) Diurnal enuresis
 (c) Continuous enuresis
 (d) Phasic enuresis

Q4. Which are the causes of enuresis?
  (a) Voluntary
  (b) Involuntary
  (c) Both (a) and (b)
  (d) None of the above

Q5. Undesirable loss of stool during day or night is known as:
  (a) Enuresis
  (b) Fecal incontinence
  (c) Encopresis
  (d) Urge incontinence

Q6. Intravaginal examination is not done in _____.
  (a) Premenstrual girls
  (b) In unmarried girls
  (c) Immediately after marriage
  (d) After menopause

Q7. Which type of psychological disorder is commonly associated with encopresis?
  (a) Attention deficit hyperactivity disorder
  (b) Autism
  (c) Mental disorder
  (d) Bipolar disorder

Q8. By which age can a child be trained by biofeedback?
  (a) 5 years
  (b) 2–3 years
  (c) 7 years
  (d) 5–7 years

Q9. A 4-year-old boy shifted with his parents to a new area and he had to change his school as well, after this the child develops bed-wetting which type of enuresis it will be?
  (a) Intentional
  (b) Unintentional
  (c) Involuntary
  (d) Stress incontinence

Q10. By what age should a child develop nocturnal bladder control?
  (a) 2–3 years
  (b) 1–2 years
  (c) 5–6 years
  (d) 3–4 years

ANSWERS

1: (a) Enuresis
2: (a) Nocturnal enuresis
3: (d) Phasic enuresis
4: (c) Both (a) and (b)
5: (c) Encopresis
6: (a) Premenstrual girls
7: (a) Attention deficit hyperactivity disorder
8: (b) 2-3 years
9: (a) Intentional
10: (c) 5-6 years

Section 4

Pelvic Floor Muscle: Fitness and Rehabilitation

"Strength does not come from winning. Your struggles develop your strengths. When you go through hardships and decide not to surrender, that is strength".
—**Arnold Schwarzenegger**

Don't let your patients surrender to pelvic floor weakness.
Strengthen them.

Chapter 15

Different School of Thoughts on Kegel and Pelvic Floor Rehabilitation

PELVIC FLOOR MUSCLE TRAINING PROTOCOLS

The different pelvic floor muscle training protocols have been given in Box 1.

Laycock Protocol: Overload Principles

- Progression: Endurance start and progress from 0–10 seconds
- Total repetitions goal can be 30–80 repetitions
- Train fast and slow fibers separately
- Build-up more hold time for progressions
- There are two options for progressions. Either add repetition once at 10 seconds or set repetition goal.

BO Intensive Protocol: Intensive Training

- Use maximum exertions of all muscles
- Target repetitions of 8–12
- Sets: 3 sets
- Frequency: 1/day
- Hold time: 8–10 seconds
- Create pelvic floor muscle (PFM) activation, hold the contraction steadily
- Then try to contract further inward with quick contraction for 3–4 times after reaching your maximum contraction, it will help extra muscle fibers to kick in.

> **BOX 1:** Different pelvic floor muscle training protocols.
>
> - Kegel exercise
> - Kegel training and protocols
> - Laycock protocol
> - BO intensive protocol
> - WebMD protocol
> - National Institute of Health (NIH) protocol
> - University of California, Los Angeles (UCLA) protocol
> - Mayo clinic protocol
> - University of Arizona protocol

WebMD Protocol

- This routine should be done on daily basis
- Position: Lying down position
- Sets: 3
- Repetitions: 10
- Hold:relax time: 5:5 seconds
- Duration: 3-6 weeks.
- Progress toward 10 seconds of hold time and standing position.

National Institute of Health Protocol

- This routine is done on daily basis
- Sets: 3-5
- Repetitions: 10
- Hold:relax time: 10:10 seconds
- Duration: For 12 weeks
- Add quick pulsed contractions for 10 times
- Maintenance is 5 min/3 times/week.

University of California, Los Angeles Protocol

- This routine is done on daily basis
- Sets: 3
- Repetitions: 10
- Hold:relax time: 5: 5 seconds.

Mayo Clinic Protocol

- This routine is done on daily basis.
- Position: Lying down position
- Sets: 3
- Repetitions: 10
- Hold:relax time: 3:3 seconds
- Progress toward sitting, standing, and walking. It is also suggested during activities of daily livings (ADLs) like brushing teeth.

University of Arizona Protocol

- This routine is done on daily basis
- Sets: 5-10
- Repetitions: 10
- Hold:relax time: 10:10 seconds
- At the end of the set, 5-10 very quick contractions.

MULTIPLE CHOICE QUESTIONS

Q1. What is the other name of overload principle?
  (a) University of California, Los Angeles protocol
  (b) Kegel's protocol
  (c) Laycock protocol
  (d) Arnold Kegel's

Q2. What type of training is BO intensive training?
  (a) Intensive training
  (b) Resistance training
  (c) Endurance training
  (d) All of the above

Q3. Which protocols have hold and relax time of 3:3 seconds?
  (a) Mayo clinic protocol
  (b) University of California, Los Angeles protocol and BO
  (c) Mayo clinic and BO
  (d) Mayo clinic and University of California, Los Angeles protocol

Q4. Which protocols have hold and relax time of 5:5 seconds?
  (a) WebMD and University of California, Los Angeles protocol
  (b) Mayo clinic and University of California, Los Angeles protocol
  (c) Mayo clinic protocol
  (d) University of California, Los Angeles protocol and BO

Q5. Which protocols have hold and relax time of 10:10 seconds?
  (a) NIH protocol and Arizona University
  (b) NIH and University of California, Los Angeles protocol
  (c) Arizona University and University of California, Los Angeles protocol
  (d) NIH and BO

Q6. Ideally in which position all the protocol should start?
  (a) Squatting position
  (b) Lying position
  (c) Standing position
  (d) Sitting position

ANSWERS

1: (c) Laycock
2: (a) Intensive training
3: (a) Mayo clinic protocol
4: (a) WebMD and University of California, Los Angeles protocol
5: (a) NIH protocol and Arizona University
6: (b) Lying position

Chapter 16
Foundation for Pelvic Floor Rehabilitation

INTRODUCTION

As we know, ideal PFM function is a balance between mobility and stability. Ability to contract, partially contract, control, and completely relax is very important for efficient functioning of PFM. Too much stability leads to hypertonus dysfunction and too much mobility leads to hypotonus dysfunction.

Millions of people are suffering from some kind of pelvic floor dysfunction (PFD).

It affects all people regardless of sex; man, woman, and even children suffer from PFD like urine incontinence, voiding problems, sexual and anorectal disturbances which may be associated with each other most of the time and can lead to serious issue later on. So, integrated diagnosis and proper treatment is required to deal with PFD.

TREATMENT

For proper treatment of PFM, these simple steps need to be taken by therapist:
- Patient education
- Muscle identification
- Movement awareness
- Muscle activation
- Treatment plan.

Education

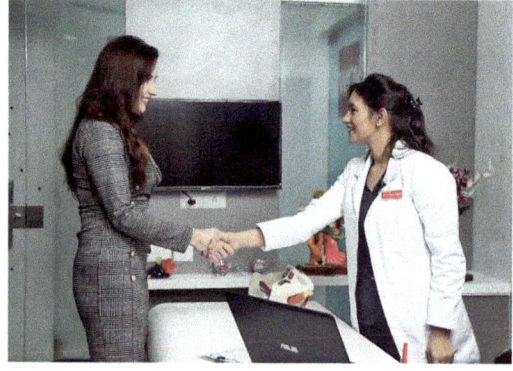

- Detailed patient education is absolute first step toward efficient pelvic floor rehabilitation.
- Practice makes the pelvic floor perfect is *not* true:
  "Only perfect practice can make the pelvic floor prefect"
- Clarity of mind is power. If the patients are confused or unclear, they will simply waste their time using and strengthening accessory muscles. However, if the patients are clear in their head about location, attachment, functions, and ways to activate them, their active correct participation will enhance the results of PFR.

Identification

Inform patient that this muscle lays inside your vagina or between your legs. It forms the base or floor and end-stop of everything inside.
- Internal identification: Self-test with finger—for proprioceptive identification, have the patient insert index finger inside vagina and try to self-palpate PFM like she is trying to stop urine.
- Indirect identification: Urine stop test—for functional test to create PFM action.
- External identification: One hand on coccyx and other on pubic symphysis—palpate movement of coccyx. You can also teach patient to put the finger on perineal body and feel the lift while contracting PFM.

Awareness

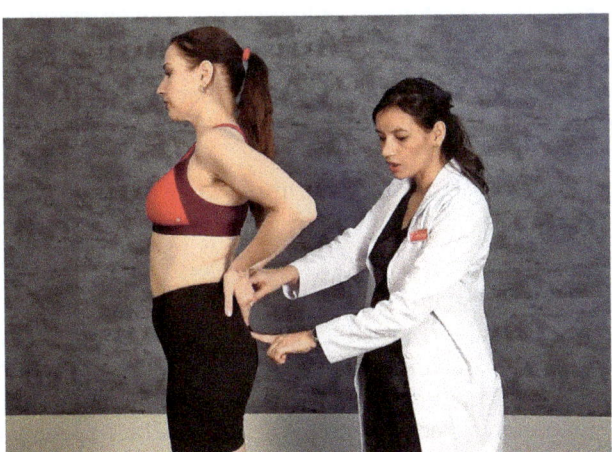

Patient can get awareness through following techniques:
- Feldenkrais method
- Cantienica.

Feldenkrais Method

Feldenkrais method is based on awareness through movement. It is a method with the intention to train the brain to bring body movements into awareness. This method can increase awareness of PFM and also directs toward functional tasks, such as weight lifting and coughing. This method encourages patients to practice awareness of PFM in differentiation from front part to back part of

PFM, from right side to left side, from isolated use to tightening of surrounding muscles. Moshe Feldenkrais quoted **"Awareness fits action to intention".**

It also suggests patient to breathe out while trying to hold urine. Breathing out forcefully is very challenging for incontinent patients. However, it can prevent the panic. It can also go with breathing and lifting pelvic floor which will increase recruitment of muscle fibers.

Through this method, differentiation is achieved first which is followed by integration as a second part of awareness to different movements like walking, breathing, coughing, etc. including contraction and relaxation during sexual activities through combination of awareness and movements. Final step is towards multiple activities of daily living (ADL) throughout the day whenever needed consciously or unconsciously.

Cantienica

Benita Cantienica in Switzerland developed this technique with the concept of sensual pelvic floor training.
- Women are taught to palpate the ischial tuberosity by bending forward. They are instructed to try to pull both the ischial tuberosities together. External self-palpation is done where a client can feel a mild gentle external shift of the ischial tuberosities due to contraction of iliococcygeus and coccygeus muscles.
- Gentle movement of greater trochanters can also be felt with PFM contraction.
- You may also suggest client for palpation of a movement underneath the fingers on the pubic bone and the coccyx.

Teach prevention of accessory muscles use: Teach patient to continue deep breathing exercise (DBE) while practice to self-palpate gluteus, rectus, hip adductors

While continuing DBE prevent bearing down or Valsalva maneuver.

Activation

Now that you can feel the muscle squeeze or lift them inside, and feel this lift every time you squeeze, try to hold it tightly for at least 2–10 seconds then let them relax completely. So, the movement will be like going up into elevator during contraction, hold there for sometime and coming down to basement as you relax completely for same seconds again. Ask them to repeat this slowly and as quick as possible to train both slow and fast twitch muscle fiber. Some basic guidelines to follow:
- Relax whole body completely
- Do not use any other muscles like buttock, thigh, and abdominal
- Keep breathing normally.

Teach Pelvic Floor Muscle Control

About 100% contraction versus relaxation or 80% contraction for submaximal or 50% contraction versus complete relaxation. Use your hand, make 100% fist, 80% fist, 50% fist, and slowly visualize PFM to do the same. Elevator exercises could be suggested especially to gain better and progressive control. Ask patient to imagine as if they are in an elevator and ask them to go to first floor, second floor, and so on while trying to increase the intensity of contractions. For teaching better contractions of engaging different fibers, ask your patient to imagine—stoping urine, closing vagina, anal wink. Practice all these contractions separately and finally together.

Treatment

In order to create individual treatment plan based on complaint and symptom and depending upon the diagnosis, treatment protocol will include combination of following (Fig. 1):
- Patient proper education or counseling
- Exercise
- Modalities
- Mobilization
- Home exercise program (HEP).

External and internal (transvaginal and transrectal), evaluation, and treatment for PFD.

Patient Education

Through awareness and detailed understanding of PFD, we can expect faster and longer lasting results

Make them feel comfortable so they can share symptoms freely with you. Give them detailed information about pelvic floor and its effects on people's life. So, detailed awareness is very important. Patient should learn and understand about what cause pelvic floor problems. How it affects quality of life and how we can treat this?

Exercise

Therapeutic exercise for PFM will include (Fig. 2):
- Pelvic floor muscle exercise for:
    - Strength
    - Endurance

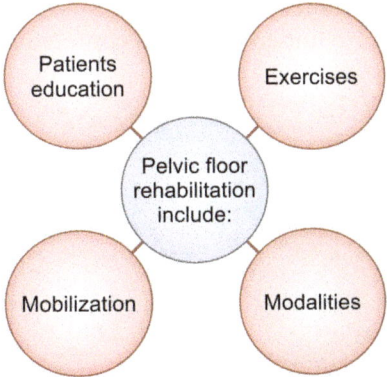

Fig. 1: Treatment plan for pelvic floor dysfunction.

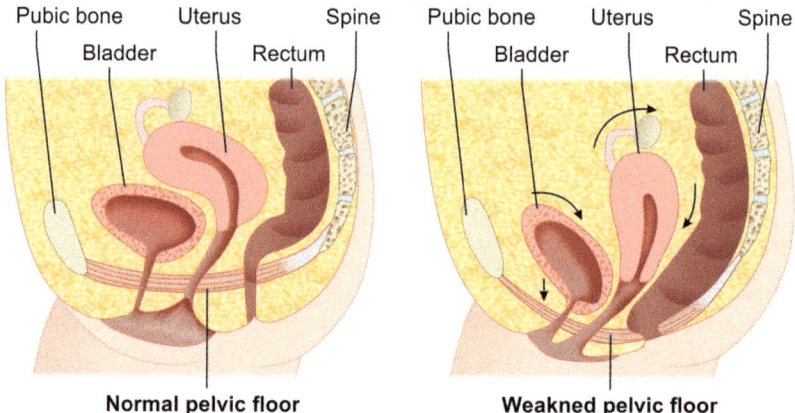

Fig. 2: Weakened pelvic floor exercise.

- - Power
- - Hypertrophy
- Coordination and functional training
- Proprioceptive neuromuscular facilitation (PNF)
- Stretching
- Postural reeducation.

Pelvic Floor Muscle Exercise

However, regardless of type of PFD, our rehabilitation protocols will not be successful, if we fail to teach our patients or clients about how exactly to perform pelvic floor muscle exercises without the use of accessory muscles. Our experience and researches suggest that 98.7% of all men or women who do pelvic floor muscle exercise are just using their accessory muscles instead of right group of PFM. Before we discuss the detailed rehabilitation of hypotonus and hypertonus types of PFD, we need to teach our patient—identification of PFM. It should be followed by pelvic floor muscle exercise, contraction, and complete relaxation techniques along with coordination training. Coordination and functional training is essential part of PF rehabilitation for both hypertonus and hypotonus types of PFD. Many pelvic floor providers focus on teaching PFM contraction and fail to focus on relaxation training. However, it is important to understand PFM contractions and relaxation, and control is evenly important.

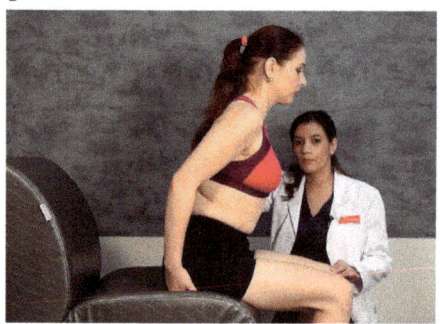

Foundation for Pelvic Floor Rehabilitation

Dr Arnold Kegel, 1940s, developed simple exercises to prepare women for childbirth. For many decades, doctors and leading medical institutions have recommended these exercises for women. World has seen the effectiveness of these exercises.

Proper instructions to teach pelvic floor muscle exercise: Most of the women who do pelvic floor muscle exercise, end up doing it wrong. It is important to give accurate instruction which can enable patients to activate right group of muscles and inhibit accessory muscles activities. Following are the keywords or instructions that can help your clients or patients to activate PFM.

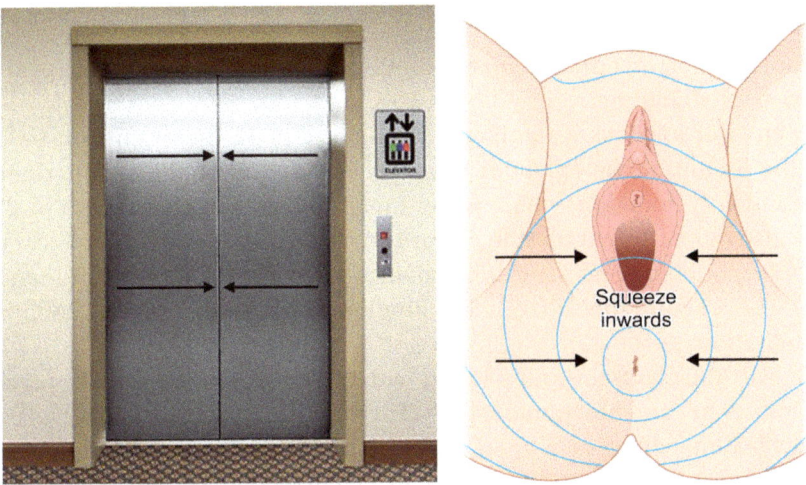

Do not say only "squeeze". Educate your clients in detail about what exactly you want them to squeeze and the way to do it.
- Close your openings and lift the floor
- Wink the anus
- Move the clitoris or penis and lift
- Pull the underwear in
- Stop urine flow
- Hold back gas
- Pull your "sits bone" together
- Pull your tailbone to your pubic bone
- Lift your perineum off the chair
- Pull up from the front as if stopping the flow of urine
- Pull up from the back as if stopping the escape of wind
- Pull up the front and back together
- Imagine the turtle pulling his head inside similarly pull the penis inside (male)
- Pull the penis (male)
- Lift the penis (male)
- Lift the testicles (male).

PELVIC FLOOR MUSCLES VERSUS ACCESSORY MUSCLES

We have always experienced that most of the people, who think they understand and do pelvic floor muscle excrcise, they do it wrong. They squeeze wrong group of muscles. They try to do pelvic floor muscle exercise and end up using their hip adductors, hip extensors, lower abs or any other group of muscle. As a responsible PFR expert, its provider's responsibility to get their patients use correct PFM. Help them also to avoid Valsalva maneuver, or bearing down activities (Fig. 3).

Functional Training

For functional or incoordination type of PF dysfunction Het's ultimate goal is reflexive rehabilitation.

Even after improving significant strength of PFM, if therapist observes that the incontinence episodes have not stopped, it could be functional or habitual dysfunction, where patient might have enough strength in the pelvic floor muscles but they do not use the strength when they need to. For example, coughing and sneezing activities for stress urinary incontinence (SUI). They require specialized rehabilitation which is functional or habitual rehabilitation.

- *In SUI:* You can train your patients with combination of especially tactile biofeedback and functional activity. For example, patient with SUI, can use tactile biofeedback and squeeze PFM. Ask them to maintain the squeeze and than artificially and intentionally cough while tactile biofeedback is sending neuromuscular signals.
- *In hypertonus:* We can be trained to relax the muscles through above mentioned rehabilitation protocol for hypertonus pelvic floor muscles. However, the same patient might generate habitual spasm of PFM in the presence of stimulus. For example, patient with dyspareunia might be able to completely relax pelvic floor muscles in routine life. However, one thought about penetration or sexual intercourse can lead to functional or hypertonus type of dysfunction and patient might demonstrate spasm just thinking about sex. You teach patients to use same tactile biofeedback and ask patient to regenerate the similar thoughts while trying relaxing muscles. Our research has shown amazing results with Het's reflexive training protocol, for functional and habitual dysfunctions. Indirectly, with the proper use of biofeedback, a provider is generating reflexive work or reflexive relaxation or pelvic floor muscles.

Proprioceptive Neuromuscular Facilitation

Proprioceptive neuromuscular facilitation is a technique aiming to stimulate the maximum numbers of motor units into activity by using three-dimensional patterns of movements. PFM activates with other group of muscles like lower abdominal muscles and glutei during voluntary exercise.

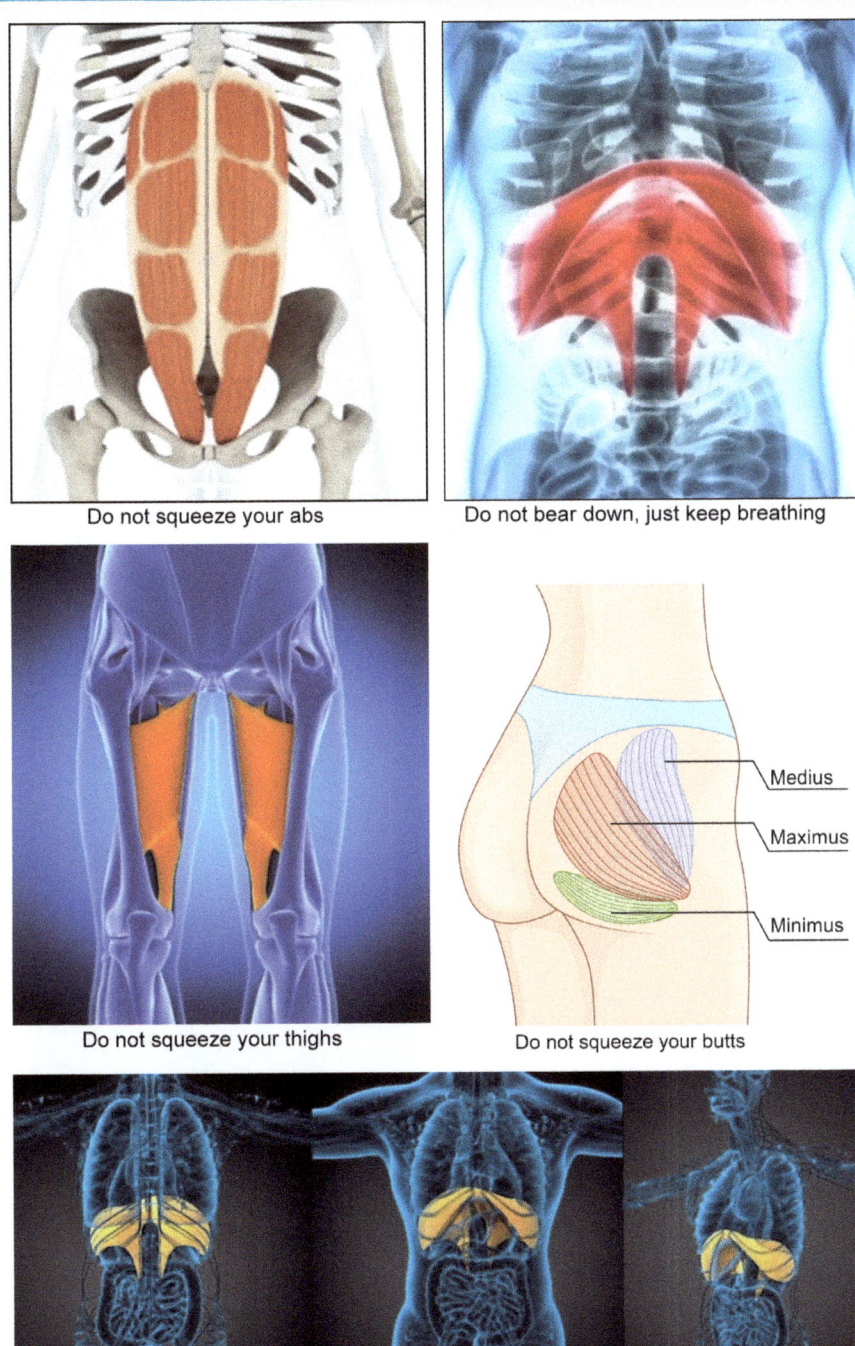

Fig. 3: Patients are likely to use accessory muscles and likely to hold their breath, while trying to do pelvic floor muscle exercise.

On electromyography (EMG) we can see increased muscle activity in the PFM:
- In response to contraction of the transverses abdominis.
- With cocontraction of the glutei.

MODALITIES

Electrotherapy Modalities Like

- Biofeedback devices like:
  - EMG
  - PF 360
- Electrical stimulation like (Fig. 4):
  - Transcutaneous electrical nerve stimulation (TENS)
  - Interferential therapy (IFT):
    » Heat and cold therapy
    » Vulvar ultrasound
- Home use devices like:
  - WOW-Woman
  - WOW Vagina-Dilate
  - WOW Vagina-Fit.

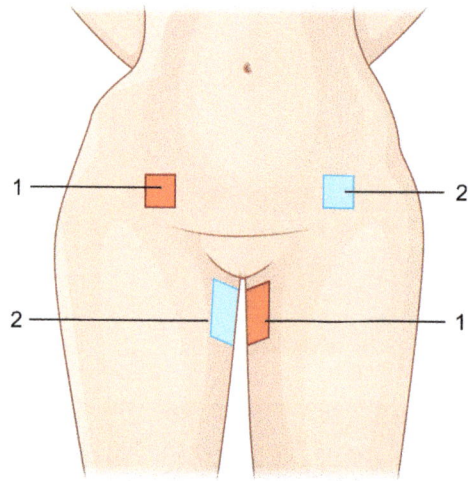

Fig. 4: Electrodes placement.

Biofeedback Devices (ICS—International Continence Society)

"Biofeedback is a technique by which information about a normally unconscious physiological process is presented to the patient and the therapist as a visual, auditory or tactile signal. The signal is delivered from the preset of measurable physiological parameter, which is subsequently used in an educational process to accomplish specific therapeutic results. The signal is generated in quantitative way and the patient is taught how to alter it and thus control the basic physiological process".

Or

Biofeedback is a process through which we can use to learn to control our body's functions. In this process we use our thoughts to control our body.

Motor Learning

Here we are using biofeedback techniques to learn or monitor the electric activity of pelvic floor muscle.

Sensory information or feedback is send to the patient through specific type of biofeedback device during or after each contraction which ultimately creates more effective PFM contraction.

Research says that just verbal instruction on how to contract PFM is not enough. To maximize the effectiveness of the contraction, biofeedback is extremely important.

Types of Biofeedback

Visual Biofeedback

Hand mirror to watch the PFMs contraction, narrowing of genital hiatus or elevation of perineum can be a simplest version of visual biofeedback.

Electromyography Biofeedback

Muscle activities are picked up using surface or internal electrodes. Electrographic biofeedback can offer visual and auditory signals. Intravaginal, intraanal, and surface electrodes are used to provide EMG biofeedback during PFM rehabilitation. Visual feedback can be given by using different graphics. Major drawback we have seen in years of experience is false biofeedback. As the sensors are too sensitive, they can detect and display accessory muscles' activities and can misguide patients or providers by showing graphical display without proper PF activation.

Manometric Visual Biofeedback

Perineometer is designed to record changes in vaginal pressure during PFM contraction.
Limitation—patient can be misguided as it can also detect and display increased abdominal pressure during activities like Valsalva maneuver, coughing, and straining.

Sonography Visual Biofeedback

Real-time abdominal and perineal ultrasound can help to clearly observe the elevation of bladder neck during a PFM contraction and descent of bladder neck during coughing or Valsalva maneuver. Perineal ultrasound can show better PFM activity than intravaginal EMG and perineometry.

Major limitation is training of the providers, cost effectiveness, and state regulations to carry portable ultrasound machines.

Tactile or Verbal Feedback

- Tactile perception is extremely effective to develop contraction awareness of PFMs. Self insertion of finger and squeezing it can also be a good method of tactile biofeedback.

- Devices like WOW-Woman and pelvic floor 360 can lead to gentle stretch reflex to PFM which creates great PF activation when associated with conscious contraction of the same muscles.

Kinesthetic Biofeedback

Weighted vaginal cones are used for a while. Different weights are used intravaginally above PFM, while women try to perform holding of the weights while standing. WOW Vagina-Fit device is one of the best assessment device which cannot only progressively strengthen PFMs but also provides great level of kinesthetic perception when the device begins to slip downward from the vagina which causes woman to activate more muscle fibers of PFM to prevent the device from slipping out.

Which Type of Biofeedback is best for PFR?

Our research and studies show some level of effectiveness of all types of biofeedback devices. However, there is a significant difference with cost, convenience, effectiveness and limitations of different types of biofeedback. We strongly recommend WOW IIPRE approved tactile based biofeedback device and PFM exercisers, pelvic floor 360 for clinical use for men, women and children. Refer to Page no. 199: Pelvic floor 360 to learn about details of benefits.

Interferential therapy/Transcutaneous Electrical Nerve Stimulation

As we are aware of the effectiveness of these modalities on improving muscle rehabilitation, now it is important to know about electrodes placement.

Heat and Cold Therapy

We can use hot pad or cold pad to increase blood circulation at pelvic floor muscle to treat spasm.

Vulvar Ultrasound

Vulvar ultrasound: Therapeutic ultrasound can be performed over water filled glove.

Vaginal Dilators

Appropriate patient education is important for correct strategies to use vaginal dilator. Forceful penetration with too big dilator without proper relaxation might cause pain and reflexive muscle spasm.

However, before we move forward, you need to understand the ultimate technology designed exclusively for pelvic floor rehabilitation PF 360. Please read and understand following technologies clearly as you will learn different ways to implement PF360 for different kind of PFD in upcoming chapters.

MOBILIZATION OR MANUAL THERAPY

A physical therapist can use external and internal hands on mobilization, manipulation, and stretching to improve blood circulation and mobility. These therapies include:
- Joint mobilization, e.g. SIJ
- Visceral manipulation
- Soft tissue mobilization—external, transvaginal, transrectal
- Trigger point release
- Myofascial release
- Deep tissue release
- Connective tissue manipulation
- Other specific technique like (Wise-Anderson and Thiele technique).

HOME EXERCISE PLAN

Suggest your patients appropriate guidelines
Simple lifestyle changes and home exercise plan can help them to manage symptoms independently on their own, after finishing the treatment sessions with therapist. We should guide them about:
- How to do pelvic floor muscle exercise correctly?
- Stretching exercises at home
- Proper relaxation techniques
- Postural correction
- Healthy toilet habits
- Use the knack trick each time during sneezing, coughing, and lifting stuff
- Do not hold urine unnecessarily
- Do not strain in bowel movement
- Do not lift heavy loads
- Avoid high intensity workout/deep squatting/jumping and skipping
- Keep healthy weight to avoid obesity
- Seek immediate care for your bronchitis
- Stop smoking.

WOW PELVIC FLOOR 360

Even the best knowledge of the world without efficient implementation cannot bring best possible results. Pelvic floor 360 will bring you great results by empowering you to provide most efficient rehabilitation for pelvic floor.

"Technology is a gift of God. After the gift of life it is perhaps the greatest of God's gifts. It is the mother of civilizations, of arts and of sciences"
—**Freeman Dyson.**

WOW! "Pelvic Floor 360"

- Pelvic floor 360 (PF360) is unique PFM exerciser especially designed to provide pelvic floor rehabilitation (Fig. 5).
- Its revolutionary technology, pelvic floor activator, and biofeedback device designed scientifically to be used in medical, paramedical or rehabilitation set up to help PFM rehabilitation.
- The simplicity and efficiency of PF360 can greatly help healthcare providers to take care of pelvic floor muscle dysfunction in male, female, and children.
- Its one of its own kind combo unit designed to provide PFM training and neuromuscular re-education through visual guidance, auditory signals, and tactile biofeedback for PFMs.
- It empowers the healthcare providers to improve pelvic floor health (strength, endurance, hypertrophy, power, control, and flexibility). Healthcare providers can choose either inbuilt programs or customized programs depending on the clinical needs.

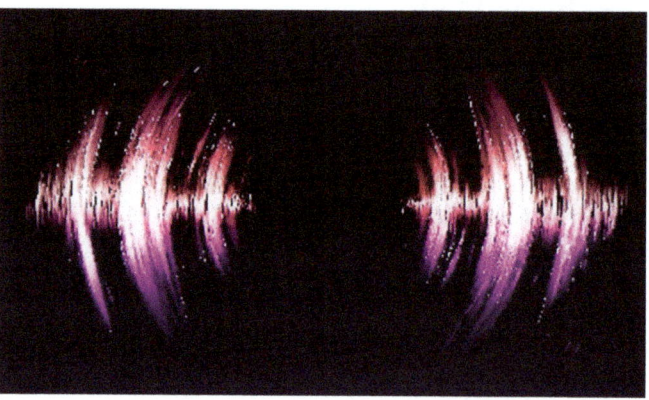

Indications

Pelvic floor 360 helps you to provide pelvic floor muscle exercises as a part of rehabilitation.

Female

- Vaginal recovery after childbirth
- Postnatal, post C-section, pre- and postsurgical and postmenopausal patients
- Hypotonus conditions like vaginal looseness, female sexual dysfunctions, stress incontinence, overactive bladder, mixed incontinence, hypermobile urethra, any pelvic organ prolapse upto grade 2 like cystocele, rectocele, enterocele, etc.
- Hypertonus conditions like PFM spasms, vaginismus, dyspareunia, pseudo UTIs, pelvic pain, interstitial cystitis, chronic pelvic pain, endometriosis, "orgasmic difficulties and other intimate health issues etc."
- Incoordination type of pelvic floor dysfunctions.

Male

- Hypotonus conditions like erectile dysfunction (ED), premature ejaculations, postvoidal dribbling, urinary incontinence, fecal incontinence, etc.
- Hypertonus conditions like pelvic trauma, pelvic pain, muscle spasm, levator ani syndrome, prostatitis, etc.
- Pre- and postprostatectomy.

Pediatric

- Early bladder and bowel control; faster and sooner potty-training.
- Conditions like enuresis, nocturnal enuresis, encopresis, urinary urgency and retention, urinary incontinence, fecal incontinence and constipation.

Contraindications

- Menstruation
- Postpartum period
- Sexually transmitted infection
- Intrauterine device
- Bacterial and viral infections and acute inflammation
- Tuberculosis
- Scleroderma
- Burns
- Eczema
- Poor healing in the treatment area
- Metal implants
- Pacemaker or automatic defibrillator
- Ablative or nonablative cosmetic intervention
- Cancer
- Active collagen diseases
- Cardiovascular diseases like vascular disease, peripheral arterial diseases, and thrombophlebitis
- Thrombosis
- Febrile condition
- Kidney or liver failure
- Any form internal rehabilitation for patients under age, etc.

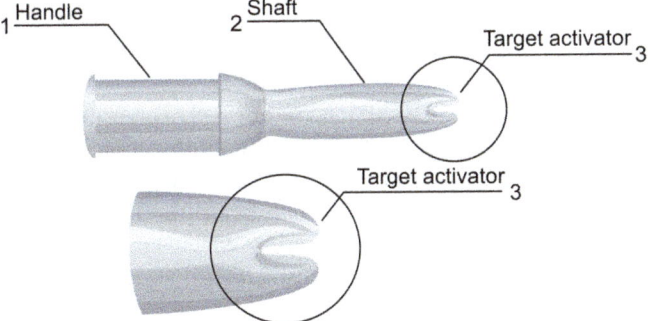

Figs. 5A and B: Showing the picture of PF360.

MODE OF APPLICATION OF PELVIC FLOOR 360 (FIGS. 6 TO 11)

1. Target activator can be applied to activate pelvic floor muscles in static way on both side of clitoris simultaneously at any angle, without touching clitoris in female patients.
2. Target activator can be applied to activate pelvic floor muscles in static way on both side of urethra simultaneously at any angle, without touching urethra in female patients.
3. Target activator can be applied to activate pelvic floor muscles at the degree of paraurethral activation in female urethra in a way where two protruded parts of target activator can cover surrounding area of urethra in dynamic circular motion from 0 to 360° without touching urethra.
4. Target activator can be applied to activate pelvic floor muscles in static way on both side of perineal body simultaneously at any angle.
5. Target activator can be applied to activate pelvic floor muscles at the degree of perineal body in a way where two protruded parts of target activator can cover surrounding area of perineal body in dynamic circular motion from 0 to 360°.
6. Target activator can be applied to activate pelvic floor muscles in static way on both side of external anal sphincter simultaneously at any angle.
7. Target activator can be applied to activate pelvic floor muscles at the degree of external anal sphincter in a way where two protruded parts of target activator can cover surrounding area of external anal sphincter in dynamic circular motion from 0 to 360°/superficial Het's ring.
8. Target activator can be applied to activate muscle fibers of different pelvic floor muscles like bulbocavernosus (BC) female muscles.
9. Target activator can be applied to activate BC reflex by targeting clitoral activation to get reflexive anal wink along with active contraction of muscles.
10. Target activator can be applied to activate multiple different muscle fibers of merging of IC and BC muscles at the same time.
11. Target activator can be applied to activate pelvic floor muscles at vaginal orifice/superficial Het's ring.
12. Target activator can be applied to activate the anococcygeal body.
13. Long shaft/rod part of PF360 can be applied to activate the whole pelvic floor muscles forming the urogenital, anorectal triangle.
14. Target activator can be applied to activate neuromuscular (pudendal nerve—region of perineal area.
15. Target activator can be applied to activate for the child such that the said stimulator compressively engages surface of a pair of paraanal/anal sphincter and perineal body.
16. The long shaft/rod part of PF 360 can be applied to activate pair of full length of bulbocavernosus muscles and merging fibers of ischiocavernosus, by flipping the penis of a patient on the abdominal wall.
17. The long shaft/rod part of PF 360 can be applied to activate (the male person) such that said stimulator compressively engages surface of a pair to activate pudendal nerve by targeting dorsal and ventral surface of the penis.

Foundation for Pelvic Floor Rehabilitation

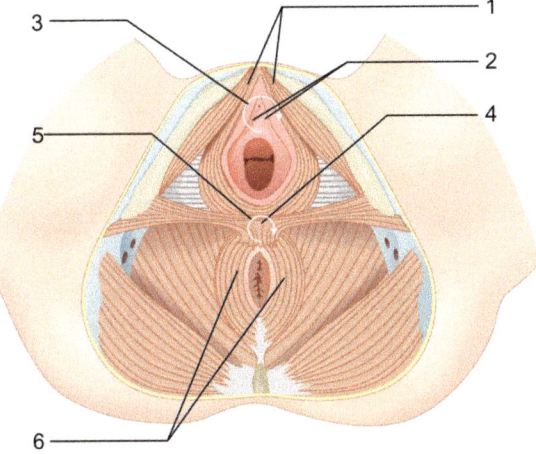

Fig. 6: Describing the points 1 to 6 in females.

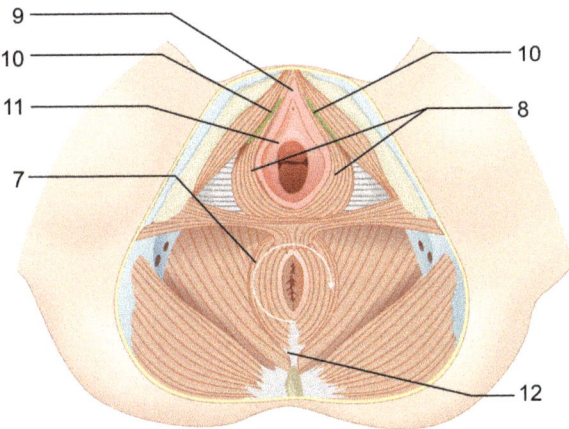

Fig. 7: Describing points 7 to 12 in females.

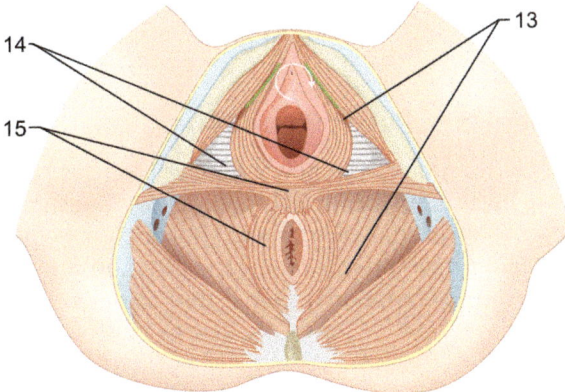

Fig. 8: Describing points 13, 14 and 15 in females.

Section 4: Pelvic Floor Muscle: Fitness and Rehabilitation

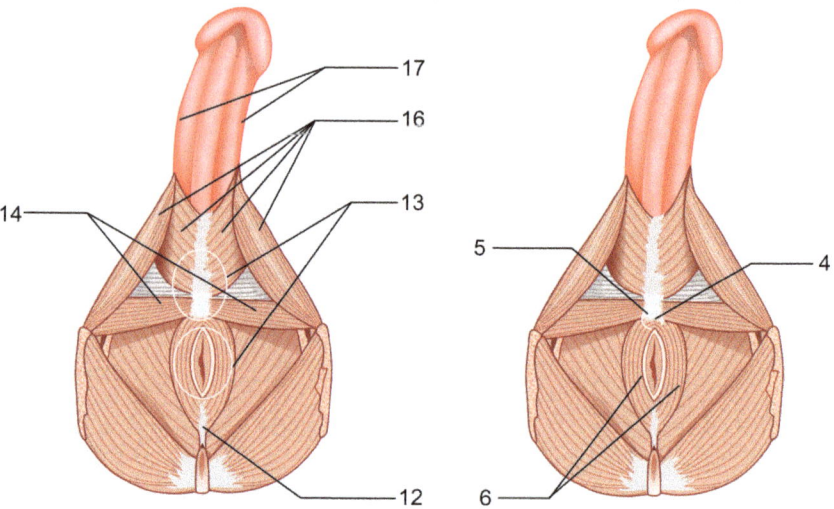

Fig. 9: Describing points 12,13,14,16,17 in males.

Fig. 10: Describing points 4,5,6 in males.

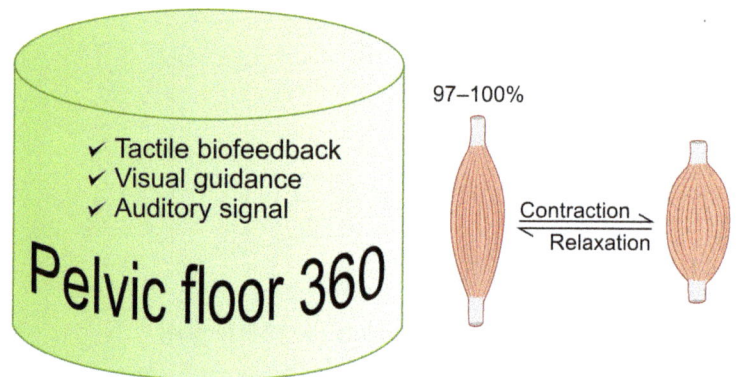

Fig. 11: Pelvic floor 360.

Medical Mechanics of Pelvic Floor 360

- *Increased O_2 consumption:* The pelvic floor 360 causes capillary dilation which leads to increase in localized blood flow. As a result it increased O_2 consumption and absorption of nutrients. Ultimately, it helps pelvic muscle regeneration. It improves muscle tone, elasticity, and contractile capacity. So, pelvic floor muscle function becomes more efficient.

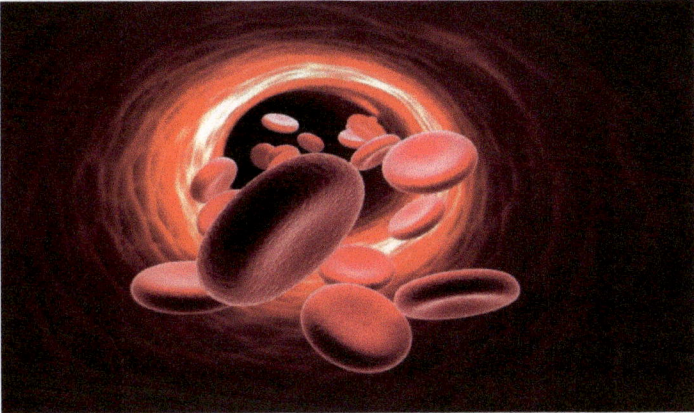

- *Stimulates the nerve endings:* Pelvic floor 360 provides 97–100% of muscle fibers activation (compared to only 40–80% in traditional strength training).

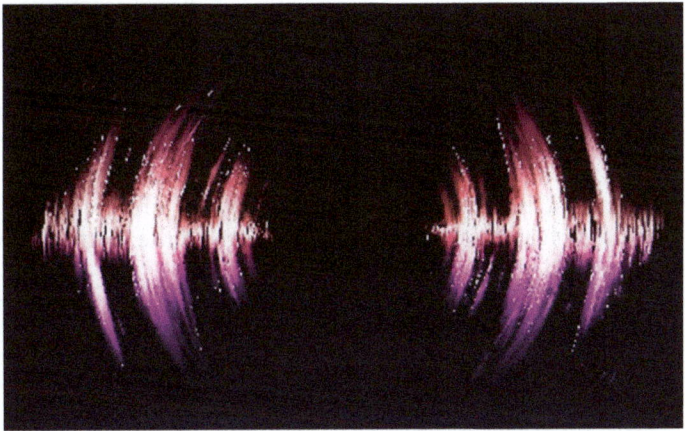

- *Improves muscle memory:* Pelvic floor 360 is designed to work through proprioceptive neuromuscular facilitation (PNF). It provides tactile biofeedback along with visual guidance and auditory training system improves muscle memory.
- Tonic vibration reflex (TVR): Pelvic floor 360 provides stretch stimulus to muscle spindle, which communicates to spinal cord through nerves and generates pelvic muscle activation. It can generate better muscle contraction through TVR. Active efforts from patients to squeeze pelvic floor muscles along with tactile feedback increase more muscle fibers recruitment (Fig. 12).

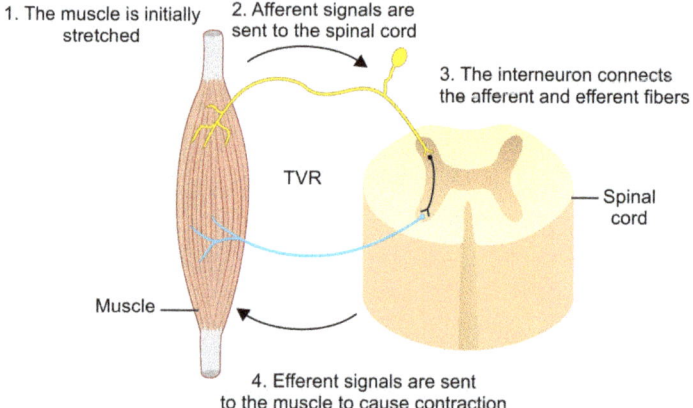

Fig. 12: Tonic vibration reflex (TVR).

PROGRESSIVE RESISTANCE TRAINING SYSTEM

PF 360 is completely noninvasive device. However, it could be used to activate targeted weak area of pelvic floor muscles. The practitioner can perform transvaginal or transrectal manual resistance training immediately followed by activation through PF360.

Rehab practitioners can insert the finger inside vagina/rectum while suggesting patient to hold. They can provide few seconds of resistance by pulling the finger out while patient is trying to hold it in.

- Patient can be trained with combination of mechanical and manual resistance to pelvic floor muscles (provider pulls the finger out while the patient is using pelvic floor muscles to hold it in).
- It is designed around key principle of exercise science to develop muscle strength through muscle facilitation and progressive resistance exercises.
- Progressive resistance training based strengthening of vaginal muscles. Agency of Health Care Policy and Research (AHCPR) concluded that the uses of resistance devices to exercise pelvic muscles are 87% more effective. However, same study showed that merely squeezing the pelvic muscles without feedback device may not be that much effective.

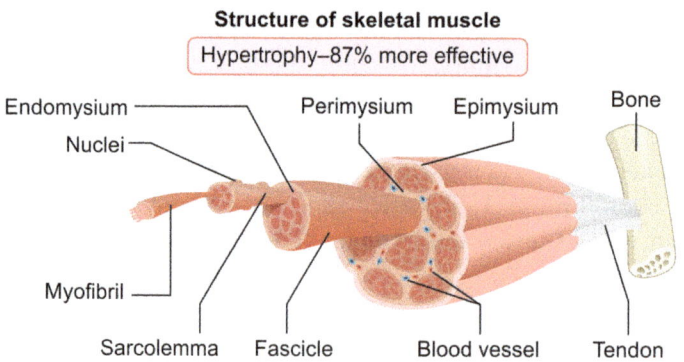

"The technology you use impresses no one. The experience you create with it is everything".
—**Sean Gerety**

Design (Technical Specifications)

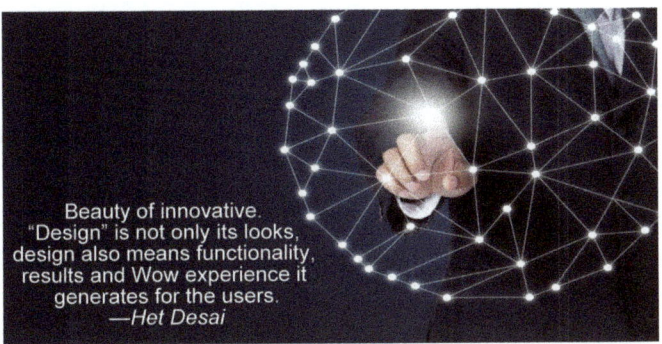

Beauty of innovative. "Design" is not only its looks, design also means functionality, results and Wow experience it generates for the users.
—Het Desai

Operational Design

- *3 in 1 combo:* One and only PFM device that can work for male, female, and children of any age.
- *Portability:* Portability of device will enable you to carry the device to different locations. If you are affiliated to multiple medical groups or hospitals, you do not have to purchase separate devices. You can carry it with you and use it for as many patients as needed.
- *User-friendly for patients:* It is extremely efficient but intellectually simplified, user-friendly device that any patient can easily use under providers guidance. Few modes of operations can be taught to the patient themselves. Like once you teach the patient to modify intensity, they will be able to do it on their own without your presence.
- *Easy to operate for providers:* Even if there are multiple programs and operations, it is scientifically designed to simplify the operations of the technology. It is extremely efficient but very easy to operate which makes it easy to train new doctors, physical therapist, and assistive staff.
- *Voice guided:* Inbuilt voice-guided exercise programs to activate sensory system through auditory signals to get best possible motor system.
- *Visual input:* Visual input is provided numerically and through dynamic graphics of muscle contraction and relaxation, which will generate more efficient muscle recruitment.
- *Tactile biofeedback:* Tactile biofeedback is provided through the activator which provides tactile biofeedback to activate correct group of PFMs. The intensity of tactile biofeedback is adjustable, where one can adjust the intensity of perceived tactile vibes through controller to customized individual need of your patients.
- *Anatomically designed shape of the activator:* The shape of the target activator is designed anatomically, to target specific group of muscle fibers to get the best possible activation of PFMs.

Mode of Application

Noninvasive

The noninvasive use of different programs of the device empowers rehabilitation specialists to provide PFMs activation without transvaginal or transrectal mode. External mode of application could be also used for pediatric, female, or male population. There are many devices designed for transrectal or transvaginal biofeedback. Unfortunately, most patients are not comfortable with invasive mode of application. Patients are even more uncomfortable, if they have to get transvaginal or transrectal electrical stimulation. As a result, it negatively affects the compliance of the patients. PF 360 is the ultimate solution to the problem. As it is completely noninvasive it does not introduce any current into the body. Patients are extremely comfortable with mode of application which positively affects patient compliance.

Time Flexible Adjustments

- *Time flexible intensity adjustments:* Complete flexibility to control intensity of vibes at any given time of treatment. For example, if you set up a patient on higher intensity at level 4 at patient comfort level, after few minutes of workout, if patient feels too intense and patient wants to turn down the intensity from level 4 to level 3, therapist can do it without stopping the workout.
- *Time flexible 5 preset workout levels:* Preset workout protocols are given to choose from. Depending on your patient's current level of pelvic floor strength, you may modify or improve level of workout. Also, flexibility to move from one type of program to another type at any given time of the treatments.

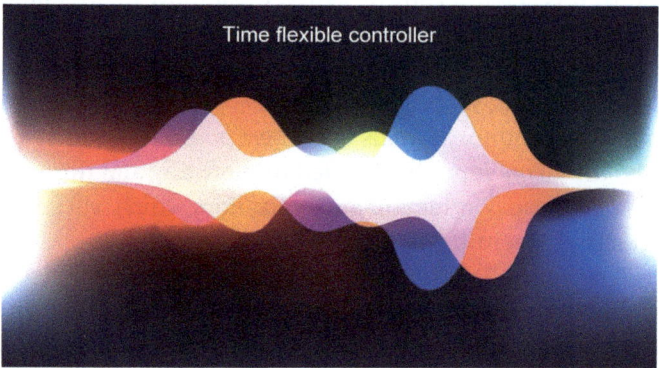

Progression

- *Objective progressions system:* System that enables patient and provider to measure progress objectively by mastering lower level and moving up to higher level of sustained hold from level 1 to level 5.
- *Mechanico-manual progressive resistance training (MPRE):* The unique shape of activator empowers the user with progressive resistance training system. MPRE is provided through manual resistance given by provider's

finger for 30 seconds and followed by target activator. The manual resistance can be progressively increased as the muscles get stronger. Alternating 30 seconds of PF 360 activation and manual resistance helps to gain most muscle fibers activation.

Protocols

- *Inbuilt protocols:* Multiple inbuilt workouts, exercise protocols, and rehabilitation programs to improve strength, endurance, hypertrophy and relaxation ability
    1. *Strength protocol:* Inbuilt program that improves strength—ability to create maximum power of the PFMs
    2. *Endurance protocol:* Inbuilt program that improves endurance, ability to work for longer duration of time of the PFMs
    3. *Hypertrophy protocol:* Inbuilt program that improves hypertrophy or size of the PFMs
    4. *SH protocol:* Inbuilt program that improves strength and hypertrophy of the PFMs
    5. *Glazer protocol:* Inbuilt program that works as antispasmodic to overtight PFMs through breakdown of chronic tightness through research-based glazer protocol
- *Manual setting:* Manually adjustable settings are designed to empower providers to customize programs as per individual needs of their patients or clients.
- *Hold time trainer:* Special adjustable setting to empower patients to improve slow twitch muscle fibers of pelvic floor muscles
- *Pulse trainer:* Special setting to empower patients to improve fast twitch muscle fibers.

How to use pelvic floor360
- Turn on the device
- Start the phone application
- Choose PF 360 from application
- You will have following options to choose from

Training protocols: Strength, endurance, hypertrophy, glazer, SH and target activation
- Choose the training type
- Place the target activator on the weaker area of PFM
- It will activate 2 muscles simultaneously as shown in diagram
- Or it will activate multiple muscle fibres of the same muscles as shown in diagram.
- For example, it can activate ichiocavernosus (IC) and BC muscles at the same time
- Or it can activate multiple different muscle fibres of IC or BC muscles at the same time
- You can place it around the urethra and it can activate tissues located on both side of urethra simultaneously, without touching urethra in female patients
- You can also change the degree of para urethral activation in female urethra in a way where two protruded parts of target activator can cover surrounding area of urethra from 0 to 360 degrees without touching urethra.

- Same protocol can be applied for other areas like paraclitoral, para-anus area or perineal body
- User can also use longer portion of activator to target elongated muscle fibres like bulbocavernosus and ischiocavernosus muscles
- Same format can be used for male patients or children as well
- This is unique non invasive targeted technology that can exercise specific targeted muscle fibres of pelvic floor muscles.

Benefits:
- Helps to activate and exercise targeted pelvic floor muscles from different angles
- Helps to activate and exercise targeted pelvic floor muscles simultaneously around the clitoris, urethra, perineal body and anus.
- Helps to activate and exercise weak muscle fibres of any individual weak muscle to take care of hypotonus pelvic floor muscles.
- Helps to relax and release muscle tightness in targeted points of hypertonus muscles
- Helps to use specialized training protocols from options in the phone app
- Latest technology we are using helps to provide visual cues and auditory biofeedback along with numbers tracking, motivation and feedback system from the app.

Sample Protocol of Pelvic Floor 360

	1	2	3	4	5
Hold—relaxation time	2:2	3:3	5:5	8:8	10:10
Reps	10 reps				
Sets	3 Sets				
Pulse—FTM on constant mode	20	30	40	50	60
Total workout time	10–15 minutes				

Variables

1. *Hold time and relaxation time*: Most of WOW group devices come with inbuilt hold time and relaxation time. Hold time means you squeeze, lift, and hold your PFM as if you are trying to stop urine. Device will empower you through tactile biofeedback. For example, if you choose program 1, it will give your tactile indication to hold the muscles for 2 seconds; and relax for 2 seconds; then repeat; also you will have visual and auditory signals which will help with proper PFM facilitation.
2. *Reps*: Its number of repetitions performed per set, means without resting in between. You may start with lower reps range and slowly progress to more repetitions as you get stronger. What if I can not do 10 reps to start with? You can take two approaches:
    i. Approach 1: Do as many reps as possible, progressively work your way up to 10

OR

ii. Approach 2: You are starting at level 1 A. Reduce the intensity of each contraction, means start with only 20-50% of your best possible intensity. It is known as submaximal level which will enable you to do 10 reps; after that, progressively add the intensity in the same rep range. For example, if you started with 30% of your best intensity, you can progressively increase to 50% after you have mastered 10 reps of 30% and so on.

3. *Sets*: Generally you will be benefited significantly if you perform 3 sets of 10 reps. You may choose to start with 1 or 2 sets depends on current ability of your PFM.
4. *Rest time*: You can rest as per recovery time of your body; may be 1 minute between the sets. Reduce the rest time between the sets as you get stronger.
5. *Pulse—FTC*: After each workout, rest for a minute or two; then perform quick flicker of contractions for above given numbers. It needs to be snap like 1 or 2 seconds—quickest possible contractions. It will train fast twitch muscle fibers of your PFM. Previous part of workout is designed to train STC slow twitch muscles fibers.
6. *Total workout time*: Most of the work out designed to be very time efficient.

Disclaimer: Wow-PF360 is not a medical device. It is a unique, noninvasive pelvic floor muscle exerciser. It should not be used transvaginally or transrectally. It should be used only externally to exercise PFM.

Safety Features Design

- *Single user:* It can be used to treat multiple user by using condom.
- *Temperature sensor safety:* Each activator has temperature sensor which will detect raise in temperature and terminate the circuit whenever temperature rises above limits, which make it much safer to use.
- *Safety fuse:* The technology is not operated by a battery. There is a safety fuse in the device which will provide best safety.
- *Results driven:* The technology is very precise and result driven. It provides all the flexibility and adjustability to customize the rehabilitation need of the individual patient. It offers best possible results in least possible time.

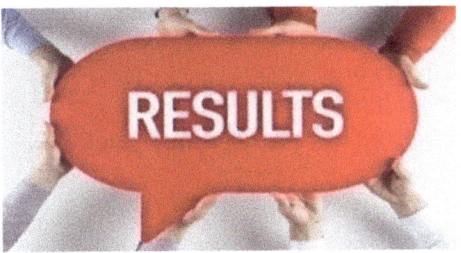

Statistics

- Approximately one-sixth women suffer from chronic pelvic pain
- More than 30 million women suffer from urinary incontinence

Section 4: Pelvic Floor Muscle: Fitness and Rehabilitation

- Every other woman is likely to have pelvic floor dysfunction
- 9/10 mothers suffer from vaginal laxity
- 50% of postmenopausal women have vaginal atrophy
- More than 43% of women in US suffer from female sexual dysfunction
- About 50 million men are likely to suffer from ED
- Almost 50% of men over age of 40 years are approximately to suffer from ED.

Clinical Research of Pelvic Floor 360

Research-based pelvic floor 360 has been researched and proven to create better peaked EMG and ultrasonic changes. It is most efficient and result driven technology as it is the end result of multiple clinical trials and many researches. Significant results were demonstrated in EMG and sonography devices.

Female Patients

- About 97% improved urine control and reduced urine leakage
- About 99% improved PFM activation on sonography, Oxford manual muscle testing, and transvaginal electromyography
- About 98% improved vaginal muscle tone and tightness
- About 96% experienced improved intimate health—libido, arousal, orgasms and pain free coitus
- About 99% patients [suffering from female sexual dysfunctions (FSD)] reported improved intimate health of FSFI (Female Sexual Functions Index) Questionnaires
- About 95% improved core stability and helped with low back pain issues
- About 98% improved overall feeling of well-being and confidence
- About 96% spouse reported improved vaginal tightness during intimacy.

Male Patients

- About 98% improved urinary leakage
- About 99% improved erectile rigidity even moderate to severe cases on ED
- About 96% experienced heightened orgasm intensity
- About 84% improved ejaculatory control
- About 80% improved ejaculatory force
- About 98% improved confidence
- About 97% reported longer lasting erections
- About 99% experienced increased intimate pleasure.

Pediatric Patients

- About 98% improved enuresis
- About 94% improved with encopresis
- About 99% satisfied parents and referring physicians
- Research based: Time-tested, reliable and valid.

"Once a new technology rolls over you, if you're not part of the steamroller, you're part of the road."
— **Stewart Brand**

Technology is nothing. What's important is that you have a faith in people, that they're basically good and smart, and if you give them tools, they'll do wonderful things with them.
— **Steve Jobs**

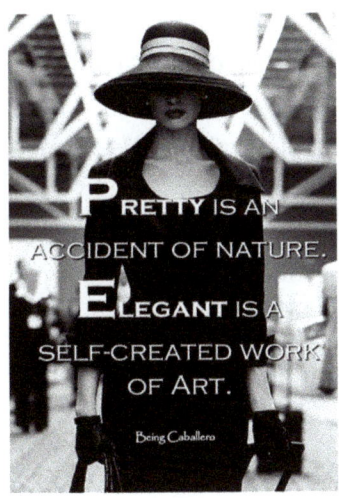

Art of pelvic floor 360 will help you create 'Elegance of pelvic floor muscles'

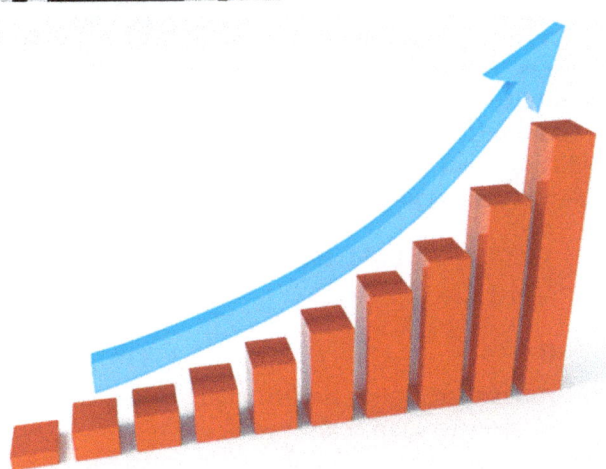

KEYPOINTS TO REMEMBER IN PELVIC FLOOR MUSCLE REHABILITATION

- Avoid Valsalva maneuver. Avoid straining and breathe holding.
- Exhale when you exert. Try to keep breathing normally when you hold the PFM contraction.
- Squeeze correct PF muscles.
- Inhibit action of accessory muscles, e.g. hip adductors, abs, gluteus, etc.
- Modify intensity, frequency, and duration of squeeze.
- Empower correct breathing pattern.

- If you hold breath, it will push down on the PFMs.
- Stay aware. BRACE before activity that can cause symptoms.

Knack it—means if you feel like coughing or sneezing, squeeze before your cough or sneeze and then try to hold PFM while you cough or sneeze, e.g. knack it before cough and sneeze for urinary incontinence.

Benefits for Doctors

Benefits for Doctors or Healthcare Providers or Physical Therapists

Pelvic floor 360 will help to:

- Expand your practice beyond basics for physical therapists, gynecologists, urogynecologists, diabetologists, sexologists, dermatologists, colorectal surgeons, proctologists, endocrinologists, psychiatrists, pediatricians and many other medical, paramedical and healthcare experts all over the world.
- Empower the doctors to provide urogenital rehabilitation or pelvic floor rehabilitation services in most cost-efficient way
- Create global recognition through global listing through WOW International Institute of Pelvic Floor Research Rehab and Education (IIPRE)
- Generate new referrals and new referral sources for your practice
- Add new dimensions to your reputation
- Provide significantly higher return on affordable investment
- Create outside the box financial gains
- Benefit American physical therapists, physical therapy assistants or medical group practices. They will be able to provide billable services through PF 360. You may also explore possibilities to get reimbursed for therapeutic exercises, neuromuscular re-education, therapeutic activities. Its provider's responsibility to check compliance with state and federal level rules and regulation—Guidelines might vary for different states of America.

WHAT ARE HOME-USED DEVICES FOR PELVIC FLOOR REHABILITATION?

WOW-Woman

- Wow-Woman—vitalize vaginal health; vaginal muscles exercise.
- Unique gift for every woman at any age.
- Revolutionary pelvic floor (-vaginal) muscle exerciser

Are you planning for pregnancy? or Did you deliver in 2 weeks or 20 years ago *pregnancy is beautiful*, but, do you know?

- Vaginal muscles are overstretched during pregnancy, labor, and childbirth
- Vagina is likely to get looser every year after childbirth
- Vaginal looseness can lead to problems like urine leakage, back pain, and intimate health issues
- As you grow older, PFMs keep getting weaker

Research says (statistics approximately): Almost every mother is likely to suffer from PFM dysfunction.

- 9/10 mothers suffer from vaginal looseness.
- About 50% loss of strength of vaginal muscle is likely to happen after delivery.

- More than 30 million women suffer from urine leakage.
- More than 55% of women are likely to suffer from female sexual dysfunctions.
- Strengthening PFMs greatly benefits intimate well-being.
- 1 in 3 women is likely to have PFD.

Benefits

- Improves tone and tightness of muscles surrounding vagina.
- Enhances fitness of vaginal muscles for healthy pregnancy.
- Optimizes vaginal recovery after childbirth.
- Promotes better urine control.
- Improves libido, sensation, orgasms, and intimate health.
- Improves sexual relations (by strengthening pelvic floor muscles). Revitalize your inner fitness and intimate wellness.
- Also, it greatly helps with conditions like vaginal looseness, urine leakage, constipation, fecal leakage, initial stage of piles or pelvic organ prolapse, menopausal changes, female sexual dysfunctions, anorgasmia, pelvic pain, pelvic floor issues, or muscles spasm.

Science

WOW-Woman is designed with clinical researches, American Guidelines and International Standards.

- Improves blood flow: Increases O_2 consumption through capillary dilatation.
- Stimulates nerve endings and promotes better activation of pelvic floor muscles.
- Provides stretch stimulation to muscle spindle and activates TVR.
- Provides tactile biofeedback, visual and auditory cues to improve muscle memory.
- As a result, it helps to improve blood flow, elasticity, tensile strength, endurance, power and flexibility of pelvic floor muscles located inside vagina.

How to use WOW-Woman?

- This device is completely noninvasive and it is home exercise device. The patient can use it in their comfortable time and without taking the clothes off.
- The patient has to sit on the WOW-Woman device in such a way that the broad part is placed anteriorly touching the anterior portion of the perineum and the narrow part will be between the gluteal folds posteriorly (the device should cover the whole of the perineal area) (Figs. 13,14,15).
- The device is connected with the WOW Group app. Once the patient sits comfortably on the device, then connect the device to the mobile app using mobile's bluetooth.
- In the mobile app there will be multiple options for workout. We recommend to start with the lowest level first.
- It is just a 3 minute noninvasive pelvic floor muscle exerciser.

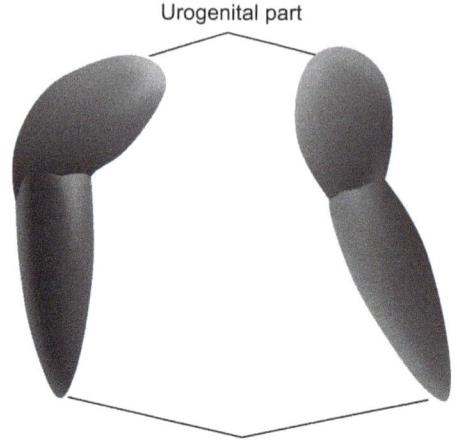

Fig. 13: Show the urogentital and anorectal part of WOW-Woman.

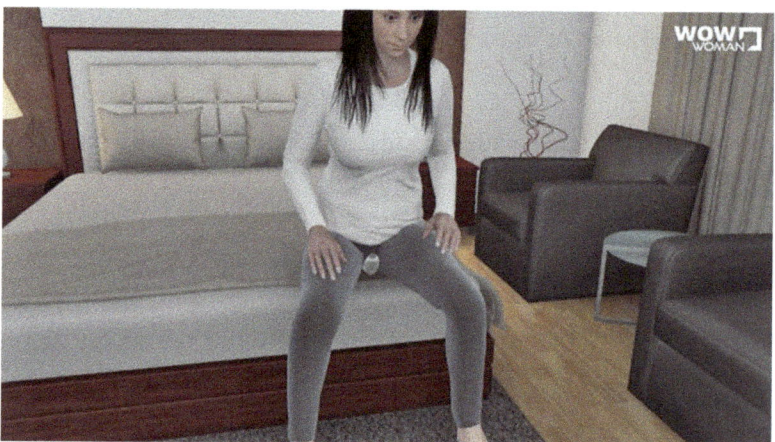

Fig. 14: Show the placement of WOW-Woman.

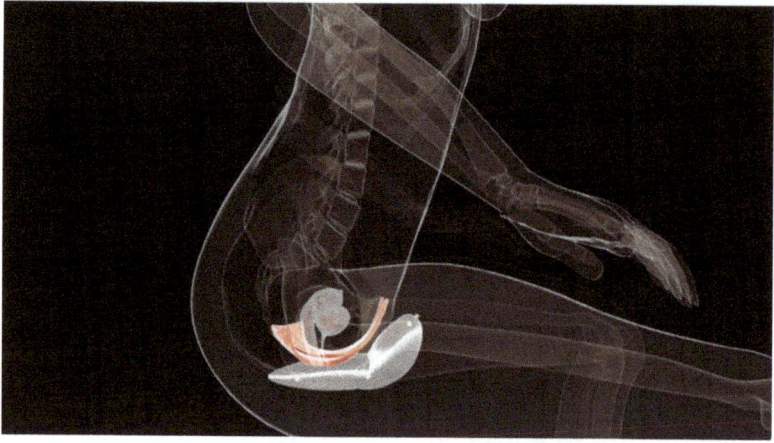

Fig. 15: Show the placement of WOW-Woman.

What makes WOW-Woman even more Special?

- Extremely time efficient: Only 3 minutes a day
- Completely noninvasive
- No need to take clothes off
- No need to insert the probe inside the vagina
- No medicine, no side effect
- Completely safe
- Smart pelvic floor muscle training
- Fancy mobile app and bluetooth technology
- Revolutionary and highly effective
- Convenient and easy to self-use
- Personal and portable
- Very high rewards at affordable cost
- Comfortable and gentle for any woman at any age
- Voice guided workouts
- Visual animations
- Medically designed
- Anatomically shaped
- Clinically tested and results driven
- Premium product at nonpremium price.

One of its own kind personal—pelvic floor exercise especially designed for women.

Testimonials

- I am so thankful to my husband for gifting me WOW-Woman. Who else will take care of my intimate health! Thanks hubby. I love you Wow-Woman so much—Renu Sharma.
- I was so embarrassed because of urine leakage during activities like coughing and sneezing. It was difficult for me to hold urine for long time during traveling. I had to go to bathroom very frequently. I was reluctant initially, but after I started using WOW-Woman. I am so happy as I do not have urine leakage anymore. Thanks to WOW-woman—Parveen Singh.
- After childbirth, I thought feeling little loose down there was normal unless my gynecologist suggested WOW-Woman. Just few weeks of use and my vagina feels toned and tight again. I feel so much confident. Thanks to my doctor who suggested WOW-Woman—Mrs Smith.
- Initially, I was hesitant to talk about this. However, I believe sex health is also a respectful part of overall well-being. After childbirth, sex became different over period of time. It was not easy to get aroused, intercourse was not as pleasurable, frequency, and intensity of climax reduced compared to before childbirth. My vaginal muscles became loose. I was not even able to tightly grip my husband's penis during sex. I was very depressed. Finally, I heard about WOW-Woman. My husband is very caring and supportive. He inspired me to get my pelvic floor muscles stronger. I have been using WOW-Woman for few weeks. I am extremely happy. I feel completely revitalized. I am interested in sex again. I can get properly aroused, intimate sensations are so much better, sex is more pleasurable and orgasms are

more frequent and intensified. I feel strong, confident, and young down there. I am very excited; WOW-Woman changed our life. My husband is also extremely happy and satisfied. I recommend WOW-Woman to every woman. It is magical—Kelly Anderson
- WOW-Woman is the best gift for any woman. She takes care of everyone else apart from herself. Thanks to WOW-Woman, it helped me to take care of her intimate health. What could be a better symbol for love and care than WOW-Woman?—Aditya Agarwal
- My wife was so happy when I gifted her WOW-Woman. It is kind of nice to see her happy like before. Our relationship is at a new spark now—Deepak Shetty
- Guess what? I am not married yet. But I love her to death. I am committed to her for rest of life. I gave my girlfriend a gift—"WOW-Woman". Do not want to wait till the time I get married. She is extremely happy that I am so caring and committed. Her happiness is my happiness. Thanks "WOW-Woman"—Krish Basu
- Every day, I treat many patients with pelvic floor dysfunctions. I have seen tears in their eyes. As a woman doctor, I can understand and respect women's intimate well-being. Before, the invention of WOW-Woman, I was also asking my patients to do pelvic floor muscle exercises after childbirth. That's what most of the doctors do. Right! It simply did not work well as most of the women end up using wrong muscles. WOW-Woman has helped so many patients. I suggest WOW-Woman to almost every single patient. It is a user friendly ultimate technology which takes care of vaginal muscles. My patients are very happy and satisfied. I have seen amazing results with WOW-Woman. Every woman and every mother should use WOW-Woman. I regularly use it for my personal health too. I have recommended WOW-Woman to all women in my family and friends. I love to use it and so you will too. Dr Sunita Patel, CEO, WOW IIPRE – International Institute of Pelvic Floor Research Rehab and Education.

Disclaimer: WOW-Woman is not a sex toy or medical device. It is a unique, noninvasive pelvic floor muscle exerciser. It should not be used for any illegal purpose. It should not be used transvaginally or transrectally. It should be used only externally to exercise PFM.

WOW VAGINA-FIT FOR TREATMENT

Treatment

The sample treatment protocol is given below. But as every patient is different, the treatment should be customized according to the need of the patient and depending upon the clinical judgement of the treating pelvic floor rehab specialist.

Although the home exercise program can be prescribed in the following way:

Follow the same hygienic protocol which is described in testing section (Chapter no. 4).

Phase 1 (Beginner)

If the patient's strength is "C", i.e. unable to hold the device in standing position then first try to hold the device in the supine position. The insertion of the device should be comfortable. If required, the patient can use lubricating gel in small amount. After the insertion ask the patient to do few counts of pelvic floor contractions. The correct pelvic floor contraction will pull the device up and into the vaginal canal.

The use of WOW Group's mobile app "She Strength" along with the device is very important for the best results as it helps to provide visual and auditory cues along with the proprioception. Patient will use one hand to hold VagniaFit inside the vagina (in supine position with knees and hips bent) and other hand to hold mobile. Initially ask the patient to do 30 counts a day. While attempting to hold Vagina-Fit the PFM contraction for upto 10 seconds. Most of the patients might not be able to hold it for 10 seconds for 30 reps. Customize the work out as per the clinical indication. Start with few seconds hold and work your way up to 10 seconds. Use of the WOW Group app will also motivate patient with better focus on duration of hold time. Use of the WOW Group mobile app will also greatly help medical practitioners to customise the home exercise program after assessing the reports generated by the app. (Also refer appendix to know more about the WOW Group Mobile App).

Continue the combine use of Vagina-Fit and Mobile app in supine position (gravity elimination position) till the time patient is able to hold the device in standing position.

Phase 2 (Intermediate)

In the standing position also the patient has to do the same exercise. Ask the patient to hold the device intravaginally by doing contraction of the pelvic floor muscles. In this phase also, use of the mobile app while doing exercise will greatly enhance benefits. Do the exercise for 40 counts a day.

The goal in this phase is that the patient should be able to hold the device by doing the pelvic floor muscle contraction for 10 seconds each rep. Progress upto 40-50 reps as per clinical need.

Phase 3 (Advance)

Once the patient is able to hold the device properly in standing then make the patient do all the 3 functional activities. (10 coughs, 10 jumps, 10 squats while holding Vagina-Fit transvaginally)

In this phase, the patient can progressively start resistance training by adding weights in Vagina-Fit.

Principles of Progression for Pelvic Floor Strengthening

Intensity of the exercise is as important as hold time or number of reps. As medical practitioners, we need to be very clear about when to make a progress? The answer is when the current challenge start being perceived as "easy" or "too easy".

Why not to Train the Failure Every Time?

Many researches on the exercise science for skeletal muscles suggest us the principle of "train till failure". Generally, it is followed by adequate rest for recovery and repair. The split training protocols like back, biceps and chest, triceps) are famous for the same reason. It gives adequate time for muscles to rest and grow before they are trained again. However, our goal to train pelvic floor muscle is not cosmetic hypertrophy. Our goal is functional outcomes. If we train them to failure every time, than they will not be ready to work when they face functional challenges. We suggest not to completely drain, fatigue or overexert the PF muscles. If they are overly trained, they may not be able to perform throughout the day especially when their performance is required during functional activities. Instead, they should be fresh and ready to progress towards Het's RR Reflexive results, the ultimate goal. Wise intensity control is extremely important.

This principle states that—when you are training a patient to do the pelvic floor muscle contractions for 3 sec hold, than do not suddenly increase the hold time upto 5, 8 or 10 seconds, instead go for a slow progression. First let the patient be comfortable to do the pelvic floor muscle contraction hold for 3 seconds and once she finds it's easy to hold for 3 seconds then only progress further to 4 seconds. Occasionally you may train them to failure. However, training to failure should not be done every time.

You may suggest more intense alternate day training (or even less frequent to some patients) who are doing weight training/resistance training for pelvic floor muscles depending on their recovery ability.

This principle can be used in all the pelvic floor exercise protocol.

Retest

Retest should be done after following the treatment session for atleast 1 month. If patient is doing intensive or resistance training daily, few days of rest time is suggested before retesting.

Common Instruction to use

- Use mild lubrication like KY gel or lubic gel. (use as minimal lubrication as necessary, as too much lubrication might lead to false reading).
- Do not use in case of pain, discomfort or tightness without doctor's advice.
- Do not use it with condom.
- After the usage, re-hygiene it for reuse and store in appropriate hygienic environment.
- Do not hold breath or bear down and do not use the accessory muscles while testing and training.

Indications

- Stress incontinence
- Urge incontinence
- Mixed incontinence

- Vaginal laxity
- Grade 1 pelvic organ prolapse
- Prepregnancy strengthening
- Postpregnancy strengthening
- Presurgical patients
- Postsurgical patients (with the advice of your doctors).

Contraindications

- Severe vaginitis
- Severe vestibulitis
- Vaginismus , infections
- Any type of pain, tightness or discomfort on insertion.
- Hypersensitivity to the material
- Before or after coital activity (intercourse)
- Pregnancy and postpartum (till the time of doctor's clearance)
- Lower urinary tract infection
- During menstrual cycle
- Grade 2 or more pelvic organ prolapse
- In case of intrauterine device
- Transrectal
- Any other medical contraindication.

Benefits

- Vagina-Fit helps to test the functionality of the pelvic floor muscles.
- Vagina-Fit helps the patient to understand the current status of the vaginal fitness or laxity.
- Vagina-Fit also helps the patient to achieve short-term achievable goal and train pelvic floor muscles.
- Vagina-Fit also helps to provide proprioceptive biofeedback to the user.
- Vagina-Fit along with the WOW Group Mobile App can be used for efficient home exercise program.
- Combination of Vagina-Fit along with WOW Group Mobile App will help to provide proprioceptive biofeedback along with visual and auditory cue.
- The combine use of Vagina-Fit and WOW Group Mobile App will also help the medical practitioners to track the progress and customise the treatment plan by assessing the reports genetrated by the mobile app.
- Vagina-Fit can also be used as a resistive training (weight training) device to strengthen the pelvic floor muscles during functional activities.
- Vagina-Fit and WOW Group Mobile App is scientifically designed for self-test and self-use which is ideal for home exercise program and maintenance therapy.

FREQUENTLY ASKED QUESTIONS

Q. When to do the pelvic floor muscle exercises?
- Generally early morning is a good time to do any muscle strengthening exercise. But you can find your own best time for it, only thing to

remember is before doing the exercise empty the bladder and bowel.
Q. If I do not get private time to use the device along with the app what should I do?
- Use of Vagina-Fit and App together will give the best result however if you cannot use it every day then you can use the device 2–3 times a week to identify and strengthen pelvic floor muscles. Other days suggest the patient to continue using the Mobile App for 30–50 repetitions per day.
Q. When will I be able to see a difference?
- A religious use of Vagina-Fit along with Mobile App can give a significant improvement within 3-4 weeks. But as every case is different the individual time can differ from person to person.

WOW VAGINA-DILATE TREATMENT

Treatment

The treatment room should be quiet, peaceful and comfortable with a soothing and relaxing environment which promotes relaxation of the patient. The WOW Vagina-Dilate should be properly washed with soap and water. It is advisable to use condom along with some water based lubricating gel for the dilator therapy treatment as it reduces the friction and can facilitate easy and pain free entry.

The patient will be in crook lying position with the legs apart and lowers off. The therapist will be standing next to the patient near her waist.

The treatment can be divided into three phases:
1. **Phase A—beginners phase** (start with the smallest diameter penetration up to the maximum depth of penetration): The dilator will be in patient's hand and patient will try to slide the dilator inside her vaginal opening, ask the patient to relax and insert the dilator, if active relaxation is not possible then you may also ask the patient to visualize her vagina as a flower or umbrella and it is getting bloomed. This kind of imagination technique can help the patients to relax.

    The most important thing is that the dilator should slide-in only when the patient is relaxing the pelvic floor muscles. You can ask the patient to slowly contract and relax the pelvic floor muscles and when the muscles relax slowly slide the dilator inside. The ridges of the dilator can be used as a short-term achievable goal for the patient.

    Once the narrow end of the dilator enters easily then ask the patient to contract and relax the pelvic floor muscles for proprioceptive input and ask the patient to relax the pelvic floor as much away from the dilator surface as possible.

    Give a gentle stretch to the vaginal orifice in all the directions to release the tightness of the muscles.

    Repeat the same protocol till the time patient is able to allow easy and pain free penetration of the narrow end upto its maximum depth.
2. **Phase B—intermediate phase:** Once the patient allowing easy and pain free penetration of the narrow end, then try with penetration with the broad end.

    In this phase the patient will try to allow the penetration of the broad end by contracting and relaxing the pelvic floor muscles. The relaxation should be complete such that the broad end enters easily. The broad end will also slide-in during relaxation only.

Once the patient allows the penetration of the broad end then ask the patient to contract and relax the pelvic floor muscles for proprioceptive input and ask the patient to relax the pelvic floor as much away from the dilator surface as possible.

Give a gentle stretch to the vaginal orifice in all the directions to release the tightness of the muscles.

3. **Phase C—functional phase:** After the patient clears phase B, then in phase C go for in and out movement at extremely slow speed and progressively building up speed for functional training. Also at this final stage of rehabilitation, you can even ask the patient to add some weights into the dilator and then go for in and out quick thrusting movement while patient is actively trying to maintain the relaxation of pelvic floor muscles. This functional training can help the patients to prevent spasm and maintain relaxation of pelvic floor muscles during unexpected thrusting movements of sexual intercourse.

APPLICATION DEVELOPED FOR THE HOME USE

WOW She Strength and WOW He Strength is downloadable mobile application of WOW Group exclusively designed to progressively train pelvic floor muscles in female and male respectively. It is designed to provide auditory cues, visual input, progressive charts and complete pelvic floor training guidelines which can be very beneficial for self-use by patients. Even the doctors, therapist and pelvic rehabilitation specialist can use these app for home rehabilitation protocol reports generated by this app can help the doctors and the users. The combination of this app and WOW Vaginal-Fit device can benefit the user/patient by providing visual and auditory cues along with proprioceptive biofeedback.

In clinical practice of pelvic floor rehabilitation specialist this app can help the clinical providers to prescribe, guide and assess the progression along with performance to customise the treatment more efficiently.

Go to app store to download WOW Group applications of She Strength/He Strength. For more information visit the website www.visionwowgroup.com.

Exclusive and Interactive App for Vaginal fitness for all women (including Pregnant Too)

WOW Vagina-Fit and WOW-Woman are revolutionary devices for PF (-Vaginal) muscles tightening. They both are extremely efficient. However, Vagina-Fit needs to be inserted tranvaginally. WOW-Woman is noninvasive and offers vaginal vibratory inputs.

WOW Group mobile app is perfect to use for every woman. Especially pregnant women, immediate postnatal women, post surgical women or any woman who cannot use any WOW Vagina-Fit or WOW-Woman. App does not require any tramsvaginal penetration, vibration or hardware.

Application is medically designed for self exercises for young girls, pregnant women, immediate postnatal mothers, postsurgical women and menopausal women as well.

Tutorial for Application

First of all you need to learn which muscles to exercise and which muscles not to use.

When the application indicates hold: Press the button and simultaneously 'squeeze' your PF (-vaginal) muscles as if you are trying to stop urine flow, (trying to stop passing of gas). Maintain the squeeze as long as possible.

Try not to use accessory muscles like butts, hips, lower abs, etc. Try to breath normally while using the app.

Visual Cues

Your left side of screen will guide your brain to squeeze the right muscles by giving visual inputs of pelvic floor contractions and relaxations.

Right side of the screen will give you an update of every single second you hold the pelvic floor contractions. It will help you to record your results and track your progress.

Auditory Cues

You will also have an option to turn on or off the auditory guide. When its on, it will also give auditory cues for holding or relaxing the muscles. It will activate your brain through your ears to send right neural signal to the right muscles. If you want to use WOW app in the public place you will have an option to turn off the voice so you can maintain the privacy.

Indirect Proprioceptive Alert

When you use the hold button on your WOW app, your mobile will vibrate for a second that will again send indirect neural signal along with visual and auditory cues to the brain. The proprioceptive (vibratory) alert and gain more concentration. Ultimately, it will make it very easy to activate pelvic floor muscles.

Results and Progress Report

When you go to the results section of WOW app, you will be able to see your results on daily, weekly, monthly and yearly bases.

You do not need to remember your performance or progress. WOW app is intelligent enough to take care of it. It will also tell you your average hold time.

If you are seeing your gynecologist or pelvic floor rehab specialist, you can also show them your weekly or monthly report from the WOW app or you can take a screen shot and send it to them. They will be able to customise your home exercise plan.

(If you are a doctor or pelvic floor specialist, make sure you use WOW app to design customised HEP for every single patient of yours and you will be amazed with the progress).

Motivational

Success is one of the best motivators. Mobile app will enable the user to measure the progress. It will record hold time, track and average the hold time. User will be able appreciate every little progress over the period of time. Combination of progress report and experience feedback will help to keep the user motivated. Motivated users will be more compliant. Higher compliance will lead to even better results.

Proper PF (-vaginal) muscle exercises will help you to strengthen PF (-vaginal) muscles which might play responsible role for better support during pregnancy, smoother childbirth, faster recovery after childbirth, better urine control, fecal control, back stabilization and sex health.

High Efficiency with Simplicity

- Turn on the app and log yourself in
- Start and complete the work out simply by pressing the hold button on app and squeezing your pelvic floor muscles
- Track your progress and enjoy awesome results.

MULTIPLE CHOICE QUESTIONS

Q1. How will a patient get proprioceptive awareness regarding pelvic floor muscles?
    (a) By doing internal identification   (b) By doing urine stop test
    (c) By external identification   (d) None of the above

Q2. Patient can do functional test of pelvic floor muscle by doing _____.
    (a) By doing urine stop test   (b) External identification
    (c) By doing internal identification   (d) All of the above

Q3. Which approaches are used to provide awareness to the patient regarding pelvic floor muscles?
    (a) Feldenkrais   (b) Kegels
    (c) Cantienica   (d) Feldenkrais and Cantienica

Q4. Who gave this quote "Awareness fits action to intention"?
    (a) Moshe Feldenkrais   (b) Arnold Feldenkrais
    (c) Moshe Cantienica   (d) Benita Cantienica

Q5. Who developed the training of sensual pelvic floor training?
    (a) Moshe Feldenkrais   (b) Arnold Feldenkrais
    (c) Moshe Cantienica   (d) Benita Cantienica

Q6. When the patient contracts pelvic floor muscles it is necessary to avoid Valsalva maneuver, what can be done to avoid it?
    (a) Contract accessory muscles
    (b) Do deep breathing exercise
    (c) Both can be done
    (d) Nothing can be done to prevent Valsalva maneuver

Section 4: Pelvic Floor Muscle: Fitness and Rehabilitation

Q7. While teaching pelvic floor muscle control focus should be on?
   (a) Only complete contraction
   (b) Only complete relaxation
   (c) Contraction at different intensities
   (d) Contraction as well as relaxation at different intensities

Q8. Teaching proper contraction and relaxation of pelvic floor muscles is an integral part of treatment of _____ :
   (a) Hypertonus dysfunction
   (b) Hypotonus dysfunction
   (c) Both (a) and (b)
   (d) None of the above

Q9. A 50-year-old female patient having significant strength of pelvic floor muscle is having frequent episodes of incontinence, which type of dysfunction it is?
   (a) Hypotonus dysfunction
   (b) Hypertonus dysfunction
   (c) Habitual dysfunction
   (d) Incoordination

Q10. If a 55-year-old male working as a laborer comes with complain of chronic low back pain (on examination you find hypomobile SI joints) and also has complaining of constipation and perineal pain, is it important to give treatment for SI hypomobility in this case?
   (a) Yes very important
   (b) No will not play a major role
   (c) Can be added later on in the treatment
   (d) It play a role but the pain will be relieved once the perineal pain subsides

Q11. Which technique can be taught to the patient in home advice in order to avoid urine leak during coughing, sneezing, etc.?
   (a) Relax pelvic floor muscle completely
   (b) Knack technique
   (c) Breath holding
   (d) Postural correction

Q12. Which type of modality is PF 360?
   (a) Pain relieving modality
   (b) Biofeedback modality
   (c) Diagnostic tool
   (d) All of the above

Q13. PF 360 can be given in all the condition except?
   (a) Enuresis
   (b) Erectile dysfunction caused by stress
   (c) Dyspareunia
   (d) Idiopathic thrombocytopenic purpura

Q14. What is the mode of application of PF 360?
   (a) Internal only
   (b) External only
   (c) Both internal and external
   (d) Only internally except for pediatric population

Q15. When you are teaching inhalation and exhalation along with contraction and relaxation of pelvic floor muscle, what line can you ask the patient to remember?
   (a) Inhale while you exert
   (b) Exhale while you exert
   (c) Inhalation or exhalation does not make any difference
   (d) Hold breath while contracting

ANSWERS

1: (a) By doing internal identification
2: (a) By doing urine stop test
3: (d) Feldenkrais and Cantienica
4: (a) Moshe Feldenkrais
5: (d) Benita Cantienica
6: (b) Do deep breathing exercise
7: (d) Contraction as well as relaxation at different intensities
8: (c) Both (a) and (b)
9: (d) Incoordination
10: (a) Yes very important
11: (b) Knack technique
12: (b) Biofeedback modality
13: (d) Idiopathic thrombocytopenic purpura
14: (b) External only
15: (b) Exhale while you exert

Chapter 17

Rehabilitation for Hypertonus Pelvic Floor Dysfunction (How to Treat Tight Pelvic Floor Muscle?)

"Your calm mind is the ultimate weapon against your challenges. So relax."
—Bryant McGill

"Sometimes the most productive thing you can do is relax."
—Mark Black

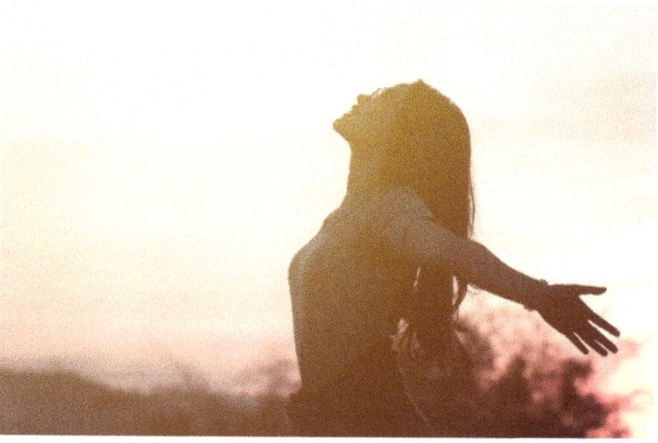

Rehabilitation of hypertonus muscles is definitely different than rehabilitation of hypotonus muscles. Main principles in treating hypertonus conditions are to promote relaxation, to break chronic tension, to loosened up and stretch tight group of muscles, release myofascial adhesion, treat trigger points and ultimately to teach better control of pelvic floor muscles.

SYMPTOMS ASSOCIATED WITH HYPERTONUS PELVIC FLOOR MUSCLE (TABLE 1)

The symptoms associated with hypertonus pelvic floor muscle have been described in Table 1.

TABLE 1: Symptoms associated with hypertonus pelvic floor muscle.

Bladder	Bowel	Pain	Sexual function
• Frequency • Urgency • Dysuria • Bladder pain • Urge incontinence	• Bloating • Constipation • Paradoxic puborectalis contractions	• Low back pain radiating to thighs or groin • Pelvic pain unrelated to intercourse • Lower abdominal wall pain	• Dyspareunia • Pelvic pain • Vaginismus

DIFFERENT REHABILITATION TECHNIQUES AND PROTOCOLS

Followings are different rehabilitation protocols to take care of tight pelvic floor muscle (PFM):

Treatment level	Proper education counseling	Exercise	Modalities	Mobilization	Home exercise program
Unintentional—unable					
Intentional—unable					
Intentional—partially able					
Intentional—superable/functionable					
Unintentional—reflexive					

Het's Protocol

Proper education and counseling needs to be given to the patients, what are the symptoms after thorough examination, depending upon their symptoms we can plan treatment.

Exercise

Therapeutic exercise and techniques for PFM will include:
- Pelvic floor exercises for relaxation
- Glazer protocol
- Paradoxical relaxation/Wise-Anderson technique.
- Coordination and functional training
- Proprioceptive neuromuscular facilitation (PNF)
- Stretching
- Postural reeducation
- Het's relaxation protocol.

Mobilization/Manual Therapy

A physical therapist can use external and internal approch for mobilization, manipulation, and stretching to improve blood circulation and mobility. These therapies include:
- Joint mobilization, e.g. sacroiliac joint (SIJ)
- Visceral manipulation
- Soft tissue mobilization: External, transvaginal, transrectal
- Pressure point release followed by warm bath
- Ischemic compression technique
- Deep tissue release.
- Thiele technique
- Trigger point release—Wise-Anderson "Sweet-Spot" principle
- Myofascial release
- Connective tissue manipulation
- Other specific technique (Wise-Anderson and Thiele technique).

Electrotherapy Modalities

These are:
- WOW Woman
- Biofeedback devices like:
  - EMG
  - PF360
- Electrical stimulation like transcutaneous electrical nerve stimulation (TENS) and interferential therapy (IFT)
- Heat therapy or hot bath
- Vulvar ultrasound
- Cryotherapy
- Internal electrical stimulation
- Vagina-Dilate.

Glazer Protocol

- Developed by Dr Howard Glazer
- Hold time—10 seconds
- Relaxation time—10 seconds
- Total repetitions—60
- Time needed—20 minutes
- Concept: As muscles strengthen, the chronic tension is broken and muscle relaxes. It might get worse during first month, but after 2-3 months pelvic floor pain will be subsided.

Paradoxical Relaxation

Paradoxical relaxation: By Wise-Anderson protocol—
- It means that accepting tension relaxes it at deepest possible level.
- When you accept something you let it be, and it creates deepest possible relaxation.
- It is a practice of conscious effortlessness.

- Patients are suggested to pay attention to sensation without putting an effort to relax it.
- Generally patients are surprised for as much number of times they find their pelvic floor uptight or stuck up. Accepting tension can produce the deepest possible relaxation.
- Practice of not thinking, attention only in sensation is paradoxical relaxation.

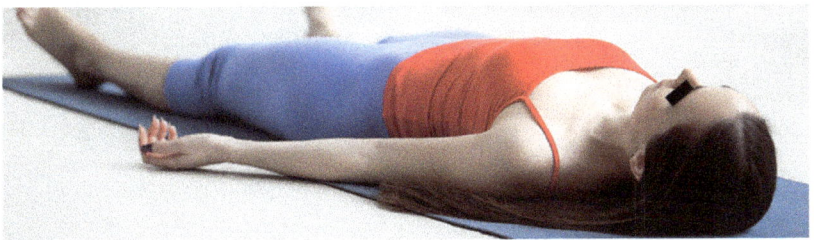

Wise-Anderson Technique

- Trigger point release–pressure application at the problem point.
- Wise-Anderson pressure principle explains the patient as "greeting the pain" which prevents self-treating patients to be overaggressive.
- The purpose of the technique is to treat protective guarding, chronic contraction or hypertonus muscle and convert them into relaxed, supple pain-free and lengthened muscle.

Sweet-spot

- Technique suggested by Wise-Anderson principle where therapist starts with neutral position means presence of finger intravaginally with no pressure application.
- It is followed by finding the taut–tender band and applying only extremely limited minimal static pressure enough to begin very first sensation of discomfort, then stopping when sensation is experienced without increasing any pressure, this spot is known as *sweet-spot* and the principle is known as *Wise-Anderson pressure principle (Fig. 1)*.
- Sometimes sweet-spot level of discomfort dissipates quickly within 15 seconds, but still pressure is not increased.
- Over a period of time, it generally requires more pressure to elicit the same pain or discomfort on tight contracted tissue as weeks or months go by.
- More pressure does not mean faster or shorter recovery time and generally it turns out to be counterproductive.

Ischemic Compression Technique

- It is also knows as pressure release technique where pressure is generated by finger of the provider and the blood is momentarily pushed out in that specific area. Feel the "taut band" inside the pelvic floor muscles, intravaginally, hold this pressure for 15–90 seconds.

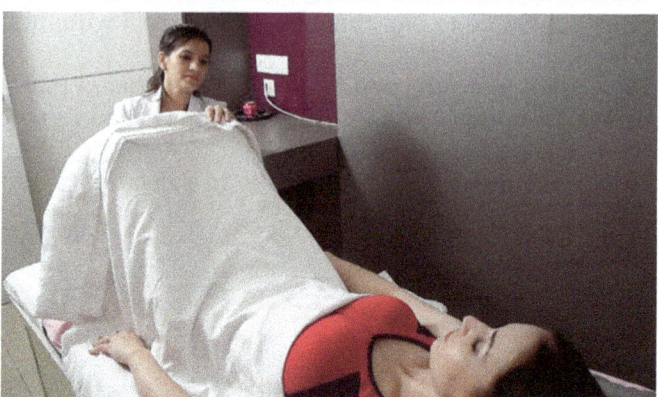

Fig. 1: Wise-Anderson "sweet-spot" principle.

- The pressure should be limited to only cause little discomfort. Some studies have suggested moderate to high pressure.
- However, we strongly believe too much pressure on the taut spot will hurt the patient and muscle will fail to release and lengthen, instead it will be counterproductive. The amount of pressure should not exceed 1/10 (0 is beginning of discomfort and 10 is intense pain).
- We believe Wise-Anderson techniques are more effective.
- External trigger points and tissues are less sensitive than internal. It is recommended to use less pressure internally.

Thiele's Technique

George Thiele, MD, published few articles about coccyx pain in 1930 and upto 1960's. His work on coccyx pain and treatment can benefit all pelvic rehabilitation providers from knowledge of his publications. Thiele's massage is a particular method of soft tissue release to the posterior pelvic floor muscles like coccygeus. Dr. Thiele, HYPERLINK "http://link.springer.com/article/10.1007/BF02633479"**in his article on the cause and treatment of coccygodynia in 1963**, mentioned that the levator ani and coccygeus muscles are tender and spastic, but the tip of the coccyx is not usually tender in patients who present with tailbone pain. The same article also mentions literature review describing interventions for coccyx pain.

Physical findings could be, slow and careful sitting with weight often shifted to one buttock, and frequent changes in the position. He also describes poor sitting posture, with pressure placed upon the middle buttocks, sacrum, and tailbone. Postural dysfunction as a proposed cause as he states "...the most important traumatic factor in coccygodynia..."

Thiele suggests putting a patient in Sims' position (left lateral side lying or recumbent position), therapist stand behind the patient and placing the gloved index finger into the rectum with the thumb over the coccyx externally. Palpate the coccyx between the thumb and index finger. The finger is moved laterally, in contact with the soft tissues of the coccygeus and levator ani. The finger

is moved with moderate pressure "...laterally, anteriorly, and then medially, describing an arc of 180° until the finger tip lies just posterior to the symphysis pubis." The massaging strokes should be carefully applied to a patient's tolerance approximately 10-15 repetitions on each side. Ask the patient to bear down during the massage strokes. Dr Thiele suggested daily thiele's techniques for 5-6 days, then every other day for 7-10 days, and gradually less often until symptoms are resolved.
- Applied intravaginally on tight bands of PFMs.
- It involves stroking and sweeping motion over the length of the muscle.
- Stroke, find trigger point and apply pressure and release where mild lengthening of the muscle is palpated.

Coccydynia: Please refer to the male section of pelvic floor rehab for hypertonus muscles.
- Transrectal assessment
- R Maigne's technique
- JY Maigen's technique
- Transrectal traction of coccyx.

Warm Compression

Warm compression or warm bath followed by trigger point release is very important.
    Movement to movement paradoxical relaxation is very effective in hypertonus muscles.

Soft Tissue Release

Mobilization of soft tissue, trigger point release, and myofascial release could be done transvaginally by trained specialist.

■ MODALITIES

Interferential Therapy or Transcutaneous Electrical Nerve Stimulation for Pain Relief

- Interferential therapy can be used as per pain and symptoms to improve blood flow and for pain relief.
- Different researches use different placement of different electrodes for PFM.
- Cross electrodes where one electrode is placed on lower abdominal wall on left side and other electrode is placed close to inguinal ligament on right side, just close to underwear.
- Other side could be placed similarly so that beat frequency can help PFM.
- We believe perfect placement of electrodes requires more research.

Vulvar Ultrasound

- Vaginal ultrasound is conducted over vulvar area.
- Instead of gel, provider might use the glove with water inside it for therapeutic ultrasound conduction.

Electromyography Biofeedback (Fig. 3)

- Normal pubococcygeus (PC) muscle resting tone 1-2 mV of electrical activity
- After few months, resting level can be achieved at 0.5-1.0 mV.

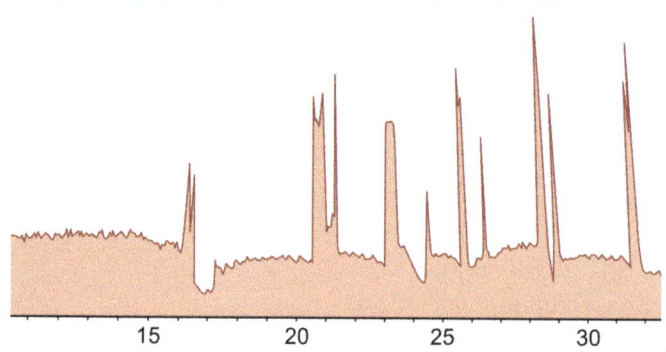

Fig. 3: Electromyography biofeedback screen.

Cryotherapy

Fill the condom with frozen peas and tie it. It generally fits between labia comfortably. You may use socks as well.

Internal Electrical Stimulation

- Intravaginal electrical stimulation has been a mode of choice of pelvic floor rehabilitation (PFR) for many providers with a theory of improving blood circulation.
- However, we have noticed that even a thought of using electric current or similar sensation inside the vagina can be a trigger to anticipation of pain for many patients with PFD.

Vaginal Dilators
(Misnomer: Vaginal Opening System) (Fig. 4)

- Many patients try to forcefully push it inside the vagina which can cause reflexive spasm of pelvic floor muscles and ultimately make it worst.
- We strongly believe the commonly known vaginal dilators should be used as vaginal relaxors which should help to promote relaxation to pelvic floor muscles. Proper patient education is extremely important to prevent forceful penetration reflexive spasm of pelvic floor.
- It uses proprioceptive way to tell the patient how much she can relax and she is in total control of it.
- However, many patients use them in a wrong manner.

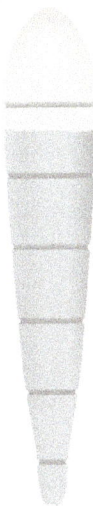

Fig. 4: WOW Vagina-Dilate.

EXERCISE TRAINING

Suggest patient to do 100% relaxation followed by only 10% squeeze to appreciate and facilitate better relaxation.

Complete Relaxation Training

Our experience says that hypertonus conditions can be greatly benefited by complete relaxation including stress releasing techniques and deep breathing exercises, relaxing music, and any other means of relaxation.

Elevator Opening Relaxation

- We have observed that visualization based training approach to the patient works really well.
- Have your patient visualize as if they are in an elevator, and elevator is going down while patient is trying to relax PFMs.
- Visualize an elevator going toward ground floor, visualize an elevator at ground floor and muscles are completely relax and finally to the basement while patient can create a little more than what she thinks is a completely relaxed state.
- At last, but not least completely opening the vagina walls, visualization of opening elevator doors.

Integrated Stretching Exercise

- Combination of conscious relaxation exercises, deep breathing exercises (DBEs), and integrated stretching exercises are very important.
- Integrated stretching exercises:

- Have patient do the stretching exercises of extrapelvic muscles like hamstrings.
- Follow the correct biomechanics
• However, the focus should be on complete opening or relaxation of PFM before, during and after the stretch, e.g. *iliopsoas and rectus femoris* (Fig. 5).

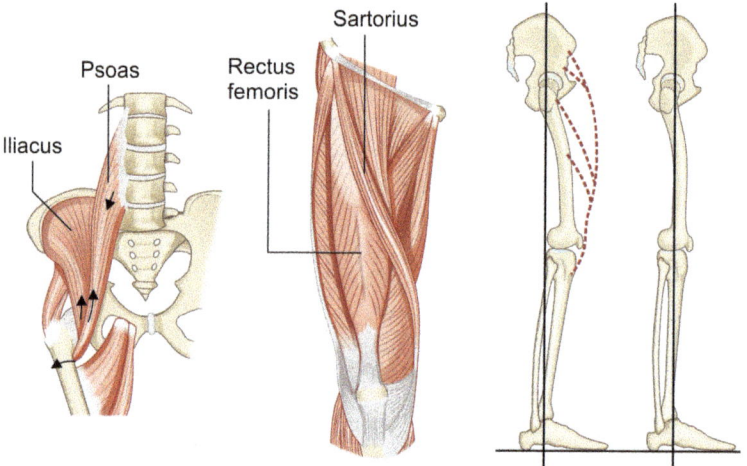

Fig. 5: Squeeze—relax—start stretch—continue to relax pelvic floor during stretch—complete stretch–squeeze partially to appreciate relaxation–repeat.

1. Integrated stretching exercise—hamstring
2. Integrated stretching exercise—tensor fasciae latae (TFL)

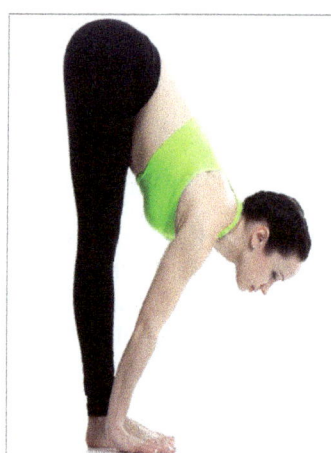

3. Integrated stretching exercise—piriformis
4. Integrated stretching of hip adductors
5. Happy baby pose

Rehabilitation for Hypertonus Pelvic Floor Dysfunction

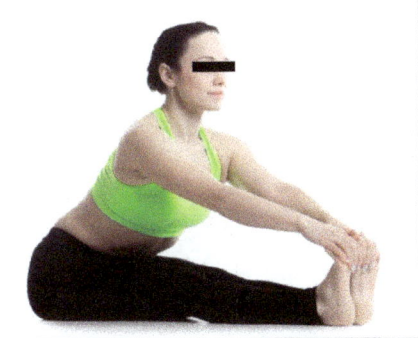

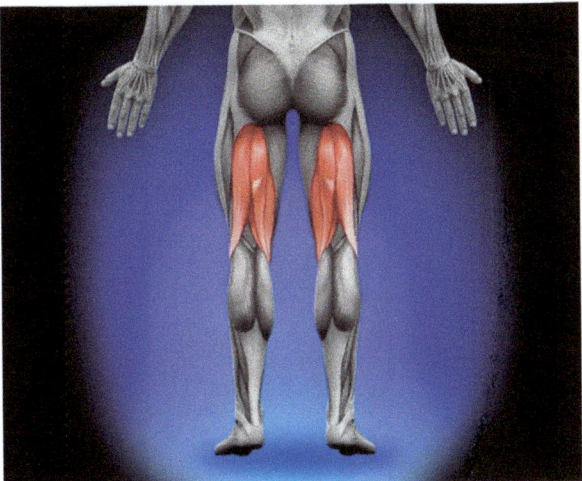

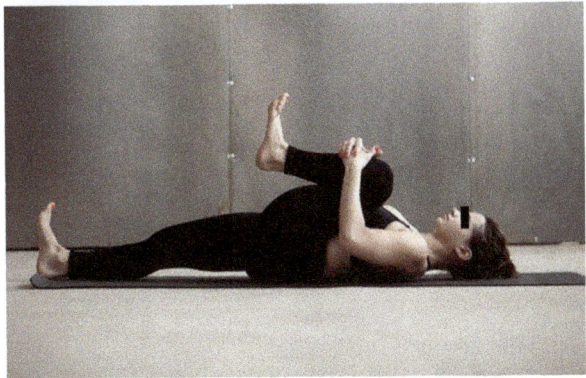

6. Deep squat stretch and deep lean backstretch
7. Half side lunge stretch
8. Deep side lunge stretch

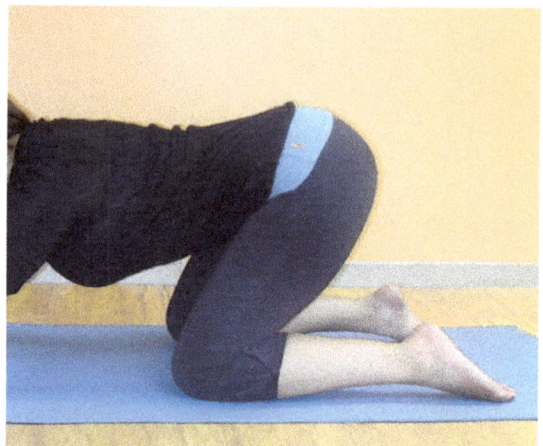
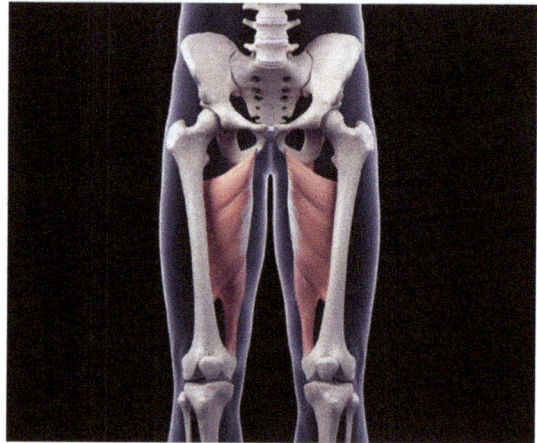
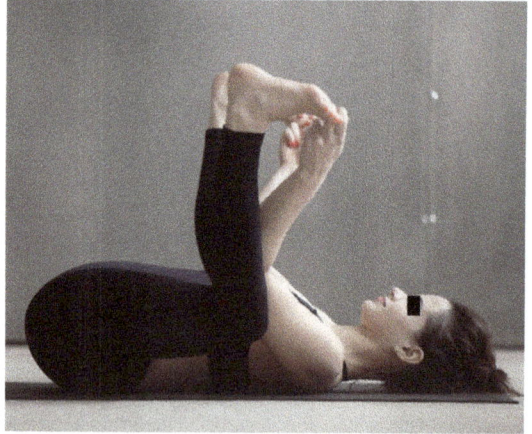

9. Integrated deep frog stretch
10. Integrated half pigeon stretch
11. Integrated reclined bound stretch

Rehabilitation for Hypertonus Pelvic Floor Dysfunction

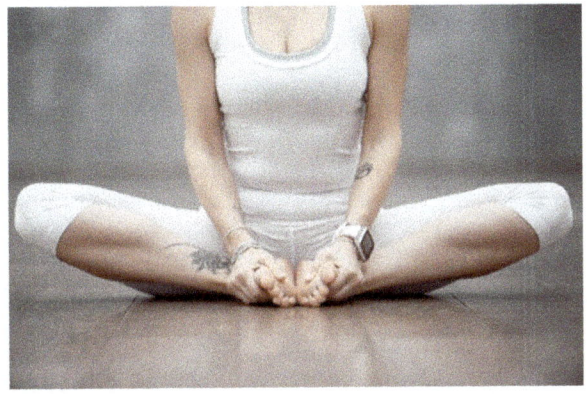

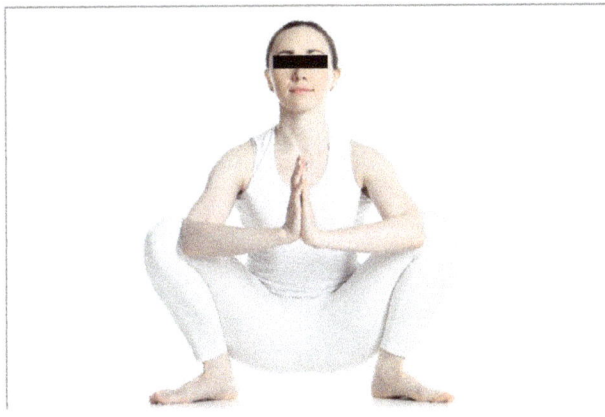

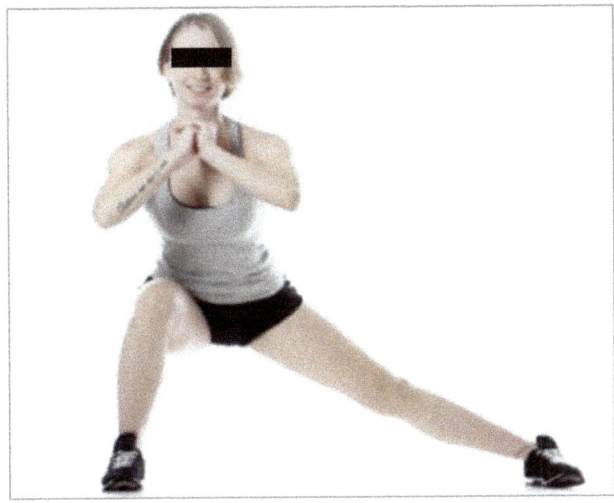

12. Deep side lunge stretch or integrated downward dog stretch
13. Integrated crescent stretch
14. Integrated warrier stretch

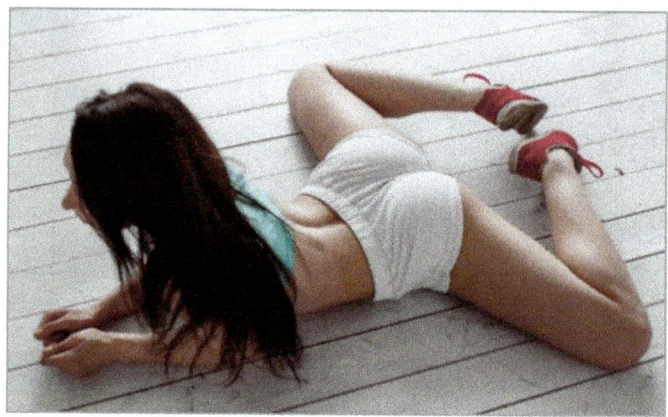

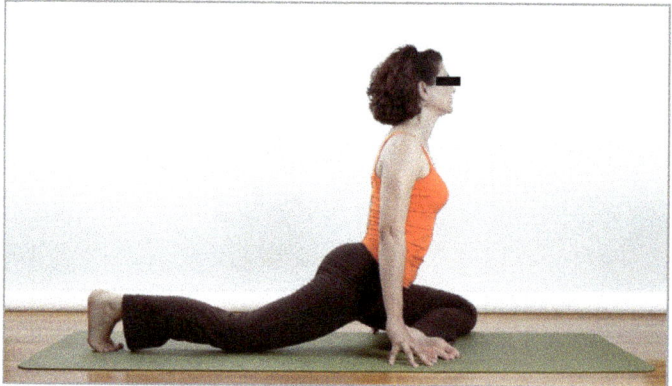

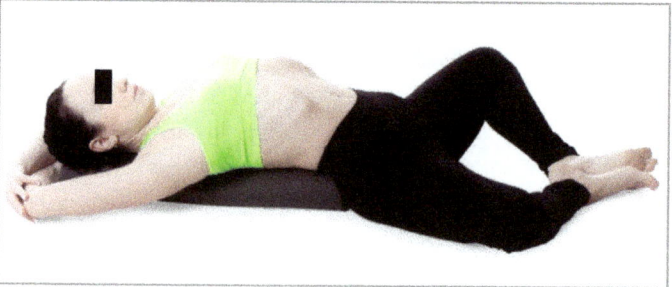

15. Integrated prayers stretch
16. Integrated warrier stretch
17. Integrated lumbopelvic stretch

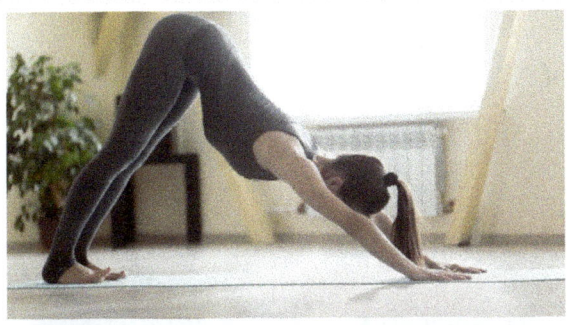

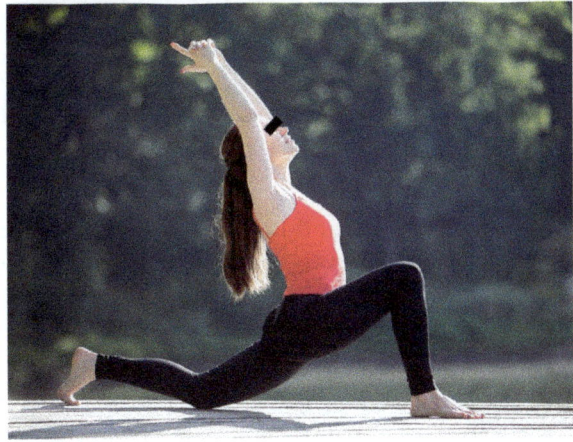

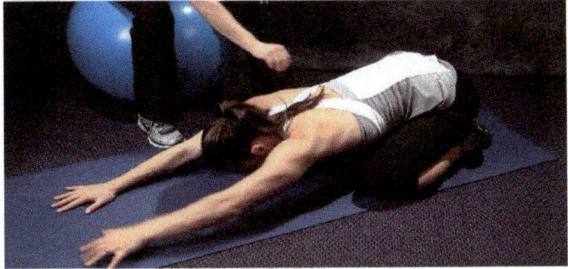

18. Integrated partial bridge stretch
19. Integrated full bridge stretch.

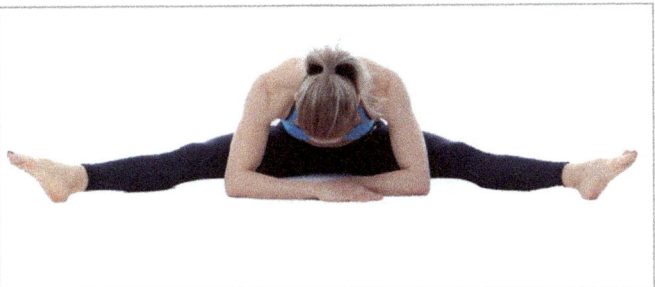

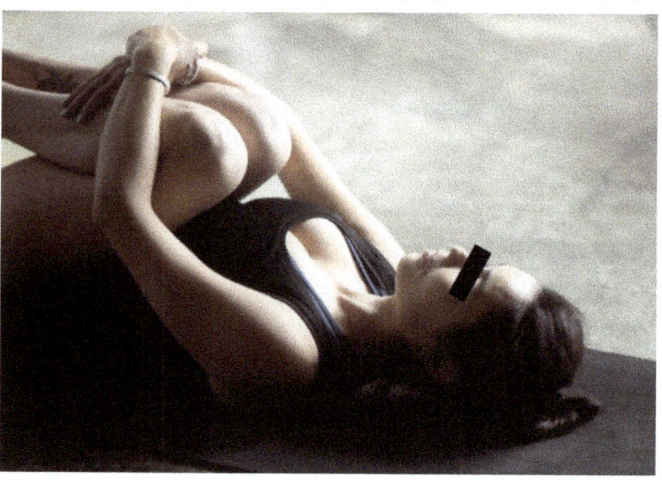

Het's RELAXATION PROTOCOL

Note: Apart from above-mentioned PFM integrated stretching exercise, provider can also use modified 4 levels of exercises that you use for hypotonus muscles (Box 1):
- Muscle identification and facilitation
- Movement training
- Plyometric or stretch and coordination training
- Functional training.

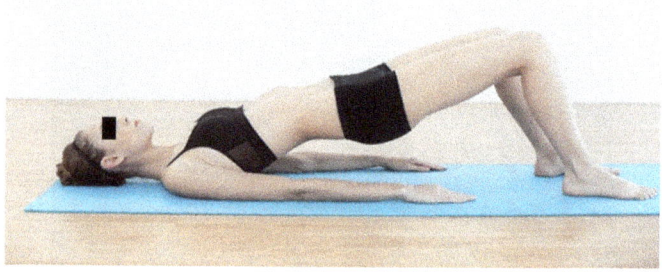

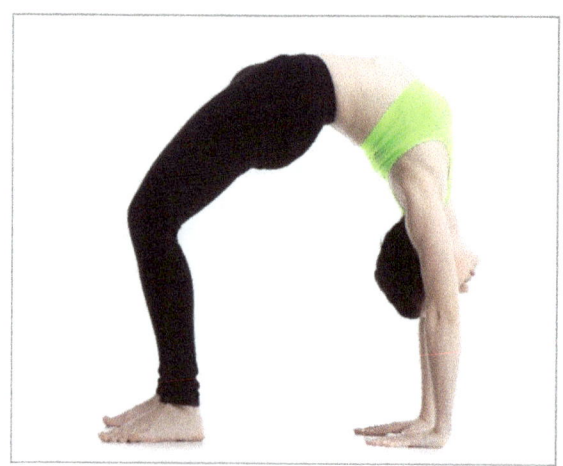

> **BOX 1:** Het's exercise protocol for hypertonus pelvic floor dysfunction.
>
> Follow each stages of Het's exercise protocol with sustained relaxation (SR):
> - SR—create sustained relaxation of pelvic floor muscle
> - Start—maintain SR and start repetition of movement or exercise
> - Continue—maintain sustained relaxation of PFM and continue exercise or integrated stretch
> - Complete—maintain sustained relaxation of PFM and complete each exercise or integrated stretch
> - Partial squeeze—create a partial squeeze of PFM at the end of each exercise to re-educate and differentiate complete relaxation, and repeat

KEYPOINTS—REHABILITATION FOR MALE PELVIC FLOOR HYPERTONUS DYSFUNCTION

Above mentioned rehabilitation techniques for rehabilitation of hypertonus muscles can be applied to male patients as well. However, approach might change to transrectal or external release.

Rehabilitation for Male Pelvic Floor Hypertonus Dysfunction

- Above mentioned PFM rehabilitation techniques including modalities, exercises, and mobilizations can be used in similar fashion for male hypertonus PFM
- When it comes to male PFM rehabilitation, transvaginal evaluation and treatments are replaced by either external treatments or transrectal treatments
- *Adapted from Stanford protocol*
- The provider can choose the trigger points on the muscle by digital palpation and also by the way it presents through referred pain
- Active trigger points refer pain on palpation
- Pressure release of holding pressure on trigger points for 60–90 seconds helps to lengthen or release it
- Skilled myofascial release is also very helpful.
- **Refer—trigger point release techniques from hypertonus pelvic floor muscle rehabilitation for women (Box 2)**
- Pubococcygeal muscles (PC)—referred pain to perineum and base of penis. Urethral pain, urgency and frequency
- Iliococcygeus muscle (IC)—referred to anterior levator, prostate, lateral wall, perineal and anal sphincter
- Levator ani (LA)—referred as *Golf Ball in the Rectum*, presents with urinary frequency and urgency
- Coccygeus: Pre- and postbowel movement pain associated with full bowel sensation and discomfort
- Anterior lower abs—pain and discomfort in bladder and lower abs
- Lateral abs—pain and discomfort in the testis, stomach, coccyx and groin
- Adductor magnus (AM)
- Gluteal—pain in tailbone, testicles, buttocks, hips, sacrum and hamstrings.

> **BOX 2:** Het's Rehabilitation protocol for hypertonus pelvic floor dysfunction.
>
> *Soft tissue release*
> - Paradoxical relaxation—Wise-Anderson technique
> - "Sweet-spot" principle of Wise-Anderson technique
> - Ischemic compression technique
> - Thiele technique
> - Warm compression
>
> *Modalities*
> - PF 360
> - IFT, TENS and other rehabilitation modalities
> - Vulvar ultrasound
> - EMG biofeedback
> - Cryotherapy
> - Transvaginal electrical stimulation
> - Vagina-Dilate
>
> *Exercise training*
> - Het's exercise protocol for hypertonus PFM
> - Glazer protocol
> - Complete relaxation training
> - Elevator opening exercise
> - Integrated stretching exercises

Het's PELVIC FLOOR MUSCLE GOALS SCALE FOR HYPERTONUS (TABLE 2)

- You might find hypertonus patients at the -1 or level -2 or somewhere in between.
- Goal for your patient is complete relaxation -3.
- Once complete relaxation, -3 is achieved; you can build up the strength to level 3, while maintaining patient's ability to relax completely.
- In other words, your patients should be able to relax completely at –3 level and contract completely at 3 level (Fig. 6).

TABLE 2: Exercise prescription according to Het's RR scale.

Assessment level/stages	Diagnosis	Exercise prescription
1	Unintentional—unable	• Het's Protocol-1 • Identification and facilitation training
2	Intentional—unable	• Het's Protocol-1 • Identification and facilitation training
3	Intentional—partially able	• Het's Protocol-2 • Movement training with pelvic floor muscle (PFM) sustained relaxation
4	Intentional—completely able	• Het's Protocol-3 • Plyometric and coordination training enhancing sustained relaxation of PFM
5	Intentional—functionable	• Het's Protocol-4 • Functional training with sustained relaxation of PFM
6	Final goal—reflexive relaxation	• Continue with exercises of Het's Protocol-4 until it becomes reflexive

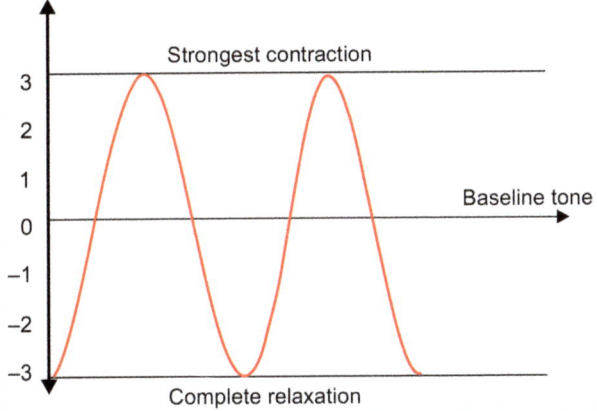

Fig. 6: Het's pelvic floor muscle goals scale for hypertonus from -1 progress towards -3.

HANDS ON TRAINING: PF 360 AND HYPERTONUS CONDITIONS

Female Patients

- Target activator of PF 360: Target activator will also help patients to learn basic relaxation.
  - You may begin with external application target activator at IC muscle and perineal body.
  - Secondary, you may target BC muscles as it is close to vaginal orifice.
  - This sequencing will help patient to prevent pain anticipation.
  - Observe externally if any group of muscles are overtight and unable to contract or relax on active efforts. Isolate them with activator.
  - Slowly progress to transvaginal or transrectal manual therapy. You may help patient to release specified areas like paraurethral, paraclitoral, perineal body, para-anus with target activator of PF 360.
  - Do not insert your finger directly inside the vagina.
  - Start slowly with the vaginal orifice and progressively insert your finger as patient become more comfortable.
  - Sometimes giving complete control in patients hand is also very effective.
  - Rhythmically move the finger in circular motion inside the vagina as patient feels more confident with relaxation techniques.
  - Progress it to clockwise and anti-clockwise approach form 12-3,3-6,6-9,9-12 O'clock positions to identify and release hypertonus pelvic floor muscles. Work on Het's ring clock for assessment and treatment purpose with combination of manual therapy and PF 360.
  - Use target activator of PF 360 simultaneously with transvaginal or transrectal manual therapy.
  - Vibratory tactile stimulus can help the patient relax better and allow for transvaginal manual therapy.

- You may use circuit training of 30 seconds of target activator application followed by 30 seconds of manual therapy. And repeat the sequence for complete course of treatment.
- 30 seconds of target activator will help patient with vibratory stimulus which will create mild twitch in muscle spindles. It will create partial contraction which will be followed by active efforts from the patient to relax. Partial contraction will help patient to appreciate better relaxation.
- 30 seconds of transvaginal or transrectal manual therapy will help patient to focus on relaxation of deep PFMs. While the first 30 seconds of target activator will focus on relaxation of superficial PFMs.
- Transvaginal or transrectal manual therapy techniques like myofascial release, trigger point release, etc. are very helpful for patients. But doing it immediately after 30 seconds of target activator application will significantly enhance the results.
- 30 seconds of time is just an example. You can customize your treatment plan in 1 minute or 2 minute of circuit as well depending on the clinical needs of the patient.
- You may also start treatment with PF 360 and target specific area for pelvic floor active release in the first half of the treatment which can be followed by transvaginal or transrectal manual therapy release.
- You can also train patients with Glazer protocol. Glazer protocol could be done noninvasively by using target activator. Glazer protocol is inbuilt program in PF360.

Male Patients

- Chronic pelvic pain can be treated with same above mentioned principles on perineal body or externally on anal sphincter.
- Transrectal manual therapy can be done in similar fashion in case of more intense spasm of PFMs.
- Coccydynia:
  - Pain at coccyx during or after sitting
  - Acute pain during transition from sit to stand
  - Pain with sitting on unstable or soft surface
  - Pain around coccyx
  - Shooting pain to legs
  - Feels like sitting on marble, knife or rod
  - Pain during intercourse or defecation
- Transrectal assessment:
  - Patient is positioned in prone.
  - Lubricated finger inserted into rectum to assess PFM tone.
  - Finger is gradually pushed upward-posteriorly which stretches the PFM.
  - Finger is pushed posteriorly until the contact is made with the coccyx.

- When therapist release the pressure of the pull, finger is expected to stay in the position with relaxed pelvic floor muscles.
  - However, If the finger is returned immediately to its initial position in the rectum by the hyper muscle tone without any conscious effort by the patient, it suggests hypertonus dysfunction of pelvic floor muscles
- Rehabilitation approach:
  - PR protocol: Protection and rest can be provided by use of donut pillow or sitting on the wheel to take the pressure off.
- R Maigne's technique:
  - Patient is positioned in prone.
  - The therapist stabilizes sacrum with one hand.
  - The finger of other hand is positioned in the rectal canal which presses coccyx into extension
  - Either the sacrum can be stabilized to the point and the coccyx is mobilized to extension

    OR

  - The coccyx is stabilized and sacrum is mobilized.
- JY Maigen's technique:
  - Patient in prone. Therapist's index finger inserted transrectally.
  - The inserted finger touches the coccyx but does not mobilize it. Just keeps gentle pressure stabilizing the coccyx
  - The external finger is on the coccyx making sure stabilization of coccyx
  - This technique helps to stretch coccygeus, the levator anus and external sphincter.
- Transrectal traction of coccyx:
  - Patient in side lying or prone
  - The therapist inserts index finger in the rectal canal and holds coccyx with finger transrectally and thumb externally. Gentle traction is given.
- Sample treatment plan:
  - Transrectal assessment
  - External SIJ joint mobilization
  - Thiele's massage and stretch to levator ani
  - Transrectal gentle traction and mobilization of coccyx with above mentioned techniques.

Reference: Comparison of three manual coccydynia treatment: Spine 2001 volume 26, JeanYves Maigen, MD and Gilles Chaterllier, MD

For example, transrectal manual therapy like Thiele's techniques for conditions like coccydynia.

Children: Only Noninvasive Methods

External target activator can be used on perineal body with similar exercises to relax PFM. Any form of invasive treatments are contraindicated for children.

Section 4: Pelvic Floor Muscle: Fitness and Rehabilitation

MULTIPLE CHOICE QUESTIONS

Q1. Bloating and paradoxical puborectalis contractions are the symptoms of which type of pelvic floor muscle dysfunction?
 (a) Hypotonus dysfunction
 (b) Hypertonus dysfunction
 (c) Incoordinated dysfunction
 (d) Visceral dysfunction

Q2. In which technique a therapist might expect an initial increase in the symptoms which will subside later?
 (a) Glazer prtocol
 (b) Thiele technique
 (c) Wise-Anderson technique
 (d) Paradoxical relaxation

Q3. How much pressure is applied to the taut band while using wise anderson pressure principle?
 (a) Minimal static pressure
 (b) Maximum pressure tolerable by patient
 (c) No pressure is applied
 (d) Intensity increases gradually

Q4. In ischemic compression technique the pressure is maintained for how many seconds?
 (a) 15–90 seconds
 (b) 2–10 seconds
 (c) 10–15 seconds
 (d) More than 90 seconds

Q5. Which technique is more effective Wise-Anderson or ischemic compression technique?
 (a) Both are equally effective
 (b) Wise-Anderson protocol
 (c) Ischemic compression technique
 (d) None is effective

Q6. Sweeping and stroking intravaginally is used in which of the following technique?
 (a) Wise-Anderson protocol
 (b) Thiele technique
 (c) Glazer protocol
 (d) None of the these

Q7. While giving treatment with vulvar ultrasound, which of the following is more preferable?
 (a) Ultrasonic gel
 (b) Glove with water inside
 (c) Coconut oil
 (d) Lignocaine gel

Q8. When treating a hypertonus pelvic floor muscle dysfunction the main focus should be on?
   (a) Complete contraction
   (b) Complete and sustained contraction
   (c) Sustained relaxation
   (d) It does not make any difference

Q9. A 35-year-old female falling in assessment level 4 (intentional completely able) should be given _____ treatment.
   (a) Identification and facilitation training
   (b) Movement training with PFM sustained relaxation
   (c) Functional training with sustained relaxation
   (d) Plyometric and coordination training enhancing sustained relaxation of PFM

Q10. When is warm bath or warm compression given?
   (a) Before the treatment
   (b) After the treatment
   (c) Between the treatment
   (d) Throughout the treatment

ANSWERS

1: (b) Hypertonus dysfunction
2: (a) Glazer protocol
3: (a) Minimal static pressure
4: (a) 15–90 seconds
5: (b) Wise-Anderson protocol
6: (b) Thiele technique
7: (b) Glove with water inside
8: (c) Sustained relaxation
9: (d) Plyometric and coordination training enhancing sustained relaxation of PFM
10: (b) After the treatment

Chapter 18

Rehabilitation for Hypotonus Pelvic Floor Dysfunction (How to Treat Weak Pelvic Floor Muscles?)

> *I have one weakness. I don't like vacations. I like to work.*
> —Shimon Peres

■ INTRODUCTION

"Weak pelvic floor says the same thing. Use them or loose them". We strongly recommend the use of pelvic floor 360 for training hypotonus muscles. Before understanding pelvic floor muscle (PFM) rehabilitation, it is important to understand following key principles of PFM training.

Main principles in treating hypotonus conditions are to promote strength, power, and endurance to have better control of PFMs.

■ Het's PELVIC FLOOR MUSCLE GOALS SCALE

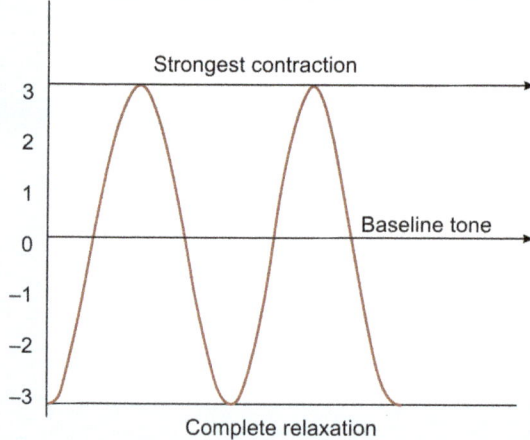

You might find your hypotonus patients at the 0 to 2 +
- Goal for your patient is strongest contraction, i.e. (+3)
- Once complete contraction (+ 3) is achieved; you can build up the relaxation also at (−3), while maintaining patients' ability to contract completely
- In other words, your patients should be able to relax completely at − 3 level and contract completely at level 3.

> **Het'S goal setting scale.**
>
> **S** Strength and relaxation: 3/-3
> **E** Endurance: 10 seconds hold/relax
> **R** Repetition: 10/10 counts
> **F** Fast twitch: 10–pulse as fast as possible

Strength

- Ability to completely contract and completely relax
- Graph from 3 to −3
- It could be applied for contraction and relaxation both
- Goal should be 3 to −3
- Suggests complete strength and relaxation of PFM.

Endurance

- Ability to hold PFM contraction for number of sec (at the same strength level)
- For example, if muscle strength is 2/3; patient can hold it for 7 seconds. But the strength becomes 1/3 after first 4 seconds
- Then the documented hold time should be 4 seconds only, 4/10
- Goal should be 10/10 at the strength level of 3/3.

Repetitions

- Number of reps at best possible hold.
- Example: If patient is able to do total 5 reps. However, she is able to do only 3 reps of 4 seconds hold, then reps range should be documented as 3/10
- Goal can be rep range 10/10 at the strength level of 3/3.

Fast Twitch or Pulses

- Number of times the patient is able to do quick 1-2 sec, hold contractions as fast as possible.
- Goal can be 10 reps pulses.
- Suggests fast twitch muscle fibers.

SAMPLE PROTOCOL

Proper education and counseling needs to be given, what are the symptoms after thorough examination, depending upon their symptom, we can plan treatment.

Strength, endurance, repetition and fast twitch (SERF)—goal

Strength = 3/3

Endurance = 3 sets of 10 reps × 10 sec hold

Power = Strength × time = 3 sets of 10 reps as fast as possible (Strength × speed)

Section 4: Pelvic Floor Muscle: Fitness and Rehabilitation

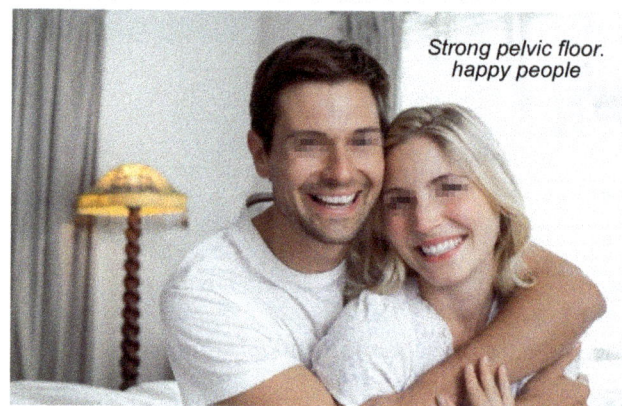

Strong pelvic floor, happy people

Het's—MANUAL MUSCLE TESTING (MMT) GRADING—PELVIC FLOOR MUSCLES

Het's—manual muscle testing grading—PFM has been described here.

Contraction	Grade 3	Strong upward and inward pull against resistance
	Grade 2	Grip with complete circumference
	Grade 1	Mild contraction (from any side)
0	Grade 0	Baseline tone
Relaxation	Grade -1	Inability to penetrate
	Grade -2	Symptomatic penetration (pain, tightness, discomfort or any other symptom)
	Grade -3	Asymptomatic penetration (easy penetration)

TABLE 1: Exercise prescription according to Het's RR scale.

Assessment level/stages	Diagnosis	Exercise prescription
1	Unintentional—unable	• Het's protocol-1 • Identification and facilitation training
2	Intentional—unable	• Het's protocol-1 • Identification and facilitation training
3	Intentional—partially able	• Het's protocol-2 • Movement training with pelvic floor muscle (PFM) sustained relaxation
4	Intentional—completely able	• Het's protocol-3 • Plyometric and coordination training enhancing sustained relaxation of PFM
5	Intentional—functionally able	• Het's protocol-4 • Functional training with sustained relaxation of PFM
6	Final goal—reflexive relaxation	• Contunue with exercises of Het's protocol-4 until it becomes reflexive

Het's EXERCISE PROTOCOL FOR PELVIC FLOOR DYSFUNCTION

Progressive four levels for hypotonus or in coordinated PFM in Table 1:
1. Identification and facilitation training
2. Movement training
3. Plyometric training
4. Functional training:
    i. Customized PFR protocol is highly essential for every patient depending of their current level of pelvic floor condition.
    ii. Following PFR protocol is designed for hypotonus conditions. It could be modified as per clinical needs of the patient.
    SC: Sustained contractions of PFM
    CR: Complete relaxation of PFM
    DBE: Deep breathing exercises
    For example, 2:2 = 2 seconds hold of SC: 2 seconds CR of PFM.
    Similarly you can progress hold time of PFM sustained contractions from 1:1, 2:2, 3:3, 5:5, 8:8, 10:10

For hypotonus muscles: Following sequence is followed, where the focus should be maintained—sustained contraction of PFMs. Clarity on sequence of training PFM.

Het's Exercise Protocol—for Hypotonus PFD.

Follow each stages of Het's exercise protocol – with SC—sustained contraction
1. **SC:** Create sustained contraction of PFM
2. **Start:** Maintain SC and start rep of movement or exercise
3. **Continue:** Maintain sustained contraction of PFM and continue exercise or movement
4. **Complete:** Maintain sustained contraction of PFM and complete each exercise or movement
5. **Partial squeeze:** Create complete relaxation of PFM at the end of each exercise to reeducate and differentiate strong contraction
6. **Repeat**

HET'S PROTOCOLS

Het's Protocol-1: Identification Training

- *Purpose:*
    - Patient awareness
    - Patient education
    - Identification of PFM
    - Facilitation of PFM
- *Indication:* Beginners
  Manual Therapy:
    - Through manual therapy. In other words, insert the finger transvaginal or transrectally and ask patient to squeeze while your finger provides proprioceptive activation of PFM. It can be done in clockwise and anticlockwise for proper muscle re-education.

- *Modality used:*
  - Noninvasively provide tactile biofeedback to PFM. It will activate tonic vibration reflex (TVR)
  - Slowly progress to active efforts to do PFM exercises with visual and auditory inputs
  - Progress them to 2:2 training protocol.
  - PF360—target activator is used noninvasively as an external applicator directly on superficial muscles:
    » Use the target activator externally on superficial muscles to activate TVR
  - Biofeedback -Electromyography (EMG)
  - Interferential therapy (IFT) and internal electrical stimulation.
- *Exercise:*
  - Start from basic 2:2 PFM.
  - PFM contraction for 2 seconds followed by 2 seconds relaxation (3:3, 5:5, 8:8, 10:10 progression hold time).
- *Exercises position:*
  - Supine position 2:2
  - Supine with pillows under hips—SC and DBE
  - Quadripod position without much movements—SC and DBE
  - Sitting position with the help of target activator of PF360. Use inbuilt program for 2:2; 2 seconds hold and 2 seconds relaxation while using auditory and visual input.
- *HEP:*
  - *Mirror biofeedback:* Teach patients to observe structures like closing of vagina—bulbocavernosus activity if visible, clitoral hood, perineal body lift, anal wink, etc. perineal body through handheld mirror for PFM contraction and relaxation.
  - *Finger palpation:* Teach your patient to try to identify PFM by putting their finger inside the vagina and try to hold the finger to palpate PFM.
  - *Stop urine flow:* Pelvic floor muscle exercise should not be performed during urination. But occasionally trying to stop urine flow can make it easy to identify correct group of PFM.
  - *Palpate accessory muscles:* Suggest patients to put other hand on abs, butt, or inner thighs to make sure they are not using wrong group of muscles.

Het's Protocol-2: Movement Training

- *Purpose:*
  - Against gravity to promote awareness, facilitation, challenged hold, and differentiation
  - Slowly progress toward 3:3, 5:5, 8:8, 10:10.
- *Indications:* Start customized training depending upon PFM strength or endurance/power
  - Add progressive functional training against gravity to promote weight bearing.

- KNACK with SC—progress your patient to brace PF with SC when getting an urge to cough, laugh, and jump. This will prepare patient for beginning of functional training.

  Manual Therapy:
  - Start with the manual therapy means transvaginal or transrectal manual therapy, ask the patient to squeeze the finger, you can even give area specific treatment so that the weaker area can be targeted more properly.
- *Modality:*
  - PF360:
    » Follow the progressive levels of Het's protocol-1
    » Start customizing in built programs of PF360 as per patients' unique needs
    » Follow all above protocols
    » Use inbuilt program from PF360
    » Opt for strength, endurance, hypertrophy or SH inbuilt programs as per your assessments.
  - *Biofeedback:* EMG can be discontinued if patient has mastered identification of PFM.
  - IFT.
- ***Exercise:*** Continue SC along with movements and DBE
  - Supine with SC:
    » Heel slides of alternate legs
    » Knee raise to chest
    » Straight legs raise
    » Bent leg abduction
    » Bridging with flat feet.
- Side lying with SC: Knee straight and hip abduction and adductions.
- Quadripod with SC:
  - Cat and camel exercise
  - Alternate knee and hip raise
  - Alternate arm and hip raise.
- Sitting with SC:
  - Bent knee raise
  - Trunk side flexion
  - Hip abduction and adduction
  - Bent knee march.
- Standing with SC:
  - Step side and back to neutral
  - Step forward and backward
  - Knee raise
  - Hip flexion, extension, abduction, circumduction
  - Front lunge
  - Side lunge
  - Step up and down.

  HEP: SC: CR -5:5, 10 × only 3 sets times a day

Het's Protocol-3: Plyometric and Coordination Training

- *Purpose:* Plyometric and coordination with increased challenge.
  Indication: Intermediate level
  Manual therapy:
    - You may progress to hold or manual resistance training transvaginally or transrectally as well. Do it either simultaneously with target activator of PF360, or you may do 30 seconds of target activator activation followed by 30 seconds of internal manual resistance training and repeat.
    - This kind of alternate training will help to activate and facilitate PFM and it will reduce the use of accessory muscles.
    - Transvaginal or transrectal manual resistance and PNF training will activate more of the deeper layers of PFM while the target activator of PF360 will activate superficial layers of PFM. Both together will create great PFR.
- *Modality used: PF360*
    - Follow similar programs in PF360 for proprioceptive training.
    - Use target activator for PNF training like hold-relax.
    - Above mentioned or similar program could be customized on PF360.
    - Depending on diagnosis of the patient you may also use any of the inbuilt programs of PF360 like strength, endurance, hypertrophy.
  IFT can also be used.

Exercise

Starting position: Swiss ball (SB)—create maximal, submaximal SC along with tabs activation and coordination with DBE.

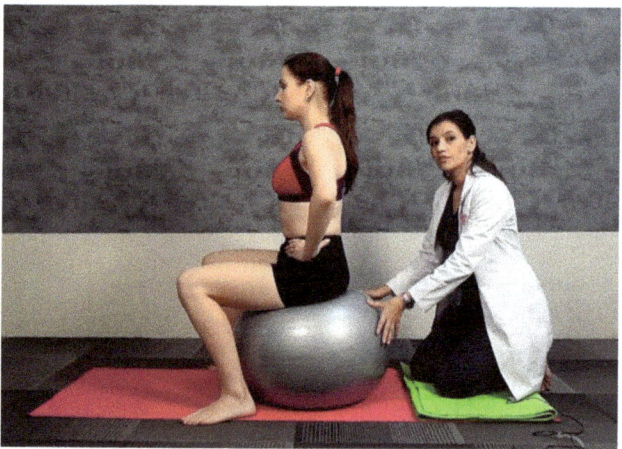

- SB under legs with SC:
    - Place the SB under legs—bend knees
    - Sit ups: Raise your head and shoulder.
- SB on abdominal and SC:
    - Hold the ball with both arms
    - Squeeze ball with both straight arms and legs while.

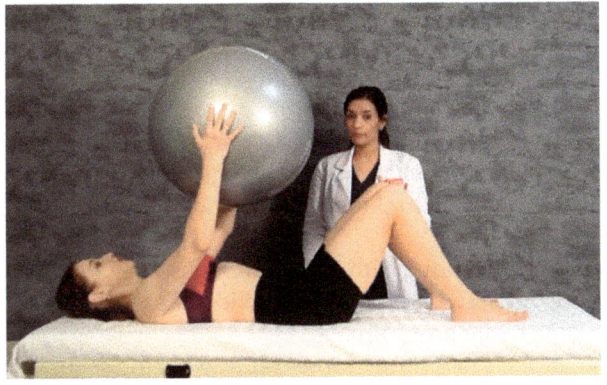

- *SB sitting:*
  - Have patient practice bouncing movements while sitting on the ball
  - Anterior and posterior pelvic tilts
  - Alternate arm and bent knee raise
  - Trunk forward or side flexion.
- *SB under legs (lying down):*
  - Straight knees—bridging
  - Bridging and SLR.
- *SB standing against the wall:*
  - Lean on the ball
  - Squeeze and squat
  - Hold the SB in the hand and do forward and side lunges.

Het's Protocol-4: Functional Training

- *Purpose:* Plyometric and coordination with increased functional activities
- *Indications:*
  - Teach patients to intentionally practice it with day to day functional activities.
  - Combine movement training and plyometric training along with functional training.

  Manual Therapy:
  - You can increase your finger resistance and even the hold time while doing the transvaginal and transrectal manual therapy.
- *Modalities:* PF360—
  - PF360 is designed in a way where you may choose inbuilt program.
  - Visualization exercise of PFM hold could be used with PF360 for functional training
  - You may follow PF360 in similar fashion to Het's protocol-3, e.g. if patient experiences leakage during coughing, suggest patient to imagine you are going to cough while target activator is used on perineal body to create proprioceptive stimulus.
- *Exercises:*
  - Sit to stand—stand to sit
  - Stand to 5-step walk relax for 5 steps

- Lifting weight.
- 5 jumps with SC
- KNACK—cough, sneeze, laugh, lift
- SC with all transfer activities
- Step up and down on the stairs or slope build up number of steps
- Lifting weight with her strength with squat or lunges
- Progressive addition to skipping rope and jumping forward, backward, and sideward
- KNACK training along with functional training
- Reaching out activities forward and sideward
- Reach outs while promoting SC
- Patient education for functional training during sexual activities.
- *HEP:*
  - For home training, you may start your patient with transvaginal weighted cones, if needed.
  - Ultimate goal of this stage of training is repeated intentional functional practice till the time final goal is accomplished and it becomes reflexive behavior. In other words, patient uses the PFM before functional activities (like cough, sneeze, laugh, etc. or sexual activities) without intention. It should happen as a reflex.

> Het's assessment level–final goal: Reflexive activation of PFM.
>
> - Patient automatically uses PFM contraction or relaxation during related functional activities
> - Patient does not try to do PFM activity intentionally
> - However, later on patient realizes that they did it. In other words, now it has become subconscious reflexive behavior to use PFM.

(PFM: pelvic floor muscle)

REHABILITATION FOR MALE HYPOTONUS PELVIC FLOOR DYSFUNCTION

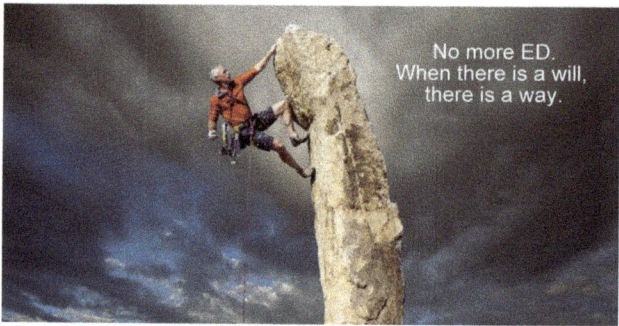

External Rehabilitation for PFM

You may use similar PFM training protocols suggested in the section of female hypotonus dysfunction.

Male PF Rehabilitation Focus

Strengthening hypertrophy of external urethral sphincter.

PFM Instructions

- Careful approach between men versus women
- Generally, men are likely to use maximum efforts; so submaxial training should be properly educated
- Goal is hypertrophy of PFM
- For any intrarectal work—wait for 6 weeks postoperative and physician consent.

PROSTATE HEALTH AND PELVIC FLOOR MUSCLE REHABILITATION

Pelvic floor muscle exercises will not prevent prostate enlargement, prostate cancer, or prostate infections, but rehabilitation devices like PF360 will increase pelvic blood flow.

Prostate health can be maintained by a healthy lifestyle and exercises that includes cardio, resistance, core, flexibility and pelvic floor training.

POSTPROSTATECTOMY REHABILITATION

- Radical prostatectomy can disturb quality of life.
- The rehab devices like PF360 enable men to prevent and recover from erectile dysfunction and urinary control issues resulting from prostate surgery.
- Just like total knee replacement (TKR) surgery, you strengthen quads and hamstring before surgery and do rehab post TKR. Similarly, it is best to start PFM rehabilitation before surgery to strengthen your pelvic floor.
- Penile erection is a neuromusculo-vascular event, happens due to nerve response, blood filling the penis and preventing the venous return is associated greatly with the fitness of PFM.
- Unfortunately, after prostate cancer treatment most men will develop dysfunctional erectile mechanisms like:
    - Poor nerve conduction to the penis
    - Poor blood flow to the penis
    - Development of venous leakage
- Oral medications and injections do not address all of these problems completely. Surgery and radiation can cause damage or disturb the nerves or muscles that help facilitate penile erections which are very close to the prostate.
- Nerve conduction is negatively affected altogether for a significant amount of time. Cavernous (penile) nerves are the road to take information from the spinal cord to the penis, which might get damaged during surgery.
- Pudendal nerves are sensory, motor, and autonomic. They are generally *not* damaged after surgery or radiation and remain intact throughout.

- Pudendal nerves become the only reliable communication pathway between the penis and spinal cord after surgery until cavernous (other penile) nerves recover.
- Pudendal nerves are responsible for penile functions like sensation, pleasure, voluntary urinary and fecal control, and rigidity of erection.
- The rehabilitation devices like PF360 activate pudendal nerve along with PFMs. Activator are designed for direct and indirect activation of PFM.
- There are millions of nerve receptors on the surface of the penis that can be activated by proper amount of activation through the activator of rehabilitation devices like PF360.
- The muscle activation and nerve stimulation can strongly activate spinal cord sensors that originate the injured cavernous nerves and get it reactivated.
- Daily disciplined repetitions of the activator induced PFM activation through rehabilitation devices like PF360 leading to regeneration of nerves and functional recovery of neuromuscular components.
- We strongly suggest to start the treatment of your patient with the rehabilitation devices like PF360 as soon as surgery is done or even 1 month before.
- When it comes to results' expectations, it is very important to realize that the benefits offered by rehabilitation devices like PF360 are cumulative and not immediate.
- It takes only few seconds to damage the nerves and muscles, but will take months for them to recover.
- While the rehabilitation devices like PF360 are safe, efficient, and cost effective. They can help erectile dysfunction in combined way of direct and indirect activation of PFM.
    - Similar placement of target activator of PF360 at junction of BC and IC muscles, at perineal body, STP muscle, and at anal sphincter.
- Section of rehabilitation for ED explains it in detail.
    - Daily use of the rehabilitation devices like PF360 leads to progressive improvement in fullness, rigidity, and spontaneous night time erections.
    - It can also help to correct poor/lack of orgasm after prostate cancer treatments.

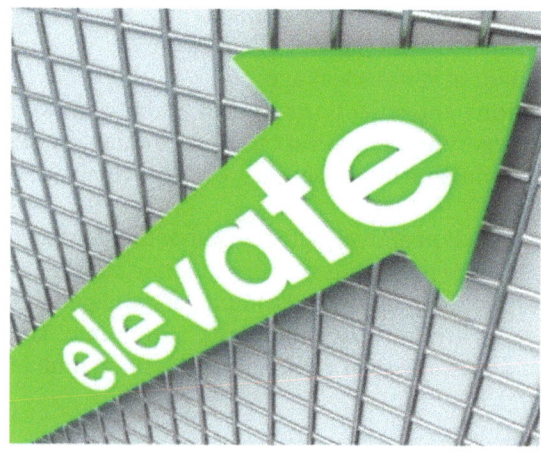

POSTPROSTATECTOMY PROTOCOL

Men can start this treatment at any stage depending on their situation. Postprostatectomy penile rehabilitation protocol is as follows:
- Begin using the rehabilitation devices like PF360 at least 1 month before surgery or radiation
- Psychological and emotional state like impatience, frustration, and anxiety will reduce effects PF360 and effectiveness on ED. So pay attention to emotional well-being of patients as well.
- The rehabilitation devices like PF360 success requires patience, disciplined frequent usage and treatment consistency.
- Suggest your patient to use the rehabilitation devices like PF360 as soon as surgery or treatment allows.

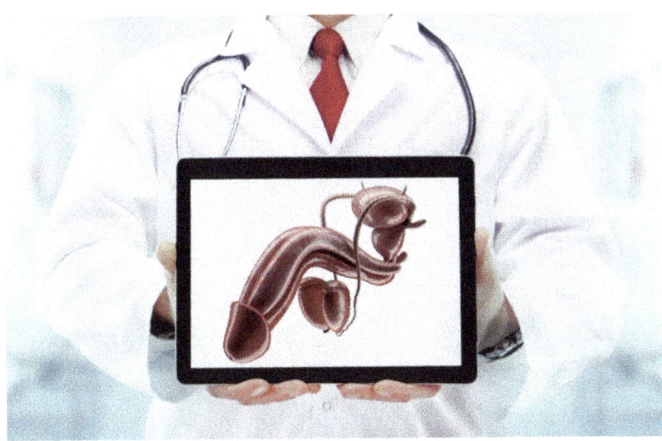

REHABILITATION FOR ERECTILE DYSFUNCTION AND PME: PFM TRAINING AND PREVENTION OF ERECTILE DYSFUNCTION

Age, sedentary lifestyle, and pathologies like diabetes, arteriosclerosis, or neuropathies that lead to decrease in muscle mass can ultimately lead to PFM weakness. Weak PFM muscle due to aging can reduce ability for penile erection and penile rigidity. There are not many clinical trials done in this area, but it clearly appears that preventive PFM strengthening can reduce the disuse atrophy. Ultimately it prevents age-related disuse atrophy of PFM.

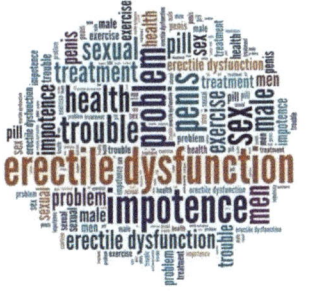
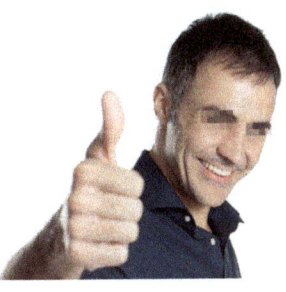

- PFM strengthening works especially for patients of:
  - ED with venous leakage issues
  - Disuse atrophy
  - Age-related ED
  - Psychological issues
- Benefits: Cost effective, no side effect, and painless.
- PFM training especially targeted toward IC and BC muscles helps to aid penile rigidity and cure or improve ED.
- Research suggests clinically and statistically raise in the intracavernous pressure during powerful contraction of IC and BC muscles.
- Contraction of IC muscle can improve pressure of the corpora cavernosum by 35.6–55.9%.

PATIENT EDUCATION ABOUT SELF-TRAINING

- Teach the patient about penile retraction and testicular lift to palpate the PFM
- BC muscle contraction can be taught by asking patient to perform a strong postvoid "squeeze-out" for final few drops.

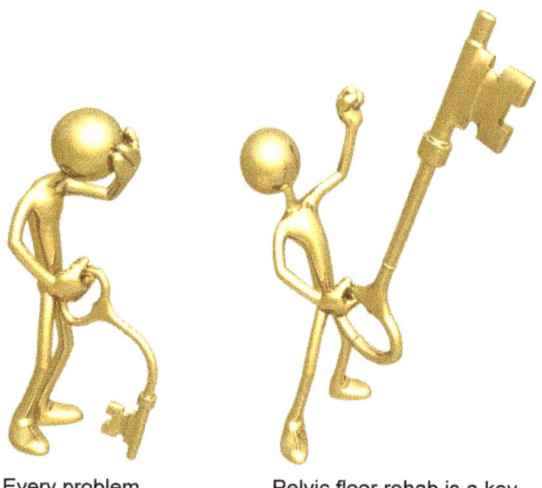

Every problem has a solution.

Pelvic floor rehab is a key to your success

Rehabilitation of ED can be done with combined application of two important factors:
1. PFM direct facilitation and indirect activation through bulbocavernosus (BC), pudendocavernosus (PC) and tonic vibrathine reflex (TVR)
2. Progressive resisted exercise (PRE).

PFM Facilitation

- The purpose of this phase is mainly to provide tactile biofeedback and PFM facilitation. You can use target activator of PF360 for direct method (directly on PB, BC and IC muscles) and indirect method (through tip of the penis by activating BC reflex associated with PFMT)

- Customize or use the inbuilt preset programs of PF360 and have patient perform workout while inhibiting use of accessory muscles through verbal, visual or tactile cues, and skilled intervention.

Progressive Resistance Exercises for IC and BC Muscles

- Resistance training is extremely important to add progressive resistance to the PFM and get to their best possible state of strength and performance.
- In women, resistance training can be managed by vaginal weights. As it could be inserted inside the vagina and PFM can try to hold them, as a woman gets stronger, amount of resistance could be increased.
- However, it is even more important in men. PFM weight training for men is little more challenging as it needs to be performed in the state of erection, which leads to amazing erections.
- BC and IC muscles are very important to improve erection angle which leads to improved solidity of erection.
- BC and IC muscles resistance training is also important to prevent premature ejaculations. Progressively increasing the hold time of resistance training of weight lifting will increase the hold time of erection and sustained contraction of BC and IC muscles will help to delay the ejaculations.
- Patients need to be taught to get themselves in the state of erection.
- Educate patients to put their finger on the tip or shaft on the penis and give gentle pressure downward. It will work as a manual resistance.
- Also, train patients to squeeze PFM to move penis upward against the resistance of his own finger.
- Educate your patients to modify resistance as necessary with the pressure of their fingers.
- Teach them to progressively increase pressure as they can easily perform targeted reps.
- Alternatively, you may also teach your patients to use some weight in a handkerchief or in a velvet bag and hang on erected penis, lift it, and relax it. Progressively, improve the weight. It will provide progressive resistance training to IC and BC muscles, which is responsible for increase of intracavernous pressure erection and solidity of erection.

INDIRECT NEUROMUSCULAR RE-EDUCATION

Indirect neuromuscular education can be done by using PF360.
- The target activator of PF360 can be used in different conditions, the placement of the PF360 target activator will depend upon the condition the patient is suffering.
- The target activator can used to activate the BC and IC muscles individually and together.
- The target activator can stimulate the full length of BC muscle if placed on the perineal are after retracting the penis and scrotum up.
- The placement of target activator on different muscles is described in the Chapter No. 16 under the heading of "mode of application".

- The treatment of BC muscle by using PF360 is described in the same chapter under the heading of "Het's BC Protocol for Male."
- Release of nitrous oxide may also help to create vasodilatation and help with penile erection by improved blood flow.
- It works through dorsal and ventral area of the pudenda nerve facilitation with the dorsal and ventral application of activator along with vibration and pressure given.
- Depending upon the severity of the symptoms of ED, in the beginning, patient may not see complete erection, he might experience only improved blood flow or fullness or heaviness in the penis due to medical release of nitrous oxide nitrous oxide along with effects of BC, TVR, and PC reflex.
- Patient education is extremely important. Realistic expectations of patients about results are even more important. Initial time might go with no results, some level of heaviness of the penis or little bit of fullness of the penis.

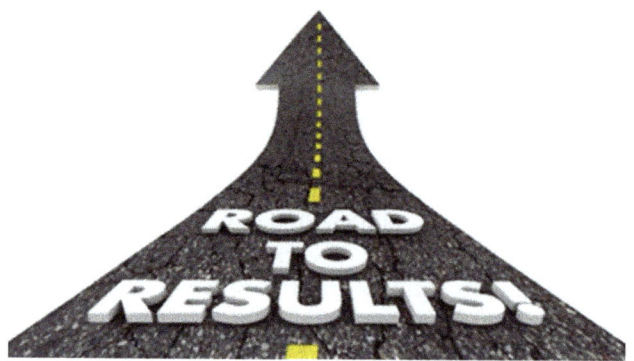

- The key to success is consistency and perseverance. Educate your patients properly about combined effect of PFM facilitation, resistance training of IC and BC muscles.
- It should be always comfortable. Suggest them to use it for 10–15 minutes daily or 3 days a week. Generally, it might take 3 months of consistent disciplined efforts with positive mindset depending upon the severity of ED. You can expect cumulative effectiveness with patient daily or at least 3/week training.
- If your patient starts expecting overnight results or rock hard erection after every training session, your patients are likely to set themselves up for the disappointment and frustration. It will create negative mindset and can possibly make their ED worst due to psychological issues.
- Constant patient education and motivation is very important along with proper progressive PFM facilitation, weight training and neuromuscular training for best possible results.
- Our researches suggest that most of the time successful results are the cumulative effect of multiple treatments.
- How to modify PFM training to delay ejaculation? Teach patient to engage PFM in sustained, long duration contraction.

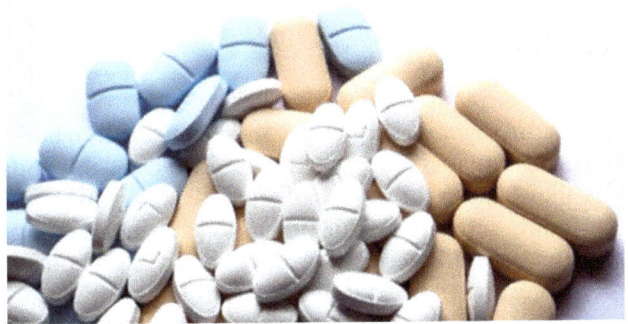

Combined with pelvic floor rehabilitation, great results.

ERECTILE DYSFUNCTION TREATMENT OPTIONS

Medications
- No clinical data to support them
- Sildenafil (Viagra)
- Tadalafil (Adcirca, Cialis)
- Vardenafil (Levitra, Staxyn)
- Avanafil (Stendra)
- Most of the medications are likely to enhance the effects of nitric oxide
- This increases blood flow and allows you to get an erection in response to sexual stimulation.

Limitations
- Possible side effects include flushing, nasal congestion, headache, visual changes, backache, and stomach upset
- Many men cannot take oral medications because of existing medical conditions or because of potentially harmful interactions with other medications
- PFM training and lifestyle management (like reduce or stop smoking and alcohol) has no side effects, improve fitness.

Other Mode of Treatment
- Vacuum device—still psychological issues happen with it due to discomfort at band, trapped ejaculation, soft base of penis
- Constriction band—have some problems with discomfort at band
- Intracavernous injections—side effect might include bruising, penile nodules, and fibrosis
- Topical therapy—side effect can lead to penile irritation and burning
- Intraurethral medicines—side effect may include penile pain, bruising, etc.
- Prosthetic implant—side effect may include risk of infection, device failure, unnatural intercourse

- Vascular surgery—risk of infection, postoperative hematoma
- Penile pump—can be used but it just temporarily helps. Also side effects are like severe penile bruising which can be scary.

Surgical Treatment

- Surgery—penile implant:
    - This treatment involves surgically placing devices into both sides of the penis. These implants consist of inflatable or bendable rods. Inflatable devices allow you to control when and how long you have an erection. The bendable rods keep your penis firm but bendable. As with any surgery, there's a risk of complications, such as infection.
    - Surgery is always the good option but should be last option due to side effects associated with surgery.

Remember: Do not take PFM rehabilitation as a treatment option. It is very important assistance to every possible treatment including surgery. Prerehabilitation and rehabilitation can offer excellent benefits to your patients.

Penile prosthesis

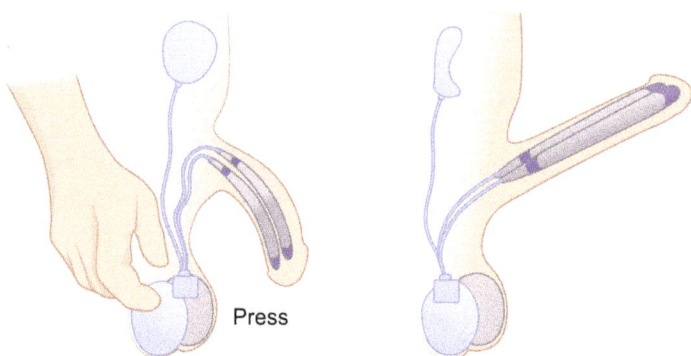

Press

PREMATURE EJACULATIONS

- Masters and Johnson have recommended a technique to prevent premature ejaculations (PE).
- Asking your patient to stay aware of the sensation of ejaculation.
- Withdraw the penis and squeeze the glans of the penis with your hand until the sensation subsides.
- It will activate BC reflex, where pressurizing the glans will lead to brisk contraction of BC and other PFM along with anal wink.
- The contraction of PFM will inhibit ejaculation.
- This technique is very effective but it can disturb the emotions of intercourse and many couple found it uncomfortable.
- It is smarter idea to slow down the pace of the intercourse, stop pelvic thrusting while the penis is still inside the vagina and perform sustained 10 seconds of solid contraction PFM or maintain the sustained PFM contraction until the ejaculatory urgency disappears. Teach your patients to mimic the same muscle control while using indirect technique of penile pressure.

- This is a technique which will allow same squeeze of PFM like suggested by Masters and Johnsons. In this technique, the squeeze happens internally so it does not cause disturbance to intercourse.
- This technique will work even better with the patients who are already using activator of PF360.
- Using the couple activator regularly and repeatedly will create neuromuscular re-education and reflexive control for the user and ultimately will be able to prevent PME without getting distracted from sexual sensations.

REHABILITATION PRINCIPLES FOR URINARY INCONTINENCE

- The rehabilitation devices like PF360 should be the first-line of treatment as its risk-free and cost-effective.
- You can apply above mentioned exact protocol (designed for women) for PFR for men. However, more work needs to be done for BC and IC muscles especially for ED.

KNACK TECHNIQUE FOR STRESS URINARY INCONTINENCE

- KNACK technique involves bracing PFM prior to the activity that can trigger stress incontinence. For example, if coughing leads to stress urinary incontinence (SUI), remember the trigger.
- Next time when your patient feels like coughing, suggest performing a sustained contraction of PFM.
- Maintain that contraction while you cough and relax PFM after that.

Overactive Bladder—PFM Tips

- As overactive bladder (OAB) happens due to involuntary contraction of the muscles of bladder which leads to urgency, frequency, and incontinence.
- First of all, teach your patients to identify the triggering factors like hand washing, key in the door, entering the shower, and rising from sitting.
- Have them perform few quick rhythm flicks or pulse of PFM contraction in high intensity prior to trigger which can prevent abnormal bladder contraction and even the urgency of urine can be avoided.
- Also squeezing the glans of the penis can activate BC reflex and cause PFM contraction which can cause relaxation of bladder muscles and prevent urgency. Also, sustained contraction of PFM can reduce the urgency.
- Quick snap contractions done in high intensity for several times will make the urgency sensation disappear.

For Postvoidal Dribbling

- Strong BC muscle can add force to expel the contents through urethra.
- The strong BC muscles can compress the deeper portion of the urethra and help to expel the urine out of the body.
- Suggest your patients to not to rush through urination process. Teach them to perform frequent contractions of PFM.

- It can be associated by milking technique, in which you teach your patient to put the thumb on top of the penis at the junction where the penis meets the scrotum.
- Have them put the middle and index fingers underneath the penis. Draw them forth toward the penile tip, which will create mechanical emptying of the urethra along with strong PFM squeeze. You can also teach the patients to shake the penis after urination along with PFM contractions, which will help to treat PVD.

HANDS ON: PF360 AND HYPOTONUS CONDITIONS

- Goal of the PFR is "strength training" of over lax or weak PFM.
- Noninvasive.
- The part of rehabilitation is completely noninvasive.
- Start with low intensity of vibrations. And level one.
- Suggest patients to do conscious relaxation while the vibration is on.
- To make it easier for patients.
- Teach them Het's scale of 0–3, where 3 means complete contraction and 0 means neutral baseline tone.
- –3 means complete relaxation (e.g. PFM relaxation during urination, passing gas or bowel movements).
- When you are treating hypotonous conditions, teach patients up training. In other words, going from 0–3.
- When you are treating hypertonus conditions, teach patients down training. Mean trying to go from baseline to relaxation training, means 0 to –3 but still avoid bear down.
- Forceful exhalation will help conscious efforts to relax PFM.
- Customize the time duration as per patients clinical needs.
- Noninvasive PF360 target activator.
- You may begin with application of PF360 target activator.
- Where you can target specific part of the PFMs which is hypoactive.
- Place it on perineal body to promote contraction.
- Observe externally which muscles are underactive and isolate them with activator.
- Slowly progress to transvaginal or transrectal rehabilitation by manual therapy or manual resistance.
- Rhythmically move the activator in circular motion on the PFM.
- Progress it to clockwise and anticlockwise approach.
- Customize use of inbuilt programs of PF360 depending on the individual need of the patient.
- You may opt from inbuilt programs like strength, endurance, hypertrophy training, etc.

Male Patients

- PFM weakness can be treated with same abovementioned principles on perineal body or externally on anal sphincter.
- Transrectal exercises can be done in similar fashion in case of weaker PFMs.

Along with use of generalized pelvic floor training, Use of target activator of PF360 to strengthen BC muscles in men can greatly help urinary incontinence because of functional anatomy of bulbocavernous muscles.

Het's BC PROTOCOL FOR MALE

Indication:
- Erectile dysfunction
- Premature ejaculation
- Urinary incontinence in male
- Postvoidal dribbling.

Purpose: Specific activation of BC muscle.

Procedure:
- Patient in supine
- Flip the penis back on abdominal wall so it will expose undersurface of penis where BC muscles are attached.
- Use target activator of PF360 to activate BC muscle at the base of the penis while patient is trying to squeeze PFM.
- Suggest patient to lift the scrotum that will allow the space to use target activator throughout the course and at the end of BC muscles towards the perineal body.

Children

Only noninvasive methods. Target activator of PF360 can be used on perineal body with similar exercises to activate PFM.

HOW TO CUSTOMIZE PELVIC FLOOR MUSCLE REHABILITATION

Endurance Training
- If patient presents with PFM strength 4/5; but endurance for hold is only 2 seconds out of 10.
- Focus on progressing the endurance time and slowly progress with number of reps.

Vaginal Laxity or Pelvic Organ Prolapse
- Patients with vaginal laxity or pelvic organ prolapse (POP) generally have low muscle tone which fails to support pelvic organs.
- So, PFR should be prioritized to build slow twitch muscle fibers.
- Work on building endurance, strength, and hypertrophy even with moderate intensity of PFM contraction. And then progressively build intensity.
- You may start with endurance training protocol in PF360.
- Start with noninvasive target activator of PF360. Start with submaximal contractions and work your way up to higher intensity.

For example, you may start with only 30% of maximum contraction and work your way up as hold time is increased.
- Fast twitch muscle fibers with high intensity could also be addressed down the road.
- Functional training: Teach your patients with laxity or POP to brace PFM during triggers like bending, straining, squatting, jumping, etc.
- Incase of more severe prolapse, you can train patients to manually reduce the POP by pushing the prolapsed body parts with her fingers and there after consciously engage the PFM
- Preoperative and postoperative prolapse rehabilitation can also work in similar fashion with target activator of PF360 as patient progresses.

For Stress Urinary Incontinence

- Strength and power training should be given the priority while managing SUI.
- Moderately intense contraction which can last for few seconds while artificially increasing intra-abdominal pressure will benefit SUI.
- For example, while using target activator, suggest patient to squeeze PFM as hard as possible, maintain the squeeze, and try to artificially cough without letting go of PFM. This will train for functional training and neuromuscular re-education (NMR) for SUI.
- Teach patients KNACK or BRACE techniques initially with PF360 activator and then without activator during functional activities.
- Train to repeat similar exercises during other triggers like jumping, etc.
- Training for power element will train the patient for speed and strength together, in other words, it will train patients on how rapidly the PFM can contract in the presence of stimulus.
- Slowly build up the progression toward endurance training too with slow twitch muscle training.

Pelvic Floor Muscle for OAB or Bladder or Fecal Incontinence

- Fast twitch muscle fibers training is extremely important and priority for OAB and fecal incontinence.
- Purpose of training is to improve inhibitory reflex between PFM and the bowel or bladder.
- When PFM becomes active, the bladder muscles-detrusor relaxes.
- So, very high intensity of PFM pulse training is the priority.
- Suggest patient to generate very quick high pulse contraction with transvaginal or transrectal.
- Progressively work on endurance training for slow twitch muscle fibers as well.
- For functional activities, suggest the patients to do strong high intensity pulse training during any kind of urge.
- They can practice few high intensity pulses before the exposure of triggers like hand washing, key in the door, running water, getting up from sitting, inside the shower, cold weather, rainy weather. It should diminish the urge.

MULTIPLE CHOICE QUESTIONS

Q1. When treating the hypotonus dysfunction the main focus should be on?
- (a) Complete relaxation
- (b) Sustained contraction
- (c) Sustained relaxation
- (d) It does not make any difference

Q2. What is the full form of SEP?
- (a) Strength, endurance and power
- (b) Speed, endurance and power
- (c) Speed, efficiency and productivity
- (d) Strength, endurance and productivity

Q3. Which are the progressive levels for treatment of hypotonus dysfunction?
- (a) Identification and facilitation training, movement training, plyometric training, functional training
- (b) Identification and facilitation training, plyometric training, movement training, functional training
- (c) Facilitation and identification training, movement training, plyometric training, functional training
- (d) Facilitation and identification training, movement training, functional training, plyometric training

Q4. What all things are covered in identification training?
- (a) Identification of pelvic floor muscle
- (b) Education of patient
- (c) Facilitation of pelvic floor muscle
- (d) All of the above

Q5. Whenever the PF360 is used in the identification training level, it activates _____ reflex.
- (a) Bulbocavernosus reflex
- (b) Tonic vibratory reflex
- (c) Cremasteric reflex
- (d) None of the above

Q6. When can you stop EMG biofeedback?
- (a) After 10 days
- (b) Once patient mastered identification of pelvic floor muscle
- (c) After 2 weeks
- (d) Once the patients hold the PFM just once

Q7. The plyometric training is given by using which exercise equipment?
- (a) Balance board
- (b) Swiss ball
- (c) Medicine ball
- (d) Proprioceptive board

Q8. What will be the benefit of giving plyometric training to pelvic floor muscles?
- (a) It will improve the coordination between pelvic floor muscles and other surrounding muscles
- (b) It will improve pelvic floor muscle strength
- (c) It will improve pelvic floor muscle endurance
- (d) It will improve pelvic floor muscle power

Q9. Which nerve is responsible for penile sensitivity?
- (a) Cavernosus nerve
- (b) Penile nerve
- (c) Pudendal nerve
- (d) Pelvic nerve

Section 4: Pelvic Floor Muscle: Fitness and Rehabilitation

Q10. Master and Johnson gave the technique of squeezing the glans of penis during sexual intercourse; this is useful in which dysfunction?
  (a) Premature ejaculation
  (b) Erectile dysfunction
  (c) Postvoidal dribbling
  (d) Penile pain

Q11. Which dysfunction can be treated by surgically placing a penile prosthesis?
  (a) Premature ejaculation
  (b) Erectile dysfunction
  (c) Postvoidal dribbling
  (d) Urge incontinence

Q12. If the female patient is having pelvic organ prolapse then the treatment aim should be on improving:
  (a) Strength of fast twitch muscle fiber
  (b) Strength of slow twitch muscle fiber
  (c) Improving coordination
  (d) Improving cocontraction

Q13. Which treatment option for erectile dysfunction has a side effect in the form of penile nodule and fibrosis?
  (a) Prosthetic implants
  (b) Oral medications
  (c) Vascular surgery
  (d) Intracavernous injections

Q14. A 60-year-old male having muscular weakness of pelvic floor muscle has complain of postvoidal dribbling for him the treatment aim should be?
  (a) Training of fast twitch muscle fiber
  (b) Training of slow twitch muscle fiber
  (c) Improving cocontraction of muscles
  (d) Improving coordination between internal sphincter muscle and external sphincter muscle

Q15. In which condition milking technique is used?
  (a) Erectile dysfunction
  (b) Postprostate surgery
  (c) Premature ejaculation
  (d) Postvoidal dribbling

ANSWERS

1: (b) Sustained contraction
2: (a) Strength, endurance and power
3: (a) Identification and facilitation training, movement training, plyometric training, functional training
4: (d) All of the above
5: (b) Tonic vibratory reflex
6: (b) Once patient mastered identification of pelvic floor muscle
7: (b) Swiss ball
8: (a) It will improve the coordination between pelvic floor muscles and other surrounding muscles
9: (c) Pudendal nerve
10: (a) Premature ejaculation
11: (b) Erectile dysfunction
12: (b) Strength of slow twitch muscle fiber
13: (d) Intracavernous injections
14: (a) Training of fast twitch muscle fiber
15: (d) Postvoidal dribbling

Chapter 19

Rehabilitation for Female Sexual Dysfunction (Woman's Sex Health and Rehabilitation)

"Sex is the driving force on the planet. We should embrace it, not see it as the enemy."
—Hugh Hefner

INTRODUCTION

- Healthy sexual function needs physical, mental and emotional well-being. Decreased mobility, alterations in sensation, decreased genital circulation and pain are some of the physical presentations that may limit sexual activity.

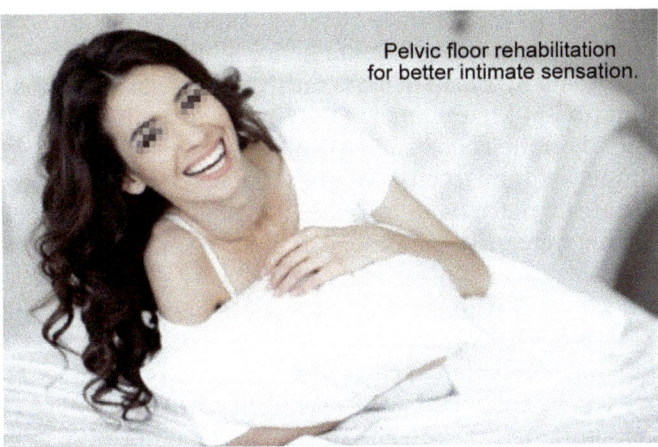

Pelvic floor rehabilitation for better intimate sensation.

- Pelvic floor rehabilitation plays an important role in facilitating optimal sexual functions by providing treatment to restore function, improve mobility, and relieve pain.

Pelvic floor rehabilitation (PFR) associated with some of the following interventions could get better results:
- *Estrogen therapy:* Localized estrogen therapy could be administered in the form of a vaginal ring, cream or tablet. Improved vaginal tone and elasticity, vaginal blood flow and lubrication results in improved sexual function.
- *Androgen therapy:* Androgens include testosterone which plays a role in healthy sexual function in women as well as men, although women have much lower amounts of testosterone. Androgen therapy for sexual dysfunction is still controversial.
- *Flibanserin (Addyi):* It was originally developed as an antidepressant. Flibanserin (Addyi) is approved by the US Food and Drug Administration as a treatment for low sexual desire in premenopausal women. A daily pill, Addyi may boost sex drive in women who experience low sexual desire. Side effects include low blood pressure, sleepiness, nausea, fatigue, dizziness and fainting, especially if the drug is mixed with alcohol. It is recommended to stop taking the drug if no improvements are noticed in your sex drive after 8 weeks.

LIFESTYLE MODIFICATIONS

- *Avoid alcohol:* Drinking too much hurts sexual responsiveness.
- *Stop smoking:* Cigarette smoking leads to restriction of blood flow throughout body. As a result, less blood reaches your sexual organs which leads to decreased sexual arousal and orgasmic response.
- *Physical activities:* Regular aerobic exercise improves body image and elevates mood. It has a positive effect on female sex health.
- *Stress control:* Being relaxed can enhance ability to focus on your sexual experiences and may lead to more satisfying arousal and orgasm.

Rehabilitation guideline for FSD—female sexual health dysfunctions directly depend on the cause and type of the sexual dysfunction. As sexual health is complicated and it can greatly be influenced by psychosomatic effect. It is the best idea if pelvic floor muscle (PFM) rehabilitation specialist work in a team with psychiatrist, psychologists, marriage or couple counselors or sexologists.
- Research says that stronger PFM have more nerve endings than weaker PFM. Clitoris has 6,000–8,000 nerve endings.
- The PFMs surround internal part of clitoris. The blood flow and sensations of clitoris can be enhanced by increasing the strength of PFM.
- It is very important to take detailed history and rule out any past experience of sexual abuse or any other cause which might be causing sexual dysfunction.
- Start with muscle awareness and identification as mentioned in earlier chapters. Work on facilitation of PFM while avoiding action from accessory muscles gives the best start. Slowly add progression with pelvic floor 360 (PF360) devices (Table 1).

Rehabilitation for Hypotonus Pelvic Floor Dysfunction

TABLE 1: Assessment or stages of female sexual health dysfunction rehabilitation*.

Assessment level/stages	Diagnosis	Female sexual health dysfunction rehabilitation
1	Unintentional — unable	• Detailed education to patient about the role of PFM in sexual well-being
2	Intentional— unable	• Start PFM rehabilitation program in nonsexual, clinical setting • If patient tried to do PFM during sexual activity at this stage, it will disappoint and discourage them
3	Intentional— partially able	• Clinically build strength, endurance, hypertrophy and power for hypotonus PFM • Flexibility and intentional quick relaxation ability for hypertonus PFM
4	Intentional— completely able	• Teach patient cocontractions of PFM along with other muscles that have significant role during sexual intercourse • For example, teach patient to activate and deactivate PFM while maintaining sustained contractions of bilateral gluteal which is used for pelvic thrusting • Similarly, teach patients to activate and deactivate PFM while maintaining sustained relaxation of gluteal muscles • PF360 the best way to create neuromuscular re-education • Also teach techniques like partial contractions or submaximal contractions
5	Intentional— functionally able	• Continue with level 4 training and let patient master it • Teach patient to functionally use PFM during foreplay, intercourse and orgasms • Teach patients to grip penis and create pulse training during intercourse and orgasms for patient with hypotonus type of PFD • Teach patients to relax and open up during penetration for hypertonus type of PFD • Simultaneously, customize PFM activation or deactivation protocol as per exact level of sexual dysfunction of each patient • Get patients to practice this over and over again till the time PFM functioning becomes automatic or reflexive for patients

*Final goal: Reflexive activation of PFM.

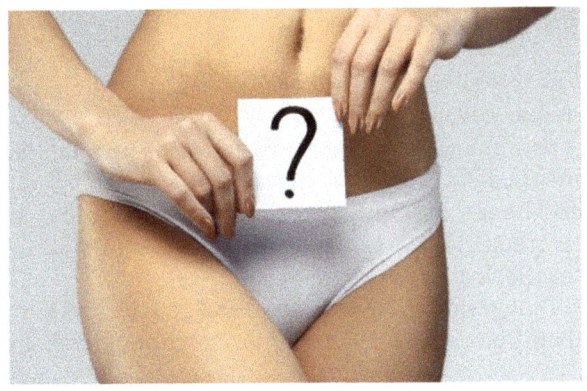

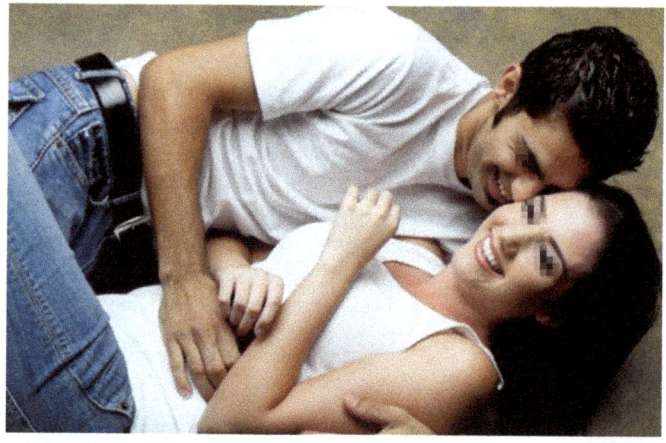

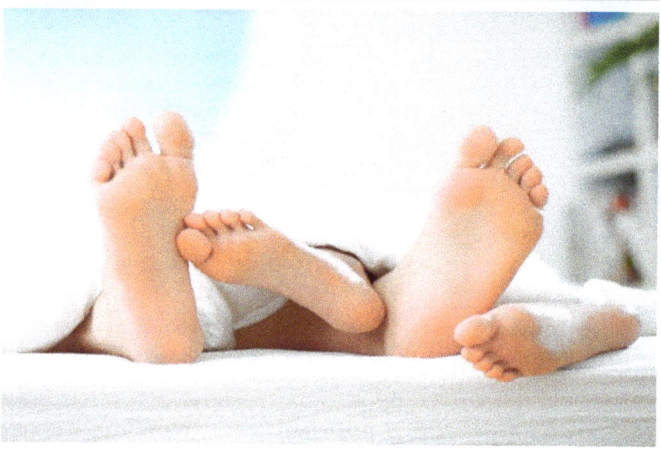

REHABILITATION FOR HYPERTONUS SEXUAL DYSFUNCTION

According to Bergeron and colleagues, the strategic goals for PFR are:
- Increase awareness and proprioception of the PFM
- Improve muscle discrimination and muscle relaxation
- Normalize muscle tone
- Increase elasticity at the vaginal opening and desensitize painful areas
- Decrease fear of vaginal penetration.

Rosenbaum has expanded the role of PFR:
- Providing behavioral therapy
- Identifying psychological components and to be further addressed with a qualified mental health professional.

Dr Howard Glazer, associate professor of psychology in obstetrics-gynecology at Cornell Medical College, strongly recommends nonpenetrative sexual practices that lead to orgasm.
- His protocol suggests couple to have sexual activity that serves emotional and sexual intimacy which leads to orgasm without having sex.

- Glazer protocol inspires everything that can increases blood flow to vulva and sexual desire at the same time keeping away from penetration to prevent further spasms.
- Clitoral stimulation, mutual masturbation, and use of PFM exercise devices like PF360 can help greatly.
- Glazer also suggests taking care of psychological issues, such as shame, sexual abuse, low self-image, low self-esteem which can lead to psychosomatic effects and pelvic floor spasms.

For rehabilitation purpose, we suggest to follow rehabilitation protocol mentioned in the chapter of "Rehabilitation for hypertonus Pelvic Floor Muscle."

Ancient-Tantric Practice for Hypertonus Pelvic Floor Muscle

Like in ancient science, tantric practice, patient is suggested to have very slow and careful penetration inside the vagina while the female have maximal control.
- After penetration, man is suggested not to move at all or move minimally just to keep the erection.
- Teach patients to be focus on patience and not to rush toward orgasm. This prevents deep thrusting effect of penis.
- As a result it can help PFM spam of female partner to relax from tighten state.
- It needs complete intellectual understanding, willingness and cooperation from both partners.
- It becomes greatly beneficial if women have maximum control over the speed, intensity and depth of penetration of penis.
- Positions like woman on top or from side or from behind has been proven greatly effective in giving control to woman and helps to minimize the irritation to vulva and PFMs.
  - In other words, also, choosing sexual positions in which female has more control will greatly help to intentionally relax the PFM. For example, female on top position.
  - In other sexual positions, developing a signal language between couple where female can guide either verbally or by putting hands on pelvis of male partner. It will prevent unexpected thrusts on spasmodic or closed muscles. It will also give female more time to relax muscles and receive penetration without much apprehension. It will also enhance trust with the male partner and will ultimately help to overcome anxiety related spasms.
  - However, very detailed couple education and understanding is required to gain proper cooperation and coordination for treatments to be effective.

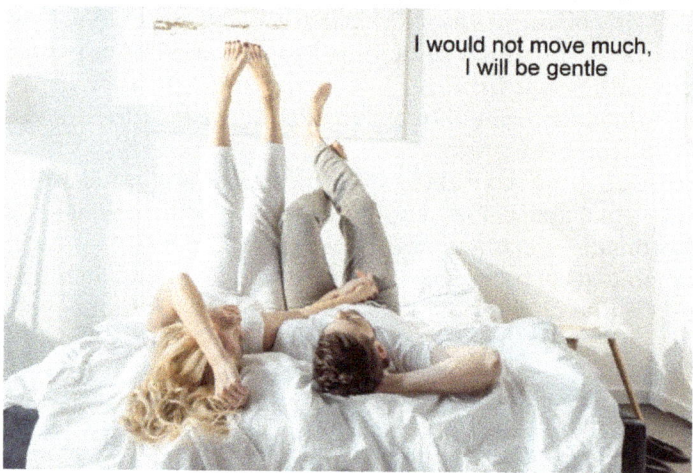

GLAZER'S PELVIC FLOOR REHABILITATION PROTOCOL

It is developed by Dr Howard Glazer.
- Hold time—10 seconds
- Relaxation time—10 seconds
- Total repetitions—60
- Time needed—20 minutes.

Concept: As muscle strengthens, the chronic tension is broken and muscle relaxes. It might get worse during first month, after that 2-3 months it takes for pelvic floor for the pain to go away completely.

Please refer to PF360. It has inbuilt Glazer protocol which can be used for hypertonus type of pelvic floor muscle dysfunction.

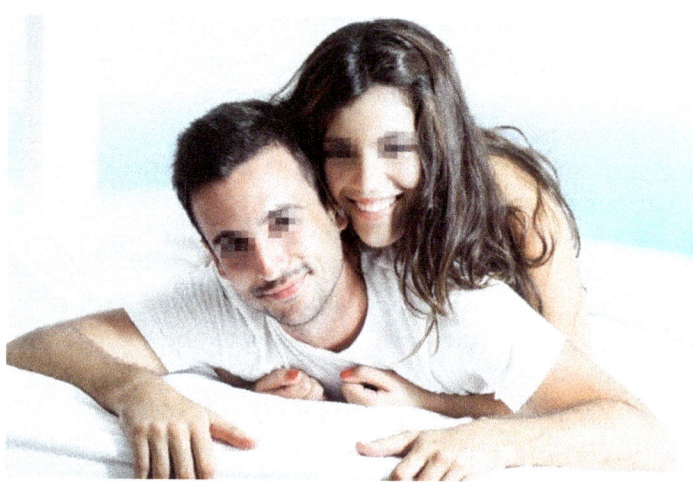

SUMMARY

- WOW Woman
- PF360 Glazer protocol
- Wise-Anderson sweet-spot release
- Trigger point release
- Intravaginal myofascial release
- Thiele's release
- R Maigne's technique
- JV Maigne's technique
- Transrectal traction of coccyx
- WOW Vagina-Dilate for dyspareunia
- Movement to movement paradoxical relaxation techniques
- Other relaxation techniques
- Lifestyle modifications
- Condom cryotherapy (CC)
- Biofeedback treatment
- Treatment ultrasound
- Interferential therapy (IFT) and modalities.
- Postural corrections—sitting and standing
- *Integrated* stretching exercises
- *Integrated* iliopsoas and rectus femoris stretch
- *Integrated* hamstring muscle stretch
- *Integrated* tensor fascia lata (TFL) stretch
- *Integrated* piriformis stretch
- *Integrated* adductor stretch
- *Integrated* yoga
- Progressive five levels for hypertonus PF muscles awareness and identification.

INFERTILITY AND PELVIC FLOOR REHABILITATION

- Wurn and colleagues have reported that in the course of treating female infertility with a manual physical therapy technique, patient is reported decreases in dyspareunia as well as improvement in all areas of sexual dysfunction including improved arousal and orgasms.
- There is not enough evidence about direct effect of PFM on fertility. However, indirectly PFM rehabilitation can help to treat the possible causative factors of infertility like endometriosis, polycystic ovary syndrome (PCOD), or pelvic pain. Also, we believe that improving plevic floor blood flow by innovative technology may greatly enhance the odds.

REHABILITATION GUIDELINES FOR HYPOTONUS SEXUAL HEALTH

- Dr Kegel observed that well-developed contractile strength of 20 mm or more of PFM, leads to nil or infrequent sexual dysfunctions.

- However, thick, inelastic, and weak contractile strength of 0–3 mm of PFM, sexual dissatisfaction was very common.
- Normally, most positions of sexual intercourse can result in direct clitoral stimulation or indirect clitoral stimulation.
- The clitoral shaft mobilizes internally in a rhythmic fashion. It happens due to traction of the penis on the inner vaginal lips which joins together to form the hood of the clitoris.
- In case of vaginal laxity and wide vaginal opening, it does not permit penis to put enough traction on the inner vaginal lips. It leads to limited clitoral stimulation and reduced sensation.
- You may implement or customize similar protocols or rehabilitation techniques depending of unique need of your patient (Please refer to chapters on Rehabilitation for Hypotonus Pelvic Floor Dysfunction).
- Your patient will report significant improvements by working with rehabilitation devices like PF360.
- As PFMs get stronger, patient will notice improved sexual sensation with more powerful intensity of orgasms.
- Stronger PFMs will create better satisfaction for the partner as well. More controlled use of the stronger PFMs will help to increase overall sexual well-being of the women.
- Reflexive training for hypotonus PFM foreplay:
  - Start PFM contractions with foreplay
  - Have your patients practice it over and over again till the time it becomes habit or subconscious
  - Exercising PFM with foreplay will increase blood flow to the genitals and promotes lubrication which enhances arousal
  - Have them experiment with quick contractions and long holding contractions.

Penetration

- Teach your patients to hold PFM during penetration and relax when he withdraws.
- However, if you are working with hypertonus condition. Make sure to teach complete relaxation while he penetrates which will reduce pain and discomfort and contract while he is in.
- Suggest the patient to squeeze PFM as hard as possible to try to grip the penis inside.
- You can provide functional training with combination of 30 seconds of functional manual therapy and 30 seconds of noninvasive target activator of PF360 activation.

Pulses

- Teach your patients to use fast twitch muscle fibers by performing quick PFM activity during sexual intercourse.

- It will also enhance sensation.
- You may provide functional training for pulse contractions with target activator of PF360.

Holding Technique
- Teach your patients to hold the penis inside with PFM and try to prevent withdrawal.
- It will work as resistance training with proprioception for PFM and simultaneously it will increase the sensation for both partners. (You can train patient for similar pelvic floor performance of PFM by using alternative method of finger hold for 30 seconds and noninvasive activation of PFMs with target activator for 30 seconds through PF360 and getting them hold it).

Orgasms
- You can teach and train patients power training along with strength, endurance, and hypertrophy training.
- Teach patients to do quickest possible contractions of PFM on noninvasive activator of PF360; studies show that PFM needs to contract at 0.8 seconds for powerful orgasms.
- Teach your patients to do the similar fastest possible PFM contractions during intercourse when she feels like climax.
- In the beginning, this kind of PFM training may distract patients during sexual intercourse.
- However, after a while it will become almost effortless, subconscious, automatic or reflexive muscle performance.

HANDS ON PF360 GUIDELINES FOR FEMALE SEXUAL DYSFUNCTION

For Female Sexual Dysfunctions: Due To Hypertonus Conditions
- For patients like vaginismus or dyspareunia, with very tight PFM use of activator will help PFMs to relax. Target activator of PF360 is ideal.
- Follow the guidelines of taking care of hypertonus conditions is mentioned earlier in the chapter.
- Apply the target activator to perineal body and let the vibration activate partial contractions and complete relaxation of PFMs. Simultaneously, suggest patient to try to do complete relaxation. Also apply the target activator on paraclitoral area, junction of ischiocavernosus and bulbocavernosus, vaginal orifice and bulbocavernosus muscle.
- Once patient is comfortable, progress toward simultaneous relaxation along with repeated in and out motion of the provider's finger transvaginally, which will re-educate active relaxation of PFM. It works best in the circuit alternate training for 30 seconds of manual therapy and 30 seconds of target activator. Target activator can be placed on perineal body, BC or IC muscles and paraclitoral area depending on clinical needs.

- Once patient feels comfortable with slow in and out movement of therapist finger, progress it to fast movement where patients will develop more control to relax and contract the muscles when the therapist finger enters and exist vaginal orifice. Again, for the best possible activation do alternate circuit training between manual therapy and PF360.
- You may also apply inbuilt Glazer's protocol of PF360 for hypetonus PFMs.
- Neuromuscular re-education can also work in sexual rehabilitation by teaching patients to practice relaxation exercises and progressively coordinate them with visualization techniques. Teach patient to open up while she visualizes penetration. Suggest them to self-insert her finger for functional training, while PF360 is on. Repeated practice will develop more automatic reflexive pattern of pelvic floor relaxation.

For Female Sexual Dysfunctions, PF360: Due To Hypotonus Conditions

- For patients with FSD due to vaginal laxity, follow guidelines of rehabilitation from hypotonus conditions.
- Follow strength, endurance, hypertrophy SH, target activation programs inbuilt in PF360 or customize it as per patient's needs
- *For orgasmic dysfunctions:*
    - Give priority to quick pulse training with highest possible intensity of target activator. You may target the BC and IC muscles with the activator of PF360 while patient is doing exercises. Target activator also allows to activate bilatral BC muscles and IC muscles through para-clitoral area simultaneously
    - PFM contracts at approximately 0.8 seconds during orgasm, more intensity we can train the muscles with combination of speed and strength (in other words, power) will generate better results with orgasmic dysfunctions
    - High intensity short pulse training is the key which mimics the functional training of orgasms
    - You may train this kind of contractions on continuous mode of PF360 as well.
- *For reduced arousal and sensations:*
    - PF360 target activator will activate BC and IC muscles and indirectly part of clitoris as well
    - Also, simultaneous manual resistance will cause hypertrophy of PFMs over the period of time
    - Use activator of PF360—vibratory biofeedback for few seconds which should be immediately followed by transvaginal manual resistance training program
    - When patient is working with the target activator of PF360. It will instantly reduce the use of accessory muscles and empower patient to use PFM. It improves immediate muscle memory of the patient. So, when it is followed by transvaginal manual resistance training program (where patient is actively trying to hold therapist's finger) instant gain of muscle memory will improve patients performance.

- Griping internally by PFMs will provide proprioceptive neuromuscular facilitation to activate right PFM.
- Simultaneous or alternate use of internal griping and PF360 will create the best outcome for patients.
- Repeated practice of PFM360 with target activator will enhance muscle memory and promote reflexive action of PFM during sexual intercourse. In other words, initially patient will consciously try to grip the penis inside but she will not be able to do so. As patient progresses, patient will be able to successfully grip it inside. And slowly it will happen automatically as a reflex. That is the ultimate goal.
- Functional training: Teach patients to focus on pulsed high intensity contractions of PFM rhythmically while thrusting. Or even couple can stop the movements and pelvic thrusting and both partners can do only high intensity pulses which will continue to provide penile stimulation even in the absence of thrusting. Even during orgasms, first teach patients to be aware of PFM contractions and progress them to create fast, high intensity PFM contractions while having orgasms.

MULTIPLE CHOICE QUESTIONS

Q1. How many nerve endings does clitoris have?
- (a) 6–8 thousands
- (b) 1–3 thousands
- (c) 5 thousands
- (d) 1 million

Q2. How can be the blood flow of clitoris improved?
- (a) Giving vasodilators
- (b) Strengthening pelvic floor muscles
- (c) Counseling
- (d) By doing only aerobic exercise

Q3. Who gave the concept of nonpenetrative sexual practices for hypertonus female sexual dysfunction?
- (a) Dr Howard Glazer
- (b) Dr Johnson
- (c) Dr Arnold Kegel
- (d) Dr Rosenbaum

Q4. Which factors causing infertility can be indirectly treated by pelvic floor rehabilitation?
- (a) Reduced sperm motility
- (b) PCOD, endometriosis, pelvic pain
- (c) Low level of female sexual hormones
- (d) None of the these

Q5. According to Dr Kegel how much mm strength of pelvic floor muscle will not lead to sexual dysfunction?
- (a) 15 mm
- (b) 20 mm
- (c) 25 mm
- (d) 10 mm

Q6. Sexual dissatisfaction can occur commonly if the pelvic floor muscles have weak contractile strength of how many mm?
- (a) 0–3 mm
- (b) 15 mm
- (c) 20 mm
- (d) 10 mm

Section 4: Pelvic Floor Muscle: Fitness and Rehabilitation

Q7. Which pelvic floor muscle activity along with foreplay can be helpful in hypotonus female sexual dysfunction?
   (a) Pelvic floor muscle relaxation
   (b) Pelvic floor muscle contraction
   (c) Pelvic floor muscle co-contraction
   (d) It would not create any effect

Q8. Contracting the pelvic floor muscle while penetration of penis and relaxing the muscles during withdrawal of penis can be useful in—
   (a) Hypotonus female sexual dysfunction
   (b) Hypertonus female sexual dysfunction
   (c) Incoordinated female sexual dysfunction
   (d) All of the these

Q9. Relaxing the pelvic floor muscle while penetration of penis and contracting the muscle while the penis is in. It can be useful in—
   (a) Hypotonus female sexual dysfunction
   (b) Hypertonus female sexual dysfunction
   (c) Incoordinated female sexual dysfunction
   (d) All of the these

Q10. What should be the contraction speed of pelvic floor muscles to have powerful orgasm?
   (a) 0.8 seconds
   (b) 10 seconds
   (c) 0.7 seconds
   (d) 0.5 seconds

Q11. Which type of training using PF360 can be used for treating orgasmic dysfunction?
   (a) Slow pulse training
   (b) Quick pulse training
   (c) Slow and sustained muscle contraction training
   (d) None of the these

Q12. In which type of female sexual dysfunction, pulsed high intensity contractions of PFM rhythmically while thrusting can be a plan of functional training?
   (a) Hypertonus female sexual dysfunction
   (b) Hypotonus female sexual dysfunction
   (c) Incoordinated female sexual dysfunction
   (d) Visceral female sexual dysfunction

ANSWERS

1: (a) 6-8 thousands
2: (b) Strengthening pelvic floor muscles
3: (a) Dr Howard Glazer
4: (b) PCOD, endometriosis, pelvic pain
5: (b) 20 mm
6: (a) 0-3 mm
7: (b) Pelvic floor muscle contraction
8: (a) Hypotonus female sexual dysfunction
9: (b) Hypertonus female sexual dysfunction
10: (a) 0.8 seconds
11: (b) Quick pulse training
12: (b) Hypotonus female sexual dysfunction

Section 5

Medical and Surgical Management

Chapter 20

Introduction of Medical and Surgical Management of Pelvic Floor Muscle Dysfunction

Akshay C Shah MD
Associate Professor
Department of Gynecology
NHL Municipal Medical College
Ahmedabad, Gujarat, India

INTRODUCTION

There are comprehensive aspects in evaluation and therapy of pelvic floor dysfunction. The goal for treating pelvic floor dysfunction is to make movements of pelvic floor muscles easier and to provide more control.

A common treatment for this condition is biofeedback. However, most of the electromyography (EMG) biofeedback has significant limitations such as misreading from accessory muscles like gluteus, hip adductors, abdominals, etc. Devices like PF 360, proprioceptive biofeedback with auditory and visual signals are greatly efficient. Other treatment options include:
- *Self-care:* To reduce strain on the specific muscle. Also relaxation techniques such as *yoga* may be helpful. Warm water bath also improves blood circulation and relaxes the muscles.
- *Medication:* Specific drug may be used for different types of pelvic floor muscle dysfunction.
- *Surgery:* Certain conditions may even require a surgery depending on the severity of the disorder. The outcomes of the surgery are benefited by preoperative and postoperative physiotherapy.

TREATMENT OF HYPERTONUS PELVIC FLOOR DYSFUNCTION IN FEMALES

Pudendal Neuralgia

Medications, such as pain killers may be useful in mild cases of neuralgia. The nerves can be blocked to relieve pain for few months by painkiller injections. These include injections like local anesthetic and steroid medication.

A newer technique of *nerve stimulation* is used nowadays in which a special device is surgically implanted under the skin to deliver mild electrical impulses to the nerve and interrupt the pain signals sent to brain.

In severe cases if something is pressing on the nerve, a decompression surgery is done to get relieve from the pain.

Tension Myalgia

Analgesics and muscle relaxants have been used frequently to treat this condition. Diazepam can help in temporary improvement.

High voltage galvanic stimulation (HVGS) is also used in which an intra-anal probe is inserted and applied to muscles in spasm.

Local injections of steroids and anesthetics are used with minimal long-lasting effects.

Botulinum toxin may also benefit these patients as it inhibits presynaptic release of acetylcholine at neuromuscular junction, resulting in decreased muscle spasm.

Coccydynia

As with others, painkillers like nonsteroidal anti-inflammatory drugs (NSAIDs) can help ease pain and reduce swelling around coccyx. In severe pain, tramadol can be used.

Corticosteroids or local anesthetic injections around the bone can reduce pain and inflammation.

In most severe cases, a partial or total coccygectomy may be done as a last resort.

Levator Ani Syndrome

Prescribing medicines such as muscle relaxants or pain medications like gabapentin and pregabalin are useful.

Trigger point injections with corticosteroid or botulinum toxin has been useful as well.

Proctalgia Fugax

Treatment options include oral diltiazem, topical glyceryl trinitrate and nerve blockers to get relieve from spasm.

Hemorrhoids

Apart from lifestyle modifications like high fiber diet and good toilet habits, sitz bath is also useful.

Topical treatment includes over-the-counter cream containing witch hazel or a numbing agent.

Oral pain relievers include acetaminophen, aspirin or ibuprofen.

Minimally invasive procedures are used nowadays on outpatient settings. In rubber band ligation, rubber bands are applied around base of hemorrhoid to cut-off its circulation. Other option is injection sclerotherapy in which a chemical solution is injected into the hemorrhoid to shrink it. Also coagulation techniques like laser, infrared or heat can be used with fewer side effects.

If all other procedures fail, hemorrhoidectomy is done, which is the most effective and a complete way to treat severe and recurring hemorrhoids. A less painful procedure, hemorrhoid stapling, is also done nowadays.

Anismus

Laxatives and newer drugs like intestinal secretagogues and serotonergic enterokinetic agents are useful which can treat constipation.

Botulinum toxin injection or surgery like myectomy may be useful.

Pelvic Inflammatory Disease

Most of the patients are usually managed on outpatient basis. This includes a combination of antibiotics for polymicrobial coverage. The drugs commonly used are:
- Ceftriaxone 250 mg single dose
- Doxycycline 100 mg BD for 14 days
- Metronidazole 500 mg BD for 14 days

To prevent reinfection, treatment of sexual partner is necessary. In severe cases, inpatient management with intravenous antibiotic therapy is advised. In rare cases, surgery may be required in cases like generalized peritonitis, pelvic abscess or tubo-ovarian abscess which does not respond to antibiotic therapy.

Endometriosis

Medications include over-the-counter painkillers. Hormone therapy is used as an expectant management. Combined oral contraceptive pills are used which mimic pseudopregnancy state. Danazol and gestrinone create a pseudomenopausal like state. Gonadotropin-releasing hormone (GnRH) analogs are very effective but when used continuously they act as medical oophorectomy due to hypoestrogenism and amenorrhea.

Laparoscopy is the best surgical management. As a conservative approach, ablation and adhesiolysis is done by electrodiatherapy or laser vaporization. Laparoscopic uterosacral nerve ablation (LUNA) is done when pain is severe. Endometriomas are treated laparoscopically by aspiration and/or cystectomy.

Definitive surgery is done only in severe cases where there is no prospect of fertility and other methods have failed. This includes hysterectomy with bilateral salpingo-oophorectomy.

Vulvodynia

Treatment therapy is not very satisfactory. Drugs like tricyclic antidepressants (TCAs), carbamazepine or gabapentin are found to be beneficial. Surgery is not indicated.

Vulvar Vestibulitis

Control of infective agent or allergen might be helpful. TCAs or gabapentin may be tried.

Rarely, surgeries like vestibulectomy, perineoplasty or laser vaporization may be done.

Interstitial Cystitis

Oral medications used are—NSAIDs (to relieve pain), TCAs (to relax bladder and block pain), antihistamines (to reduce urgency and frequency and other symptoms) and newer drugs like pentosan polysulfate sodium (restores the inner surface of bladder and protects from substances that irritate it).

Drug like dimethyl sulfoxide is instilled in bladder through a catheter. Local anesthetic may also be added. The drug is allowed to stay in bladder for 15 minutes before patient is asked to void the urine.

Surgery is rarely used but includes fulguration or resection in which instruments are inserted through the urethra to burn or cut any ulcers, respectively. Rarely, bladder augmentation is done by putting a patch of intestine on bladder to increase bladder capacity.

Urethral Syndrome

Drugs like benzodiazepines, amitriptyline, antibiotics, and estrogen replacement therapy provide symptomatic relief. Cryosurgery is also useful. Progressive urethral dilatation is the treatment of choice.

Constipation

Apart from lifestyle modifications, over-the-counter laxatives are useful. These include stimulants, lubricants, stool softeners, fiber supplements, osmotics, saline laxatives, chloride channel activators and 5-hydroxytryptamine 4 (5-HT4) agonists. Surgery is not used commonly.

Inflammatory Bowel Disease

Goal of treatment is to reduce the inflammation that triggers the signs and symptoms. Medications include anti-inflammatory agents like corticosteroids and aminosalicylates. Immunosuppressant drugs like azathioprine, mercaptopurine, cyclosporine, and methotrexate are also used. Tumor necrosis factor-alpha (TNF-α) inhibitors and other biologic therapies are also used nowadays.

Antibiotics are added in case of superinfection. Iron, calcium and vitamin D are also used as supplements.

Surgery for ulcerative colitis includes removing entire colon and rectum (proctocolectomy). With this either an ileal stoma (permanent opening on abdomen) or an ileal pouch anal anastomosis is done.

Surgery for Crohn's disease is less useful as chances of recurrence are high. Surgery includes removal of damaged portion and then reconnecting it with healthy sections.

Irritable Bowel Syndrome

Routinely fiber supplements, pain relievers, laxatives, antidiarrheal agents, anticholinergic drugs, TCAs and selective serotonin reuptake inhibitors (SSRI) antidepressants are used. Medications used specifically for irritable bowel syndrome (IBS) are alosetron (relaxes colon and slows movement through lower bowel), eluxadoline (reduces muscle contractions and fluid secretions in intestine and increases muscle tone in rectum), rifaximin (decreases bacterial overgrowth), lubiprostone and linaclotide (eases passage of stool).

TREATMENT OF HYPOTONUS PELVIC FLOOR DYSFUNCTION IN FEMALES

Vaginal Laxity

Laser and radiofrequency based devices are used for vaginal rejuvenation. Radiofrequency devices emit focused electromagnetic waves generating heat targeting cellulite, laxity and noninvasive fat removal. Minimally ablative fractional laser therapy based on fractional photothermolysis is safe, precise and efficient method in field of plastic surgery.

However, further researches should be done to measure longevity of results gained.

Urinary Incontinence

Urge incontinence or overactive bladder: First of all, psychosomatic problems are to be ruled out. Also, other medical problems (neurological, diabetes, etc.) should also be ruled out.

Bladder retraining should be practiced.

Aim of medical therapy is to inhibit bladder contractility and increase bladder neck and urethral resistance. Anticholinergic drugs like oxybutynin, tolterodine, fesoterodine, darifenacin, trospium reduce detrusor irritability. Drugs with antimuscarinic activity like tamsulosin, silodosin, terazosin are also used with minimal side effects.

Intravesical use of capsaicin will improve the symptoms.

Surgery in the form of denervation—to interrupt nervous pathways is rarely used. Other surgical options include—augmentation cystoplasty (to increase bladder capacity) or urinary diversion (ileal conduit).

Genuine Stress Incontinence

Conservative therapy includes pelvic floor muscle training and biofeedback therapy.

Medical management includes estrogens in postmeopausal women and sympathomimetic drugs like imipramine which improves the tone of urethra and bladder neck.

Paraurethral implants (Teflon) increase functional strength of urethra. Periurethral injection of glutaraldehyde cross linked bovine collagen is also effective.

Surgery varies depending on individual patient and severity of symptoms. *Retropubic cystourethropexy (colposuspension)* restores normal anatomy of urethrovesical junction and to prevent hypermobility of bladder neck. Burch colposuspension is considered to be gold standard. Endoscopic bladder-neck suspension is also used. *Retropubic midurethral sling* procedures are of two types: (1) tension-free vaginal tape (TVT) and (2) transobturator tape

(TOT). In TVT, synthetic mesh is passed vaginally in "U" shaped manner under midurethra to either side along the back of pubic bone to skin incision on either side. In TOT, a tunnel is created out to the obturator foramen on either side. The tape is left tension free under midurethra to act as a natural hammock supporting urethra. Microsling surgeries are also used nowadays. In *pubovaginal sling* operations, autogenous sling–rectus sheath or fascia lata or inorganic sling–silastic, Marlex or Gore-Tex are used.

Urethral bulking agents like bovine collagen, Teflon, calcium hydroxyapatite are injected transurethrally under cystoscopic guidance. These agents create obstructive effect at the level of bladder neck.

Kelly's cystourethroplasty is a common surgery performed plicating the pubocervical fascia along the proximal urethra and bladder neck.

Salvage procedures include implantation of artificial sphincter and urinary diversion.

Overflow Incontinence

If obstruction is the cause, surgical treatment of obstruction is to be done. In case of nonobstructive causes, continuous catheter drainage is done followed by intermittent clamping and then removal.

Pelvic Organ Prolapse

Preventive measures like pelvic floor rehabilitation during pregnancy and avoiding strenuous activities are advisable. Estrogen replacement therapy is useful in mild cases in postmenopausal women. Pelvic floor exercises (Kegel's exercise) are useful to strengthen the muscles. Pessary treatment relieves symptoms by stretching hiatus urogenitalis, thus preventing descent.

Surgical management for different types of prolapse is as follows:
- *Cystocele: Anterior colporrhaphy* is done. In this, relaxed portion of anterior vaginal wall is cut and bladder is pushed upward and permanently supported by endopelvic fascia and pubocervical fascia. If required, paravaginal defect repair is also done.
- *Rectocele: Colpoperineorrhaphy* is the operation done to repair the prolapse of posterior vaginal wall. In this, the repair is extended by tightening the pararectal fascia.
- *Enterocele:* High perineorrhaphy is done up to the cervicovaginal junction along with correction of enterocele, in which sac of enterocele is obliterated with purse string suture.
  Pelvic floor repair includes anterior colporrhaphy and colpoperineorrhaphy. Restoration of perineal body is essential in this repair to maintain the normal vaginal axis.
- *Uterine prolapse: Fothergill operation* is done when reproductive function is to be preserved. In this, preliminary dilatation and curettage is done. This is followed by low amputation of cervix and then plication of Mackenrodt's ligaments is done in front of cervix to facilitate shortening and raising of cervix in its normal position. Following this pelvic floor repair is done.
  If a woman's family is completed and has uterovaginal prolapse, *vaginal hysterectomy* with pelvic floor repair is done.

If there is prolapse congenitally or in a nulliparous woman, *Purandare's sling operation (cervicopexy)* is done. Through abdominal route, strips of rectus sheath are passed extraperitoneally and stitched to anterior surface of cervix by silk so that the cervix is pulled up mechanically.

Vaginal Vault Prolapse

Vaginally, repair of vaginal vault with pelvic floor repair can be done. In *LeFort's colpocleisis*, after denudation of vaginal mucosa, successive purse string absorbable sutures are placed from above downward to appose the vaginal walls. In *sacrospinous colpopexy*, vaginal vault is fixed to coccygeus sacrospinous ligament complex through pararectal space.

Abdominally, in *sacral colpopexy*, vaginal vault is suspended to anterior longitudinal ligament in front of third sacral vertebra.

TREATMENT OF PELVIC FLOOR DYSFUNCTION IN MALES

Erectile Dysfunction

Drugs like sildenafil are used to increase the penile blood flow. Caverject and papaverine are injectable drugs injected directly into penis to cause an erection. Yohimbine is an effective dietary supplement. Testosterone replacement therapy is useful in men with low testosterone levels.

Mechanical treatment involves use of vacuum erection device with a constriction ring.

Surgical therapy includes use of implants and correction of vascular blockage to restore erectile capacity.

Premature Ejaculation

Behavioral therapy is most commonly useful. Drugs known to delay ejaculation like SSRIs are also useful.

Postvoidal Dribbling

Surgery is indicated for organic problems like strictures and congenital diverticuli. Pelvic floor muscle exercises are effective for functional problems.

Benign Prostatic Hyperplasia

Medications are used most commonly. These include:
- Alpha-blockers: These include alfuzosin, doxazosin, tamsulosin. They relax bladder neck muscles and muscle fibers in prostate, making urination easier.
- 5-α-reductase inhibitors: Drugs like finasteride, dutasteride shrink prostate by preventing hormonal changes that cause prostate growth. Combination of drugs is very effective.

Minimally invasive procedures or surgery removes part of prostate to relieve symptoms. These include:
- Transurethral resection of prostate (TURP)

- Transurethral incision of the prostate (TUIP)
- Transurethral microwave thermotherapy (TUMT)
- Transurethral needle ablation (TUNA)
- Laser therapy includes photoselective vaporization of prostate (PVP) and Holmium laser ablation of prostate (HoLAP).

Newer procedures like prostatic urethral lift, embolization and open or robot-assisted prostatectomy are also used.

Prostate Cancer

In slow growing cancer, supportive care and monitoring for changes is advised.
- In aggressive types, multipurpose therapy is applied. Medications include hormone-assisted therapy, bone health, chemotherapy, and urinary retention medication. Radiation therapy, brachytherapy, and teletherapy are also used. Surgical options include laparoscopic radical prostatectomy or radical retropubic prostatectomy.
- Pelvic floor rehabilitation can be a great asset before and after surgery for every single patient. Pelvic floor rehabilitation is not an optional treatment, but it is a complementary and supportive treatment for every patient and use of innovative devices like PF360 which is an external, noninvasive, anatomically shaped to cover pelvic floor muscles, pelvic floor muscles compressive exercising device for pelvic floor muscles.
- Apart from preoperative and postoperative cases, pelvic floor rehabilitation could be a great asset to:
  - Patients with mild symptoms who are not right match for the surgery
  - Patients who want to delay the surgery
  - Patients who cannot opt for the surgery due to personal or socioeconomic reasons.
- Combination of medical or surgical treatment along with pelvic floor rehabilitation can bring great benefits to patients by increasing strength, flexibility, power, endurance and hypertrophy of the muscles. Well-functioning pelvic floor muscles will improve sphincteric, sexual, supportive, and stabilization functions for patients.

Appendix

WOW IIPRE "INTERNATIONAL INSTITUTE OF PELVIC FLOOR RESEARCH, REHAB AND EDUCATION"

IIPRE is an International Institute exclusively designed for Research, Rehabilitation and Education of Pelvic Floor and related conditions for therapists, medical and paramedical professionals. Millions of women, men and children all over the world silently suffer from different types of pelvic floor dysfunctions. There is huge demand for pelvic floor rehabilitation specialists all over the world. IIPRE will empower the IIPRE certified professionals to be "Game Changers" in the world of rehabilitation by mastering rehabilitation beyond basics (urogential/Anorectal rehabilitation).

Statistics Says

Approximately

- More than 34 million women suffer from urinary incontinence.
- Nine out of ten mothers suffer from vaginal laxity or some other form of pelvic floor dysfunctions (PFDs).
- One out of six women suffers from chronic pelvic pain (CPP).
- More than 50 million men in America are likely to suffer from erectile dysfunction (ED) or premature ejaculation (PME). Statistics for India is even higher.
- Almost every single men or women are likely to suffer from PFD during their lifetime.

Most of the rehabilitation specialists are completely unaware of their own potential to get super-specialization in the world of rehabilitation. Majority of rehabilitation specialists are just busy practicing basic therapy like ortho, neuro, pediatric, cardiac and women's health rehabilitation. Unfortunately, most of the people who practice women's health are also limited to external exercises. Transvaginal and transrectal evaluation and rehabilitation is extremely sensitive and result oriented.

IIPRE is created to benefit millions of people and empower practices of healthcare providers like physical therapists, nurse practitioners, occupational therapists and other medical and paramedical professionals like doctors of osteopathic medicine, DO; Doctor of chiropractic, DC; nurse midwifes; nurse

practitioners ARNP; physical therapy and occupational therapy assistants, doctors of medicine, MD; registered nurses, RN; physician assistants, PA.
- IIPRE is designed to provide a complete overview of the clinical assessment and management of pelvic floor dysfunctions. IIPRE will also train you with needful details about the functional anatomy, causes of pelvic floor dysfunctions, associated pathologies, types of pelvic floor muscle dysfunctions (hypertonus, hypotonus incoordination) and sexual dysfunctions in female along with different pelvic floor dysfunctions in male and pediatric populations.
- The courses and workshops of IIPRE are designed to teach different efficient techniques of pelvic floor evaluation methodologies and treatment options for pelvic floor muscles conditions.
- You will learn the unique role of pelvic floor rehabilitation specialists for conditions like stress urinary incontinence, urge urinary incontinence, vaginal laxity, pelvic organ prolapse, sexual dysfunctions, pelvic pain and pelvic floor muscles spasms in female.
- IIPRE will also train you for pelvic floor rehabilitation for conditions like erectile dysfunction, premature ejaculations, post voidal dribbling, prostatitis, postprostatectomy rehabilitation and pelvic pain in male, along with enuresis and encopresis like conditions in children.
- IIPRE workshops and fellowship/internship program will also teach you details about multiple types of biofeedbacks, different modalities, evaluation techniques, rehabilitation protocols and other treatment options along with different types of rehabilitation devices or pelvic floor muscle exercisers.
- IIPRE workshop and fellowship/internship will also train you with transvaginal/transrectal evaluation, diagnosis and treatments for PFR.
- IIPRE courses are designed to simplify the complexity of pelvic floor muscles which will provide interested certified professionals with scientific and clinical fundamentals of pelvic floor rehabilitation.
- For further details on recent IIPRE workshop and courses visit the website www.visionwowgroup.com/iipre

Het's PROVIDER PROTECTION (HPP) GUIDELINES

- Because of the extreme sensitivity of the subject related to transvaginal and transrectal skills, Only female physical therapists will be certified for transvaginal/transrectal evaluation, diagnosis, and treatment only for female patients. Only male physical therapists will be certified for transrectal evaluation, diagnosis, and treatment for only male patients.
Disclaimer:
This book is designed exclusively for medical and paramedical professionals only. We highly recommend the readers to spread awareness about pelvic floor dysfunctions among society. However, please DO NOT teach or train the principles of this book to medical or paramedical students or professionals (without professional training, exam, appropriate certifications and written permission from IIPRE "International Institute of Pelvic floor research, rehabilitation and education".) It will be complete responsibility of practitioners or readers to obtain certifications and written permission from IIPRE to enable to teach the

concepts of this book, to medical or paramedical students and/or professionals. This may not be used for any illegal purposes. Practitioners or readers will be hold directly responsible for all legal consequences or liabilities. WOW IIPRE has set very high quality standards which should not be compromised at any cost (due to sensitivity of subject related to tranvaginal/transrectal skills). With all respect ,WOW IIPRE holds the right to blacklist and or take legal actions by initiating legal proceedings.

COMMON PELVIC FLOOR DYSFUNCTION— RELATED CONDITIONS

- Chronic pain: General
- Chronic prostatitis
- Constipation, unspecified
- Cystocele: Lateral
- Damage to pelvic joints or ligaments
- Detrusor sphincter dyssynergia
- Diastasis recti
- Dysfunctional voiding
- Dyspareunia
- Erectile dysfunction
- Incomplete bladder emptying
- Incontinence: Fecal
- Incontinence: Female stress
- Incontinence: Male stress
- Incontinence: Mixed
- Incontinence: Urge
- Interstitial cystitis
- Levator ani syndrome
- Low back pain (lumbago)
- Unspecified back
- Muscle incoordination
- Muscle and tissue atrophy
- Nocturnal enuresis
- Overactive bladder syndrome
- Painful episiotomy
- Painful scar
- Pelvic pain: Female
- Peripheral nerve injury: Pudendal nerve
- Rectocele
- Spasm of muscle
- Sprain or strain of pelvis
- Unspecified disorder
- Urinary frequency
- Urinary prolapse
- Vaginismus
- Vulvodynia or vestibulitis
- Others.

Following are multidisciplinary facets for pelvic floor rehabilitation:
a. **Prenatal rehabilitation:**
   The focus of this program is to evaluate and proactively take care of any type of PFD that exists in prenatal women. Every pregnant patient is an ideal candidate for pelvic floor training before and during pregnancy.

   Pelvic floor rehabilitation helps to create solid foundation to carry healthy pregnancy. It will improve strength, flexibility, endurance and power for pelvic floor muscles (PFMs) to handle upcoming childbirth. Pelvic floor rehabilitation during pregnancy can greatly empower your patients for more efficient pregnancy, labor and childbirth.

b. **Postnatal rehabilitation:**
   Our research says approximately 9 out of 10 mothers have postnatal vaginal laxity. Every single postnatal patient should be privileged with PFR for vaginal laxity. It will greatly help to gain best possible vaginal recovery after childbirth. It will create healing of PFMs along with progressive toning and tightening of vagina. It will help new mothers to prevent urinary incontinence or intimate health issues.

c. **Vaginal tightening rehabilitation:**
   Vaginal laxity can happen in many women due to age, pregnancy, childbirth, pudendal nerve damage, disused pelvic floor atrophy, etc. Vaginal laxity can be one of the major causes for urinary incontinence, pelvic organ prolapse or reduced sexual sensations. Toning and tightening of vaginal—PFMs could help to prevent and treat vaginal laxity. Introducing vaginal tightening program in your practice will bring awareness among patients.

d. **Incontinence rehabilitation:**
   Postnatal vaginal laxity or weak PFMs fail to create complete closure of the sphincters which can lead to urinary or fecal incontinence. Approximately more than 34 million women suffer from urinary incontinence. Incontinence rehabilitation involves much more than suggesting the patients to do Kegel exercises. Studies show that approximately 98.7% of women who try to do Kegel, end up using accessory muscles like hip adductors, lower abdominals, gluteus, Valsalva maneuver, etc. WOW IIPRE affiliated pelvic rehabilitation practitioners can perform transvaginal and transrectal evaluation and management techniques like pelvic floor biofeedback, transvaginal or transrectal rehabilitation like proprioceptive neuromuscular facilitation (PNF) and ultimate pelvic floor exercises, activation and facilitations with exclusive underpatent pelvic floor devices like PF360 which greatly can improve the functionality of PFMs. Pelvic floor rehabilitation program could be executed for mild to moderate cases of stress urinary incontinence, urge incontinence and mixed incontinence. Apart from the medical management of urinary incontinence, building strength, endurance, power and hypertrophy of PFMs can greatly benefit patients. Pelvic floor rehabilitation will enhance benefits for postsurgical patients as well. Promoting functional strength of PFMs can also greatly enhance the recovery and longevity of results for your patients.

e. **Menopausal vaginal rehabilitation:**
   Menopause causes ovaries to stop producing estrogen which also leads to PFD. Incontinence, prolapse and sexual problems are common with menopause.

Pelvic floor rehabilitation can help menopausal women to take care of urinary frequency and urgency along with improving bladder control and intimate health issues.

f. **Posthysterectomy vaginal rehabilitation:**
Hysterectomy could be considered blessings for patients who are suffering from the conditions like severe endometriosis, uterine fibroids, cancer, etc. One in five women is likely to go for hysterectomy. Vaginal hysterectomy can directly interfere with functioning of PFM. One of the most common side effects of hysterectomy is hormonal changes. The ovaries are epicenter of estrogen and progesterone. Production of this hormone is reduced by posthysterectomy or oophorectomy which leads to vaginal thinning and dryness. Posthysterectomy women are at increased risk of POP after a hysterectomy. Reduced ligamental support and new vacant space in the pelvis can leave remaining organs more vulnerable to slipping out. Preoperative rehabilitation and postoperative PFR can empower great recovery to the patients.

g. **Pelvic pain rehabilitation:**
Many women who suffer from pelvic pain might come across similar triggers. Almost one out of five women is likely to have pelvic pain. Pelvic floor rehabilitation for hypertonus or incoordination type of PFMs is extremely important. Sharing their experiences with other patients who are also getting PFR, while going through pelvic pain rehabilitation might help them to learn about triggers from other patients. This will help them to cope with emotional release and ultimately help to get better results with physical release as well. From ages many medical professionals have primarily focused on contractile component of pelvic floor muscles only, however active relaxation and releasing muscle tension can help patients with CPP which can be accomplished by specialized techniques like myofascial release, trigger point release, etc. along with proper technologies like WOW Vagina-Dilate, WOW Woman and PF360.

h. **Prolapse rehabilitation (pre- and postsurgical):**
Weak pelvic floor leads to overstrained suspensory ligaments and ultimately pelvic organ prolapse.

Pelvic floor rehabilitation might not be able to completely treat prolapse. However, it could greatly benefit for FSD, FSDs associated with prolapse. Taking care of pelvic floor fitness before and after surgery can significantly help to improve results of pelvic organ prolapse and quality of life concerns.

i. **Gynecological surgery—pre- and postrehabilitation:**
In any corner of the world, every single patient receives pre- and postoperative knee rehabilitation before and after knee replacement surgery. Similarly, before and after gynecological surgery, PFR is very important to improve strength, endurance, power, hypertrophy and flexibility of PFMs which will ultimately benefit patients by improving sphincteric, sexual, stabilization and supportive functions of PFMs. Pelvic floor rehabilitation also helps to prevent spasmodic hypertonus dysfunction of PFMs and related vicious cycle due to surgical or scar pain.

j. **Postvaginal rejuvenation rehabilitation:**
Many women are very sensitive when it comes to appearance of their private body parts. Plastic surgeries like vaginal rejuvenation are getting more famous.

This program is designed to add value to the appearance by providing additional functional beauty to the private body parts. Steve Jobs said "Design is not only how it looks like or feels like, but design is how it works like." Gynecologists and esthetic gynecologists are ultimate designer of perineal area. Designing perineal area is also improving functionality of perineal area and PFMs. Postsurgical PFR will help your patients with much better functional recovery, higher self-esteem, more confidence and satisfaction.

k. **Female sexual dysfunction rehabilitation:**
Most of the postnatal or menopausal women might observe significant reduction in their sexual well-being. Sexual well-being is essential part of well-being for any woman and her partner. Too tight PFMs can cause pelvic pain and lead to painful intercourse which hurts the sex life and relationship. Also, too weak PFMs can cause vaginal laxity and lead to reduced sensation along with reduced intensity of orgasm. Both types of PFDs can lead to reduced libido, sensations, orgasms and regressed relationship. Intimate health enhancement rehabilitation will help to create proper balance with stability and mobility of PFM along with perfect coordination which will increase sensations, libido, orgasm and overall well-being of women.

Female sexual dysfunction affects millions of women all over the world. Any disorder related to female sexual desire, arousal, orgasm and/or sexual pain can be classified under FSD. Sexual arousal is associated with vaginal lubrication, depends on intact sympathetic nervous system. Arousal can be significantly reduced by pain or even anticipation of pain. The pain or discomfort creates anxiety and fear which leads to reduced libido, arousal response and can reduce vaginal lubrication. Vaginal lubrication can also be decreased by estrogen deficiency, pain medication, anticholinergic, antidepressant, and antihistamine medications. Poor lubrication causes vaginal dryness and microtrauma to vaginal tissue and pain. Conditions like dyspareunia and vaginismus create pain with sexual activity. Pain or anticipation of pain can lead to spasmodic contraction or hypertonus PFMs. Hypertonus or spasmodic PFMs make it more difficult to penetrate. Pelvic floor rehabilitation for hypertonus PFMs can bring great results for patients. Similarly, too weak or lax PFMs can lead to hypotonus type of PFD. It can negatively affect arousal, sensation, and intensity of orgasm. Weaker grip can also create negative effect on the grip over penis during intercourse. Pelvic floor rehabilitation is extremely important and commonly missed treatment approach for FSD. It is important to treat sexual dysfunction at earliest possible as it can cause low self-confidence, low self-esteem, personal distress, negative experience, relationship disputes, husband's or partner's disappointment and can negatively affect quality of life concerns for the couple.

l. **Pelvic cancer and PFR:**
Some of the studies like Bernard et al. (2016) studied the effects of radiation therapy on the structure and function of the PFMs of patients with cancer in the pelvic area. Surgery, chemotherapy or radiation therapy can lead to PFDs like urinary incontinence, dyspareunia, and fecal incontinence. "Pelvic floor rehabilitation physiotherapy is effective even in gynecologic cancer survivors who need it the most."

m. **Breast cancer and PFR:**
   Issues like pelvic floor problems, lack of control of the bladder and/or bowel, burning, itching, overwhelming urge, frequency, painful urination, leaking urine, recurring urinary tract infection, vaginal dryness, urinary incontinence during sex, difficult or discomfort with intercourse, painful sex and sexual dysfunction may arise either during or after treatment for breast cancer. These are important quality of life issues and they should not be ignored. Reasons behind this problem could be related to estrogen or the after effects of chemotherapy and/or radiation. Drug therapy can suppress estrogen production if tumor was estrogen driven, chemotherapy can lead to early menopause and radiation can affect tissues as well. As a result, it leads to dryness of the vagina which may cause pain when attempting intercourse; pain can lead to tension and tightness in the PFMs which can lead to an inability to have intercourse. Symptoms of prolapse can worsen, and PFMs can weaken—both of which can lead to loss of control of the bladder and/or bowel. Also, poor body image and self-esteem can lead to psychosomatic dysfunctions along with PFDs. PFR in oncological setup is highly recommended.

n. **Diabetes and PFR:**
   Huge number of patients all over the world are affected by diabetes. Patients with diabetes commonly experiences urinary incontinence or difficulty controlling. It could be due to obesity, diabetic neuropathic affecting nerves of bladder, pudendal nerve neuropathy. Also there could be significant issues with sexual well-being due to pudendal nerve neuropathy. Every diabetologist can expand their practice and benefit their patients with PFR.

o. **Erectile dysfunction and premature ejaculation rehabilitation:**
   Approximately 50% men over the age of 40 years suffer from ED. PFR program at psychiatrist's clinic can greatly help patients with ED. Drug, injections and surgical interventions are great. However, well integrated PFR for ED and PME is completely free from side effects and can greatly help patient recovery. Specialized rehabilitation for muscles like bulbocavernosus and ischiocavernosus can help to improve blood flow to penis which can help with erection. It can also help to reduce venous return which can help to gain harder and longer lasting erections.

p. **Prostate rehabilitation:**
   Prostate health can be greatly improved by improving pelvic blood flow. Prostate rehabilitation program can help patients with preprostatectomy rehabilitation and postprostatectomy rehabilitation from consequences like ED, urinary incontinence, postvoidal dribbling, etc. All oncologists and urologists can greatly benefit their patients by incorporating with pelvic floor rehabilitation.

q. **Bed-wetting or enuresis or encopresis rehabilitation:**
   Parents will love to be free from diaper-related issues like changing diaper frequently, diaper rashes, etc. Children will be more confident by gaining better and faster control over their bladder and bowel. Starting early potty training program at your practice could benefit many children. Pelvic floor facilitation at early age can help your patients. Research says that more than 10% of pediatrician visits are for incontinence. Children who suffer from enuresis or encopresis types of problems can progressively lead to psychosomatic dysfunctions.

All pediatricians can start PFR for children to help them gain better control. Their self-image, self-control and self-worth get damaged at early age which affects almost all dimensions of their life. So PFR program for this condition is very important.

r. **Geriatric PFR:**
Geriatric homes, geriatric groups and assisted living facilities can adopt PFR centers which will greatly benefit senior population with quality of life concerns. Most of the geriatric population suffer from urinary or fecal incontinence. Unfortunately, the only help they are aware of is adult diapers. Diapers can only hide the problems. They do not solve it. Geriatric specialist can greatly benefit their patients by starting PFR center under their roof. Pelvic floor rehabilitation program can be greatly beneficial for geriatric population.

s. **Colorectal PFR:**
When it comes to PFR, many medical professional only think about genitourinary rehabilitation. Anorectal rehabilitation is also very important part of PFR especially if patient has gone through any form of colorectal surgery. Preoperative and postoperative PFR can be extremely beneficial for patients. Medical professionals like colorectal surgeons can expand the level of the care by offering their patients pre- and postoperative or procedural PFR.

t. **Bariatric PFR:**
If you are a group of bariatric surgeons or associated with medical or paramedical professionals who provide obesity care, chances are very high that most of your patients might have some level of PFD. Extra body weight can lead to PFDs. Patients can be greatly benefited by PFR programs along with obesity management.

u. **Cardilology and PFR:**
The incidence of atherosclerosis is increasing nowadays, surprisingly the diameter of coronary artery is approx 5 mm and that of penial artery is approx 1mm. The chances of blocking of penial artery before the coronary is high due to its small diameter, this can lead to development of sexual dysfunction prior to the development of coronary symptoms, the interventional cardiologists are doing stenting is the penial artery, but PFR can work as an adjunct therapy for improving the overall quality of life of these patients.

The following practitioners can provide a complete care to their patients by developing pelvic floor rehabilitation clinic
1. Gynecologist
2. Urogynecologist
3. Urologist
4. Psychiatrist
5. Oncologist
6. Neurologist
7. Pain medicine
8. Sexologist
9. Proctologist
10. Gasteoenterologists
11. Colorectal surgeons

12. Endocrinologist
13. Bariatric surgeons
14. Diabetologist
15. Onco surgeon
16. Pediatricians
17. Plastic surgeon
18. Cosmetic gynecologist
19. Geriatric medicine
20. Cardiologists
21. Physical therapist
22. Occupational therapist
23. Chiropractors
24. Osteopathic medicine
25. Midwifes/nurses
26. Advanced registered nurse practioner (ARNP)
27. Registered nurses (RN)
28. Physician assistants (PA)

And other medical or paramedical practitioners who deals directly or indirectly with pelvic floor related conditions.

APPLICATION DEVELOPED FOR THE HOME USE

WOW She strength and WOW He strength is downloadable mobile application of WOW Group exclusively designed to progressively train pelvic floor muscles in female and male respectively. It is designed to provide auditory cues, visual input, progressive charts and complete pelvic floor training guidelines which can be very beneficial for self-use by patients. Even the doctors, therapist and pelvic rehabilitation specialist can use these app for home rehabilitation protocol reports generated by this app can help the doctors and the users. The combination of this app and WOW Vagina-Fit device can benefit the user/patient by providing visual and auditory cues along with proprioceptive biofeedback.

In clinical practice of pelvic floor rehabilitation specialist this app can help the clinical providers to prescribe, guide and assess the progression along with performance to customise the treatment more efficiently.

Go to app store to download WOW Group applications of She Strength/He Strength. For more information visit the website www.visionwowgroup.com.

Resources and References

Doctors, who are sincerely interested in learning more details about pelvic floor and related research, please refer to following medical research.
- "Clitoris". Inner Body. N.p., n.d. Web. 27 Feb. 2017.
- "Egg Cell". Egg Cell - Biology-Online Dictionary. N.p., n.d. Web. 26 Feb. 2017.
- "Fallopian Tube". Inner Body. N.p., n.d. Web. 26 Feb. 2017.
- "Female External Genital Organs - Women's Health Issues". Merck Manuals Consumer Version. N.p., n.d. Web. 28 Feb. 2017.
- "It's as good as Viagra, without the cost and the side effects." — Dr. Grace Dorey, The New York Times July 2014
- "Labia Majora". Inner Body. N.p., n.d. Web. 27 Feb. 2017.
- "Medical Definition of Ovary." Medicine Net. N.p., n.d. Web. 28 Feb. 2017.
- "Sign up for Our Newsletter Get Health Tips, Wellness Advice, and More". Healthline : Power of Intelligent Health. N.p., n.d. Web. 26 Feb. 2017.
- "Sign up for Our NewsletterGet Health Tips, Wellness Advice, and More." Healthline: Power of Intelligent Health. N.p., n.d. Web. 27 Feb. 2017.
- "The Clitoris and Female Orgasm — All Things Vagina". All Things Vagina. N.p., 22 Jan. 2017. Web. 27 Feb. 2017.
- "What Is the Function of the Labium Minora?" Reference. N.p., n.d. Web. 28 Feb. 2017.
- "Corpus Cavernosum of Clitoris." Wikipedia. N.p., n.d. Web 20 May 2017.
- "Doctor: Pubic Hair Exists for a Reason."Alternet. N.p., n.d. Web 20 May 2017.
- "The Perineum." Teach Me Anatomy. N.p., n.d. Web 27 Feb 2017.
- "Uterus." InnerBody. N.p., n.d. Web 20 May 2017.
- "Vulvar Anatomy." Improving Wom zen's Health. N.p., n.d. Web 20 May 2017.
- 76% of men experienced significant improvement in erectile function. —British J Urol. 2005
- Abrams P, Cardozo L, Fall M, et al. The standardisation terminology of lower urinary tract function: report from the Standardisation Sub-committee of the International Continence Society Neurourol Urodyn. 2002;21:167-78.
- Abrams PA, Blaivas JG, Stanton SL, et al. Standardization of the lower urinary tract function [abstract]. Neurourol Urodyn. 1998;7:403.
- Addison R. Cranberry juice: the story so far. J Assoc Chart Physiother Women's Health. 1997;80:21-2.
- Agency for Health Care Policy and Research. (1996). Overview: Urinary Incontinence in Adults, Clinical Practice Guideline Update. [online]. Available from www.ahrq.gov/clinic/uiover [Accessed December 2018].
- Albaugh J, Lewis JH. Insights into the management of erectile dysfunction: Part I. Urol Nurs. 1999;19:241-7.
- Allen RE, Hosker GL, Smith ARB, et al. Pelvic floor damage and childbirth: A neurophysiological study. Br J Obstet Gynaecol. 1990;97:770-9.

- Amarenco G, Le Cocquen A, Bosc S. Stress urinary incontinence and genitor-sexual conditions. Prog Urol. 1996;6:913-9.
- American Association of Sexuality Educators, Counselors and Therapists. www.aasect.org.
- American College of Obstetricians and Gynecologists. www.acog.org (search for "Urinary incontinence").
- American College of Sports Medicine Position Stand. 1990. The recommended quantity and quality of exercise for developing and maintaining cardiorespiratory and muscular fitness, and flexibility in healthy adults. Med Sci Sports Exerc. 1990;22:265-74.
- American Physical Therapy Association 800 – 999 – APTA, ext. 3229.www.womenshealthapta.org.
- American Urological Association Foundation. www.urologyhealth.org.
- Amrams P, Cardozo L, Fall M, et al. The standardisation of terminology of lower urinary tract function: report from the standardisation sub-committee for the International Continence society. Neurourol Urodyn. 2002;21:167-78.
- Andersen KV, Bovim G. Impotence and nerve entrapment in long distance amateur cyclists. Acta Neurol Scand. 1997;95:233-40.
- Arias E, MacDorman MF, Strobino DM, et al. Annual summary of vital statistics—2002. Pediatrics. 2003;112:1215-30.
- Ashton-Miller JA, DeLancey JOL. The knack: use of precisely-timed pelvic muscle contraction can reduce leakage in SUI. Neurourol Urogyn. 1996;15:392-3.
- Ashton-Miller JA, Howard D, Delancey JOL. The functional anatomy of the female pelvic floor and stress continence control system. Scand J Urol Nephrol. 2001;207:1-7.
- Astin JA, Shapiro SL, Eisenberg DM, et al. Mind body medicine: state of the science, implications for Practice. J Am Board Fam Pract. 2003;16(2):131-47.
- Aydin S, Ercan M, Caskurlu T, et al. Acupuncture and hypnotic suggestion in the treatment of non-organic male sexual dysfunction. Scan J Urol Nephrol. 1997;31:271-4.
- Aytac JA, McKinlay JB, Krane RJ. The likely worldwide increase in erectile dysfunction between 1995 and 2025 and some possible policy consequences. BIJU Int. 1999;84:50-6.
- Bachmann GA, Phillips NA. Sexual dysfunction. In: Stress JF, Metzger DA, Levy BS (Eds). Chronic pelvic pain. Philadelphia: WB Saunders; 1998. pp. 77-90.
- Baker PK. Musculoskeletal problems. In: Steege JF, Metzger DA, Levy BS (Eds). Chronic Pelvic Pain. Philadelphia: WB Saunders; 1998. pp. 215-40.
- Ballard DJ. Treatment of erectile dysfunction: can pelvic muscle exercises improve sexual function? J Wound Ostomy Continence Nurs. 1997;24:255-64.
- Barber MD, Kuchibhatla MN, Pieper CF, et al. Psychometric evaluation of 2 comprehensive condition-specific quality of life instruments for women with pelvic floor disorders. Am J Obstet Gynecol. 2001;185(6):1388-95.
- Barber MD, Lambers A, Visco AG, et al. Effect of patient position on clinical evaluation of pelvic organ prolapsed. Obstet Gynecol. 2000;96(1):18-22
- Basmajian JV. Muscles alive—their functions revealed by electromyography, 3rd edition. Baltimore: Williams and Wilkins; 1974.
- Basson R, Berman J, Burnett A, et al. Report of the international consensus development conference on female sexual dysfunction: definitions and classifications. J Urol. 2000;163(3):888-93.
- Bates B. A Guide to Physical Examination and History Taking, 6th edition. Philadelphia: JB Lippincott Company, 1995. pp. 361-76, 417-26.

- Beachy EH. Bacterial adherence: adhesion receptor interactions mediating the attachment of bacteria to mucosal surfaces. J Infect Dis. 1981;143:325-45.
- Beji NK, Yalcin O, Erkan HA. The effect of pelvic floor training on sexual function of treated patients. Int Urogynecol J Pelvic Floor Dysfunc. 2003;14:234-8.
- Benet AE, Melman A. The epidemiology of erectile dysfunction. Urol Clin North Am. 1995;22:699-709.
- Bennett JK, Foote JE, Green BG, et al. Effectiveness of biofeedback/electrostimulation in treatment of post-prostatectomy urinary incontinence. [Paper presented at Urodynamics Society Conference, New Orleans, April 1997].
- Berger Y. Urodynamic studies. In: Fitzpatrick JM, Krane RJ (Eds). The bladder. Edinburgh: Churchill Livingstone; 1995. pp. 119-28.
- Berman L. It's You!: How to Take Charge of Your Life and Create the Love and Intimacy You Deserve. New York: DK Publishing; 2010.
- Bernstein IT. The pelvic floor muscles: muscles thickness in healthy and urinary-incontinent women measured by perineal ultrasonography with reference to the effect of pelvic floor training. Estrogen receptor studies. Neurourol. 1997;16:137-75.
- Bo K, Borgen JS. Prevalence of stress and urge urinary incontinence in elite athletes and controls. Med Sci Sports Exerc. 2001;33(11):1797-802.
- Bo K, Finckenhagen H. Vaginal palpation of pelvic floor muscle strength: Inter-test reproducibility and comparison between palpation and vaginal squeeze pressure. Acta Obstet Gynecol Scan. 2001;80:883-7.
- Bo K, Kvarstein B, Nygaard I. Lower urinary tract symptoms and pelvic floor muscle exercise adherence after 15 years. Obstet Gynecol. 2005;105(5):999-1005.
- Bo K, Larsen S, Oseid S, et al. Knowledge about and the ability to perform correct pelvic floor muscle exercises in women with urinary stress incontinence. Neurourol Urodyn. 1988;7(7):261-2.
- Bo K, Talseth T, Holme I. Single blind, randomised controlled trial of pelvic floor exercises, electrical stimulation, vaginal cones, and no treatment in management of genuine stress incontinence in women. BMJ. 1999;318:487-93.
- Bo K, Talseth T. Change in urethral pressure during voluntary pelvic floor muscle contraction and vaginal electrical stimulation. Int Urogynecol J. 1997;8:3-7.
- Bo K. Is there still a place for physiotherapy in the treatment of female incontinence? EAU Update Series. 2003;1:145-53.
- Bo K. Pelvic floor muscle training is effective in treatment of stress urinary incontinence, but how does it work? Int Urogynecol J. 2004;15(2)76-84.
- Bo K. Pelvic floor muscles exercise for the treatment of stress urinary incontinence: an exercise physiology perspective. Int Urogynecol J Pelvic Floor Dysfunct. 1995;6:282-91.
- Bo K. Reproducibility or instruments designed to measure subjective evaluation of female stress urinary incontinence. Scand J Urol Nephrol. 1994;28:97-100.
- Bo K. Techniques. In: Schussler B, Laycock J, Norton P, Station S (Eds). Pelvic floor re-education: Principles and Practice, 3rd edition. London: Springer, 1997. pp. 134-9.
- Bodel PT, Contran R, Kass EH. Cranberry juice and antibacterial action of hippuric acid. J Lab Clin Med. 1959;54:881-8.
- Bordo S. The Male Body: A New Look at Men in Public and in Private. US: Farrar, Strauss and Giroux; 1999.
- Bosco C, Colli R, Introini E, et al. Adaptive responses of human skeletal muscle to vibration exposure. Clin Physiol. 1999;19(2):183-7.

- Bourcier AP, Juras JC, Villet RM. Office evaluation and physical examination. In: Bourcier AP, McGuiter EJ, and Abrams P (Eds). Pelvic Floor Disorders. Philadelphia: Elsevier Saunders, 2004. pp. 133-48.
- Bradford A, Meston CM. Behavior and symptom change among women treated with placebo for sexual dysfunction. J Sex Med. 2010;8(1):191-201.
- Brigham and Women's Hospital. (2011). Urinary incontinence. [online] Available from https://www.brighamandwomens.org/obgyn/urogynecology/diagnosis-treatment-and-prevention-of-urinary-incontinence [Accessed January 2019].
- Brink C, Sampselle C, Wells T, et al. A digital test for pelvic muscle strength in older women with urinary incontinence. Nurs Res. 1989;38(4):196-9.
- Britton JP, Dowell AC, Whelan P. Prevalence of urinary symptoms in men aged over 60. Br J Urol. 1990;66:175-6.
- Brocklehurst JC. Urinary incontinence in the community: analysis of a MORI Poll. Br Med J. 1993;306:832-4.
- Brubaker L, Benson JT, Bent A, et al. Transvaginal electrical stimulation for female urinary incontinence. Am J Obstet Gynaecol. 1997;177:536-40.
- Bump RC, Mattiasson A, Bø K, et al. The standardization of terminology of female pelvic organ prolapsed and pelvic floor dysfunction. Am J Obstet Gynecol. 1996;175:10-7.
- Bump R, Norton P. Epidemiology and natural history of pelvic floor dysfunction. Obstet Gynecol Clin North Am. 1998;25(4):723-46.
- Bump RC, Hurt WG, Fantl JA, et al. Assessment of Kegel pelvic muscle exercise performance after brief verbal instruction. Am J Obstet Gynecol. 1991;165:322-9.
- Bump RC, McClish DM. Cigarette smoking and urinary incontinence in women. Am J Obstet Gynecol. 1992;167(5):1214-8.
- Bump RC, Norton PA, Zinner NR, et al. Mixed urinary incontinence symptoms: urodynamic findings, incontinence severity, and treatment response. Obstet Gynecol. 2003;102(1):76-83.
- Bump RC, Norton PA. Epidemiology and natural history of pelvic floor dysfunction. Obstet Gynecol Clinic North America. 1998;4:723-46.
- Burgio KL, Locher JL, Goode PS, et al. Behavioral vs. drug treatment for urge urinary incontinence in older women in a randomized controlled trial. JAMA. 1998;280:1995-2000.
- Burio KL, Stutzman RE, Engel BT. Behavioural training for post-prostatectomy urinary incontinence. J Urol. 1989;141:303-6.
- Burrows LJ, Shaw H. Contemporary management of pelvic organ prolapse. Menopause Management. 2008:23-30.
- Butler RN, Lewis MI, Whitehead ED. Love and sex after 60: how to evaluate and treat the impotent older man. A roundtable discussion: Part 2. Geriatrics. 1994;49:27-32.
- Cantieni B. Tiger feeling. The sensual pelvic floor training for her and him. 2000.
- Cardozo L. Detrusor instability. In: Stanton S (Ed). Clinical gynaecologic urology. St. Louise; CV Mosby; 1984. pp. 193-203.
- Center for Sexual Health Promotion, Indiana University. Results of the National Survey of Sexual Health and Behavior (NSSHB). J Sex Med. 2010;7(5):243-373.
- Chalker R. The Clitoral Truth: The Secret World at Your Fingertip. New York: Seven Stories Press; 2000.
- Chambless DL, Sultan FE, Stern TE, et al. Effect of pubococcygeal exercise on coital orgasm in women. J Consult Clin Psycho. 1984;52:114-8.
- Chang PL, Tsai LH, Huang ST, et al. The early effect of pelvic floor muscle exercise after transurethral prostatectomy. J Urol. 1998;160:402-5.
- Chiarelli P, Brown W. Perineal elevation – the reliability testing of a new measure of pelvic floor muscle function. In: Continence Foundation of Australia 8th National Conference on Incontinence Foundation of Australia; 1999.

- Chiarelli P, Cockburn J. Promoting urinary continence in women following delivery: randomised controlled trial. Br Med J. 2002;324(25):1241-7.
- Chiarelli P. Female urinary incontinence in Australia: prevalence and prevention in postpartum women [doctoral thesis]. Newcastle (Australia): University of Newcastle; 2001.
- Claes H, Bijnens B, Baert L. The hemodynamic influence of the ischiocavernosus muscles on erectile function. J Urol. 1996;156:986-90.
- Claes H, Van Kampen M, Lysens R, et al. Pelvic floor exercises in the treatment of impotence. Eur J Phys Med Rehabil. 1995;5:135-40.
- Claes HIM, Vandenbroucke HB, Baert LV. Pelvic floor exercise in the treatment of impotence [abstract]. J Urol Suppl. 1996a;157:786.
- Clark AL, Gregory T, Smith VJ, et al. Epidemiological evaluation of reoperation for surgically treated pelvic organ prolapse and urinary incontinence. Am J Obstet Gynecol. 2003;189:1261-7.
- Colpi GM, Negri L, Nappi RE, et al. Perineal floor efficiency in sexually potent and impotent men. Int J Impot Res. 1999;11(3):153-7.
- Colpi GM, Negri L, Scroppor FI, et al. Perineal floor rehabilitation: a new treatment for venogenic impotence. J Endocrinol Invest. 1994;17:34.
- Concell K, Guess MK, La Combe J, et al. Evaluation of the role of pudendal nerve integrity in female sexual function using noninvasive techniques. Am J Obstet Gynecol. 2005;192(5):1712-7.
- Costello K. Myofascial syndromes. In: Steege JF, Metzger DA, Levy BS (Eds). Chronic Pelvic Pain. Philadelphia: WB Saunders; 1998 pp. 251-66.
- Cullen PJ, Heit M. Urinary incontinence in women: Evaluation and management. Am Fam Phys. 2000;62(11):2433-44.
- Davidson PJT, Van den Ouden D, Schroeder FH. Radical prostatectomy: prospective assessment of mortality and morbidity. Eur Urol. 1996;29:168-73.
- Davison SL, Bell RJ, La China M, et al. Sexual function in well women: Stratification by sexual satisfaction, hormone use, and menopause status. J Sex Med. 2008;5(5):1214-22.
- Davison SL, Bell RJ, La China M, et al. The relationship between self-reported sexual satisfaction and general well-being in women. J Sex Med. 2009;6(10):2690-7.
- Dean N, Wilson D, Herbison P, et al. Sexual function, delivery mode history, pelvic floor muscle exercises and incontinence: A cross-sectional study six years postpartum. Aust NZ J Obstet Gynaecol. 2008;48(3):302-11.
- DeLancey J. Functional anatomy of the pelvic floor and urinary continence mechanism. In: Schussler B, Laycock J, Norton S (Eds). Pelvic floor re-education: principle and practice, 3rd edition. London: Springer; 1994. pp. 9-21.
- Denmeade SR, Lin XS, Isaacs JT. Role of programmed (apoptotic) cell death during the progression and therapy for prostate cancer. Prostate. 1996;28:251-65.
- Denning J. Male urinary continence. In: Norton C (Ed). Nursing for continence. Beaconsfield, UK: Beaconsfield Publishers; 1996. pp.153-69.
- Denson M, Houser E. Improving the symptoms and quality of life of patients with overactive bladder and urinary incontinence. Brochure. The Urology Team, PA; 2006.
- Derouet H, Nolden W, Jost WH, et al. Treatment of erectile dysfunction by an external ischiocavernosus muscles stimulator. Eur Urol. 1998;34:355-9.
- Desai KM, Gingell JC. Hazards of long distance cycling. Br Med J. 1989:1072-3.
- Dietz H, Clarke B. The urethral pressure profile and ultrasound imaging of the lower urinary tract. Int Urogynecol J. 2001;12(1):38-41.
- Dietz H, Wilson P, Clarke B. The use of perineal ultrasound to quantify levator activity and teach pelvic floor muscle exercise. Int Urogynecol J Pelvic Floor Dysfunct. 2001;12:166-9.

- DiNubile NA, Patrick W. Frame Work. US: Rodale Books; 2005.
- DiNubile NA. Strength training. Clin Sports Med. 1991;10;33-62.
- Dixon J, Dorey G, Eve B, et al. Postprostatectomy incontinence. J Assoc Chart Physiother Women's Health. 1997;80:35-8.
- Dixon JS, Gosling JA. The anatomy of the bladder, urethra and pelvic floor. In: Mundy AR, Stephenson TP, Wein AJ (Eds). Urodynamics: principles, practice and application, 2nd edition. Edinburgh: Churchill Livingstone, 1994. pp. 3-14.
- Djavan B, Madersbacher S, Klinger HC, et al. Outcome analysis of minimally invasive treatments for benign prostatic hyperplasia. Tech Urol. 1999;5:12-20.
- Djurhuus JC, Matthiesen TB, Ritting S. Similarities and dissimilarities between nocturnal enuresis in childhood and nocturia in adults. BJU Int. 1999;84(Suppl 1):9-12.
- Donnellan SM, Duncan HJ, MacGregor RJ, et al. Prospective Assessment of incontinence after radical retropublic prostatectomy: objective and subjective analysis. Urology. 1997;49:225-30.
- Dorey G, Siegel A, Nelson P. The effect of a pelvic floor muscle training program using active and resisted exercises on male sexual function: a randomised controlled trial. Semantic School. 2015.
- Dorey G, Speakman MJ, Feneley RC, et al. Pelvic floor exercises for erectile dysfunction. BJU Int. 2005;96(4):595-7.
- Dorey G. Conservative treatment of erectile dysfunction, 1: anatomy/physiology. Br J Nurs. 2000;9:691-4.
- Dorey G. Conservative treatment of erectile dysfunction, 2: clinical trials. Br J Nurs. 2000;9:859-63.
- Dorey G. Conservative treatment of erectile dysfunction, 3: literature review. Br J Nurs. 2000;9:859-63.
- Dorey G. Conservative treatment of male urinary incontinence and erectile dysfunction. London: Whurr; 2001.
- Dorey G. Is smoking a cause of erectile dysfunction? A review of the literature. Br J Nurs. 2001;10:455-65.
- Dorey G. Partners' perspective of erectile dysfunction: literature review. Br J Nurs. 2001;10:187-95.
- Dorey G. Pelvic floor exercise for erectile dysfunction. London: Whurr. 2003.
- Dorey G. Pelvic floor exercises after radical prostatectomy. Brit J Nurs. 2013;22(9):S4-6.
- Dorey G. Physiotherapy for male continence problems. Physiotherapy. 1998;85:556-63.
- Dorey G. Physiotherapy for the relief of male lower urinary tract symptoms: a Delphi study. Physiotherapy. 2000;86:413-26.
- Dorey G. Randomised controlled trial of pelvic floor muscle exercises and manometric biofeedback for erectile dysfunction. Br J Gen Pract. 2004;54:819-25.
- Elbadawi A. Pathology and pathophysiology of the detrusor in incontinence. Urol Clin North Am. 1995;22:499-512.
- Elving LB, Foldspang A, Lam GW, et al. Descriptive epidemiology of urinary incontinence in 3,100 women aged 30-59. Scan J Urol Nephrol Suppl. 1989;125:37-43.
- Emberton M, Neal DE, Black N, et al. The effect of prostatectomy on symptom severity and quality of life. Br J Urol. 1996;77:233-47.
- Emmaus PA, Sapsford R, Hodges PW. Contraction of the pelvic floor muscles during abdominal manoeuvres. Arch Phys Med Rehabil. 2001;82:1081-8.
- Fabra M, Porst H. Bulbocavernosus-reflex latencies and pudendal nerve SSEP compared to penile vascular testing in 669 patients with erectile failure and sexual dysfunction. Int J Impot Res. 1999;11:167-75.

- Fall M, Lindstrom S. Electrical stimulation: a physiological approach to the treatment of urinary incontinence. Urol Clin North Am. 1991;18:393-407.
- Fantl JA, Wyman JF, McClish DK, et al. Efficacy of bladder training in order women with urinary incontinence. J Am Med Assoc. 1991;265(5):609-13.
- Fayed L. There are two - internal and external Os. Very well. N.p., n.d. Web. 26 Feb. 2017.
- Feldenkrais M. Awareness thought movement. Health exercises for personal growth. Hammondsworth, UK: Penguin Books; 1977.
- Feldman HA, Goldstein I, Hatzichristou DG, et al. Importance and its medical and psychological correlates: results of the Massachusetts Male Aging Study. J Urol. 1994;151:54-61.
- Feneley RCL. Post-micturition dribbling. In: Mandelstam D (Ed). Incontinence and its Management. London: Croom Helm; 1986.
- FitzGerald MP, Kitarinos R. Rehabilitation of the short pelvic floor: background and patient evaluation. Int Urogynecol J. 2003;14:261-8.
- FitzGerald MP, Kotarinos R. Rehabilitation of the short pelvic floor. Int Urogynecol J. 2003;14:269-75.
- Freidman R. Electrical stimulation effective for urinary incontinence. American Urogynecologic Society. Doctor's Guide. 2002.
- Frewen W. Role of bladder training in the treatment of the unstable bladder in the female. Urol Clin North AM. 1979;6:273-7.
- Ganz PA, Rowland JH, Desmond K, et al. Life after breast cancer: understanding women's health-related quality of life and sexual functioning. J Clin Oncol. 1998;16(2):501-14.
- Gearhart SL, Pannu HK, Cundiff GW, et al. Perineal descent and levator ani hernia: a dynamic magnetic resonance imaging study. Dis Colon Rectum. 2004;47(8):1298-304.
- Gee WF, Ansell JS, Bonica JJ. Pelvic and perineal pain of urologin. In: Bonic JJ (Ed). The Management of Pain, volume 2. Philadelphia: Lea and Febiger, 1990. pp. 1368-94.
- Geirsson G, Fall M. Maximal function electrical stimulation in routine practice. Neurourol Urodyn. 1997;16:559-65.
- Gentile A. Skill acquisition: action, movement and neuromotor processes. In: Carr J, Shepherd R, Gordon J (Eds). Movement science: Foundations for physical therapy in rehabilitation. Rockville, MD: Aspen Systems; 1987.
- Getliffe K, Dolman M. Promoting continence: A clinical and research resource. Oxford, UK; 2007.
- Gibbons JM. Valvar vestibulitis. In: Streege JF, Metzger DA, Levy BS (Eds). Chronic pelvic pain. Philadelphia: WB Saunders; 1998:181-7.
- Gill BC, Kim D. Medscape. (2018). Injectable bulking agents for incontinence. [online]. Available from https://emedicine.medscape.com/article/447068-overview [Accessed January 2019].
- Glazener CM. Sexual function after childbirth: Women's experiences, persistent morbidity, and lack of professional morbidity. BJOG. 1997;104:330-35.
- God's Doodle: The Life and Times of the Penis by Tom Hickman Square Peg, Random House, 2012.
- Gordon D, Groutz A, Sinai T, et al. Sexual function in women attending a urogynecology clinic. Int Urogynecol J Pelvic Floor Dysfunct. 1999;10(5):325-8.
- Gorman MO (2009). Good sex gives women a sense of a higher purpose. Rodale News: Prevention Healthy Living Group. [online]. Available from www.rodale.com/sexual-satisfaction-women?page=0%2C0 [Accessed December 2018].

- Gosling JA, Dixon JS, Critchley HO, et al. A comparative study of the human external sphincter and periurethral levator ani muscle. Br J Urol. 1981;53:35-41.
- Grambert SR. Alcohol abuse: medical effect of heavy drinking in late life. Geriatrics. 1997;52:30-7.
- Gray M. Genitourinary disorders. St. Louis: Mosby Year Book; 1992.
- Gray ML. Neurophysiology of the bladder. [Paper presented at the Fourth National Multispecialty Nursing Conference, Orlando, Florida, 1998].
- Guess M, Connell K, Schrader S, et al. Decreased genital sensation in competitive women cyclists. J Sex Med. 2006;3(6):949-1101.
- Guyton AC. Textbook of Medical Physiology, 7th edition. Philadelphia: Saunders; 1986. pp. 1013-4.
- Hagen S, Stark D, Maher C, et al. Conservative management of pelvic organ prolapse in women. Cochrane Database Syst Rev. 2006;(4):CD003882.
- Handa VL (2003). Report from the 24th Annual Scientific Meeting of the American Urogynecological Society. Medscape Ob/gyn ⊠Women's Health 8:2 [online] Available from www.medscap.com/viewarticle/461719_print [Accessed December 2018].
- Hannestad YS, Rortveit G, Hunskaar S. Help seeking and associated factors in female urinary incontinence: The Norwegian EPINCONT study. Scand J Prim Health Care. 2002;20:102-7.
- Harewood GC, Coulie B, Camilleri M, et al. Descending perineum syndrome: audit of clinical and laboratory feature and outcome of pelvic floor retraining. Am J Gastroenterol. 1999;94(1):126-30.
- Harrison SCW, Abrams P. Bladder Function. In: Sant GR (Ed). Pathophysiologic Principles of Urology. Boston: Blackwell Scientific; 1994. pp. 93-121.
- Haslam J. Biofeedback for the assessment and re-education of the pelvic floor musculature. In: Laycock J, Haslam J (Eds). Therapeutic management of incontinence and pelvic pain. London: Springer-Verlag; 2002. pp. 75-81.
- Haslam J. Evaluation of pelvic floor muscles assessment, digital, manometric and surface electromyography in females [M.Phil. Dissertation]. Manchester: University of Manchester; 1999.
- Haslam J. Physiotherapy: EMG/biofeedback. [Paper presented at the Second International Conference of the Association for Continence Advice, Edinburgh, 1998].
- Hayden LJ. Chronic testicular pain. Aust Fam Phys. 1993;22:1357-65.
- Hay-Smith E, Bo K, Berghmans L, et al. Pelvic floor muscles training for urinary 2003(1):Oxford: Update Software.
- Hay-Smith EJ, Berghmans LC, Hendriks HJ. Pelvic floor muscle training for urinary incontinence in women. Cochrane Database Syst Rev. 2001;(1):CD001407.
- Henry Gray, Warren H. Lewis. Anatomy of the Human Body, 20th edition. Philadelphia: Lea and Febiger; 1918
- Henry M, Parks A, Swash M. The pelvic floor musculature in the descending perineum syndrome. Br J Surg. 1982;69:470-2.
- Hilton P. Urinary incontinence during sexual intercourse: a common, but rarely volunteered, symptom. Br J Obstet Gynaecol. 1988;95(4):377-81.
- Hirakawa S, Hassouna M, Deleon R, et al. The role of combined pelvic floor stimulation and biofeedback in post-prostatectomy urinary incontinence [abstract]. J Urol. 1993;149:235A.
- Hodges PW, Richardson CA. Inefficient muscular stabilization of the lumbar spine associated with low back pain. Spine. 21;22:2640-50.
- Holland JM, Feldman JL, Gilbert HC. Phantom orchialgia. J Urol. 1994;152:2231-3.

- How Deep Is the Average Vagina? New Health Advisor. N.p., 31 July 2015. Web. 26 Feb. 2017.
- http://me./webmd.com/kegel-exercis-treating-male-urinary-incontinence
- http://surgery.arizona.edu/sites/surgery.arizona.edu/files/pdf/Kegel%20Exercises.pdf
- http://urology.ucla.edu/workfiles/prostate_Cancer/Kegel_Exercise_for_Men.pdf
- http://www.fmpe.org/en/documents/handout_ui_exercises.pdf
- http://www.nlm.nih.gov/meslineplus/ency/article/003975.htm
- Hulme JA. Research in geriatric urinary incontinence: pelvic muscle force field. Top Geriatric Rehabil. 2000;16(1):10-21.
- Hutchinson MR, Tremain L, Christiansen J, et al. Improving leaping ability in elite rhythmic gymnasts. Med Sci Sports Exerc. 1998;30(10):1543-7.
- Intili H, Nier D. Self-esteem and depression in men who present with erectile dysfunction. Urol Nurs. 1998;18:185-7.
- Iribarrent IM, de Tejada IS. Vascular physiology of penile. In: Textbook of erectile dysfunction. Oxford: Isis Medical Media; 1999. pp. 141-8.
- Jackson J, Emerson L, Johnston B, et al. Biofeedback: a noninvasive treatment for incontinence after radical prostatectomy. Urol Nurs. 1996;16:50-4.
- Jarrow JP, Nana-Sinkam P, Sabbagh M, et al. Outcome analysis of goal directed therapy for impotence. J Urol. 1996;155:1609-12.
- John D. Pelvic dysfunction in men: diagnosis and treatment of male incontinence and erectile dysfunction by professor grace. US: Wiley and Sons; 2006.
- Jones R. Neuromuscular adaptability: therapeutic implications. J Assoc Physiother Obstet Gynaecol. 1994;75:12-7.
- Jozwik M. The physiological basis of pelvic floor exercises in the treatment of stress urinary incontinence. BJOG. 1998;105:1046-51.
- Kaplan SA, Santarosa RP, D'Alisera PM, et al. Pseudodyssynergia (contraction of the external sphincter during voiding) misdiagnosed as chronic nonbacterial prostatitis and the role of biofeedback as a therapeutic option. J Urol. 1997;157:2234-7.
- Kawanishi Y, Kishimoto T, Kimura K, et al. Spring balance evaluation of the ischiocavernosus muscle. Int J Impot Res. 2001;13(5):294-7.
- Kawanishi Y, Nergi L, Nappi RE, et al. Perineal floor efficiency in sexually potent and impotent men. Int J Impot Rec. 2001;13(5):294-7.
- Kegal AH. Physiologic therapy for urinary incontinence. JAMA. 1951;146:915-7.
- Kegel AH. Progressive resistance exercise in the functional restoration of the perineal muscles. Am J Obstet Gynecol. 1948;56:238-48.
- Kegel AH. The nonsurgical treatment of genital relaxation. West Med Surg. 1948;31:213-6.
- Kegel AH. The physiologic treatment of poor tone and function of the genital muscles and of urinary stress incontinence. West J Surg Obstet Gynecol. 1949;57(11):527-35.
- Kho HG, Sweep CG, Chen X, et al. The use of acupuncture in the treatment of erectile dysfunction. Int J Impot Res. 1999;11:41-8.
- Kincade JE, Dougherty MC, Busby-Whitehead J, et al. Self-monitoring and pelvic floor muscle exercises to treat urinary incontinence. Urol Nurs. 2005;25(5):353-63.
- Kirby R, Carson C, Goldstein I. Anatomy, physiology and pathophysiology. In: Kirby R (Ed). Erectile Dysfunction: A Clinical Guide. Oxford: Isis Medical Media; 1999. pp. 11-28.
- Kirby R. An Atlas of Erectile Dysfunction. New York; The Parthenon Publishing Group; 2004.

- Kisner C, Colby L. Therapeutic exercise: Foundational concepts. In: Kisner C, Colby L (Eds). Therapeutic exercise: Foundation and techniques. Philadelphia: FA Davis Co; 2002. pp. 3-33.
- Klein MC, Gauthier RJ, Robbins JM, et al. Relationship of episiotomy to perineal trauma and morbidity, sexual dysfunction, and pelvic floor relaxation. Am J Obstet Gynecol. 1994;171:591-8.
- Kosch SG, Curry RW Jr, Kuritzky L. Evaluation and treatment of impotence: a pragmatic components. Fam Pract J. 1988;7:162-74.
- Kraemer WJ, Adams K, Cafarelli E, et al. Progression models in resistance training for healthy adults. Med Sci Sports Exerc. 2002;34:364-80.
- Krauss DJ, Lilien OM. Transcutaneous electrical nerve stimulation for stress incontinence. J Urol. 1981;125:790-3.
- Kuncharapu I, Majeroni BA, Johnson DW. Pelvic organ prolapse. Am Fam Physician. 2010;81(9):1111-7.
- La Pera G, Nicastro A. A new treatment for premature ejaculation: the rehabilitation of the pelvic floor. J Sex and Marital Therapy. 1996;22(1):22-6.
- Lake B. Acute back pain. Treatment by the application of Feldenkrais Principles. Aust Fam Physician. 1985;14(11):1175-8.
- Laumann EO, Paik A, Rosen RC. Sexual dysfunction: in the United State: Prevalence and predictors. JAMA. 1999;281:1174.
- Lavoisier P, Courtois F, Barres D, et al. Correlation between intracavernosus and contraction of the ischiocavernosus muscles in man. J Urol. 1986;136:936-9.
- Lawrence WT, Mac Donagh RP. Treatment of urethral stricture disease by internal urethrotomy followed by intermittent "low friction" self-catheterisation. JR Soc Med. 1988;81:136-9.
- Laycock J, Haslam J. Therapeutic management of incontinence and pelvic pain: pelvic organ disorders. Evaluation of Prolapse. London: Springer-Verlag; 2002. p.198.
- Laycock J. Clinical Evaluation of the Pelvic floor in Pelvic Floor Re-education, Principles and Practice. London: Springer Verlag; 1994. pp. 42-8.
- Laycock J. Pelvic floor assessment; the PERFECT scheme. Physiotherapy. 2001;87(12):631-42.
- Laycock J. Pelvic muscles exercises: physiotherapy for the pelvic floor. Urol Nursing. 1994;14:136-40.
- Leaver RB. Cranberry juice. Prof Nurse. 1996;11:525-6.
- LeCraw D, Wolfs S. Electromyographic biofeedback (EMGBF) for neuromuscular relaxation and re-education. In: Gersh M (Ed). Electrotherapy in rehabilitation. Philadelphia: FA Davis Company; 1993:291-327.
- Lewis RW, Mills TM. Risk factors for impotence. In: Carson CC, Kirby RS, Goldstein I (Eds). Textbook of Erectile Dysfunction. Oxford: Isis Medical Media; 1999. pp. 141-8.
- Lien KC, Mooney B, DeLancey JO, et al. Levator ani muscle stretch induced by simulated vaginal birth. Obstet Gynecol. 2004;103:31-40.
- Light JK, Rapoll E, Wheeler TM. The striated urethral sphincter: muscles fiber type and distribution in the prostatic capsule fiber types and distribution in the prostatic capsule. Br J Urol. 1997;79:539-42.
- Lilius HG, Oravisto KJ, Valtonen EJ. Origin of pain in interstitial cystitis. Scand J Urol Nephrol. 1973;7:150-5.
- Luber K, Boero S, Choe J. The demographics of pelvic floor disorders: current observations and future projections. Am J Obstet Gynecol. 2001;184:1496-501.
- Lukban JC, Whitmore KE. Pelvic floor muscle re-education treatment of the overactive bladder and painful blander syndrome. Clin Obstet Gynecol. 2002;45(1):273-85.

- Maatita M, Bhaumik J, Davies AE. Sexual function after using tension-free vaginal tape for the surgical treatment of genuine stress incontinence. BJU Int. 2002;90:540-3.
- Mahajan ST, Elkadry EA, Kenton KS, et al. Patient-centered surgical outcomes: The impact of goal achievement and urge incontinence on patient satisfaction one year after surgery. Am J Obstet Gynecol. 2006;194(3):722-8.
- Mahony DT, LAferte RO, Blais DJ. Integral storage and voiding reflexes. Neurol. 1977;9:95-106.
- Malmgren-Olsson EB, Branholm IB. A comparison between three physiotherapy approaches with regard to health-related factors in patients. Disabil Rehabil. 2002;24(6):308-17.
- Malmsten UGH, Molander I, Norlen LJ. Urinary incontinence and epidemiological study of men aged 45 to 99 years. J Urol. 1997;158:1733-7.
- Mambert-Dias A, Vasavada SP, Bourcier AP. Pelvic floor dysfunction: investigations and conservative treatment. Rome: Casa Editrice Scientifica Internationale; 1993. pp. 303-10.
- Mamberti-Dias A, Bonierbale-Branchereau M. Therapy for dysfunctioning erection: four years later, how do things stand? Sexologique. 1991;1:24-5.
- Mant J, Painter R, Vessey M. Epidemiology of genital prolapse: Observations from the Oxford Family Planning Association Study. Br J Obstet Gynaecol. 1997;104:579-85.
- Marthol H, Hilz MJ. Female sexual dysfunction: a systematic overview of classification, pathophysiology, diagnosis and treatment. Fortschr Neurol Psychiat. 2004;72(3):121-35.
- Mathewson-Chapman M. Pelvic muscle exercise/biofeedback for urinary incontinence after prostatectomy: an education program. J Cancer Educ. 1997;12:218-23.
- Mayo Clinic Staff. (2010b). Uterine Prolapse: Preparing for Your Appointment. Mayo Foundation for medical Education and Research. [online] Available from www.mayoclinic.com/health/Uterine - prolapse/DS00700/DSECTION = preparing - for - your - appointment [Accessed December 2018].
- Mayo Clinic Staff. (2018). Kegel Exercises: A How to Guide for Women. Mayo Foundation for Medical Education and Research. [online]. Available from www.mayoclinic.com/health/kegel-exercises/WO00119 [Accessed December 2018].
- Mayo Clinic. Kegel exercises for men: Understand the benefits. [online]. Available from http://www.mayoclinic.com/health/kegel-exercises-for-men/MY01402 [Accessed January 2019].
- McNevin N, Gabriele W, Carlson C. Effects of attention focus, self-control and dyad training on motor learning: Implications for physical rehabilitation. Phys Ther. 2000;80(4):373-85.
- Meadows E. Treatment for patient with pelvic pain. Urolog Nurse. 1999;19(1):33-5.
- Meaglia JP, Joseph AC, Change M, et al. Postprostatectomy urinary incontinence: response to behavioural training. J Urol. 1990;144:674-6.
- Medical Definition of Vaginal Introitus. MedicineNet. N.p., n.d. Web. 28 Feb. 2017.
- Medical News Today. (2006). Kegel Exercises Reduce Urinary Incontinence in Women, Study Confirms. [online]. Available www.medicalnewstoday.com/erticles/37110.php [Accessed December 2018].
- MedlinePlus
- Mellion MB. Common cycling injuries: management and prevention. Sports Med. 1991;11:52-72.
- Menston CM, Hull E, Levin RJ, et al. Disorders of orgasm in women. J Sex Med. 2004;1(1):66-8.

- Messelink B, Benson T, Berghmans B, et al. Standardization of terminology of pelvic floor muscle function and dysfunction: report from the pelvic floor clinical assessment group of the International Continence Society. Neurourol Urodyn. 2005:24;374-80.
- Meston CM. Validation of the Female Sexual Function Index (FSFI) in women with female orgasmic disorder and in women with hypoactive sexual desire disorder. J Sex Marital Ther. 2003;29(1):39-46.
- Mezey MD, Rauckhorst LH, Stokes SA. Health assessment of the older individual. New York: Springer Publishing Company; 1980.
- Mikhalidis DP, Ganotakis ES, Papadakis ES, et al. Smoking and urological disease. J R Soc Health. 1998;118:210-2.
- Millard RJ. After-dribble. In: Miller RJ (Ed). Bladder control: a simple self-help guide. Sydney: Williams and Wilkins; 1987. pp. 89-90.
- Miller J, Aston-Miller J, DeLancy J. The Knack: Use of precisely-timed pelvic muscle contraction can reduce leakage in SUI. Neurol Urodyn. 1996;15:302-93.
- Miller J, Kasper C, Sampselle C. Review of muscle physiology with application to pelvic muscle exercise. Urol Nurs. 1994;14(3):92-7.
- Miller JM, Perucchini D, Carchild L, et al. Pelvic floor muscle contraction during a cough and decreased vesical neck mobility. Obstet Gynecol. 2001;97(2):255-60.
- Miller JM. Criteria for therapeutic use of pelvic floor muscle training in women. JWOCN. 2002;29(6):301-11.
- Miodrag A, Castleaden CM, Vallance TR. Sex hormones and the female urinary tract. Drugs. 1988;36:491-504.
- Moen DV. Observation on the effectiveness of cranberry juice in urinary infection. Wis Med J. 1962;61:282-3.
- Moller LA, Lose G, Jorgensen T. The prevalence and bothersomeness of lower urinary tract symptoms in women 40-60 years age. Acta Obstet Gynecol Scand. 2000;79:298-305.
- Moore H. Caffeine Which? [London]. 1990;314-7.
- Moore KN, Dorey G. Conservative treatment of urinary in men: a review of the literature. Physiother. 1999;85:77-87.
- Moore KN, Griffiths DJ, Hughton A. A randomized controlled trial comparing pelvic muscles exercises with pelvic muscles exercise plus electrical stimulation for the treatment of post-prostatectomy urinary incontinence. Br J Urol. 1999;83:57-65.
- Muller N. Keeping the vital pelvic floor healthy. J Active Aging. 2005:34-6.
- Muller N. What American understand and how they are affected by bladder control problems: Highlights of recent nationwide consumer research. Urologic Nurs. 2005;25(2):109-15.
- Muller N. What Americans understand. 2005.
- Munarriz R, Kim NN, Goldstein I, et al. Biology of female sexual function. Urol Clin N Am. 2002;29:685-93.
- National Association for Continence. www.nafc.org/media/media kit/facts - statistics.
- National Institute of Diabetes and Digestive and Kidney Diseases. Urinary incontinence in women. NIH Publication. 2007;8(4132):3.
- National Institute of Health, Medline Plus. (2010). Orgasmic dysfunction. [online]. Available from www.nlm.nih.gov/medlineplus/ency/article/001953.htm [Accessed December 2018].
- National Institute of Health, Medline Plus. (2011). Urge incontinence. [online]. Available from www.nm.nih.gov/medlineplus/ency/article/001270.htm [Accessed December 2018].

- National Institute of Health, Medline Plus. Causes of sexual dysfunction. [online]. Available from www.nlm.nih.gov/medlineplus/femalesexualdysfunction.htm [Accessed January 2019].
- National Institute of Health, Medline Plus. Urinary incontinence. [online] Available from www.nlm.nih.gov/medlineplus/urinaryincontinence.html [Accessed January 2019].
- National Institutes of Health (NIH) Consensus Conference. Impotence. NIH Consensus Development Panel on Impotence. JAMA. 1993;270:83-90.
- National Institutes of Health State-of-the-Science Conference Statement: Prevention of fecal and urinary incontinence in adults. Ann Intern Med. 2008;148(6):449-58.
- National Kidney and Urologic Diseases Clearinghouse. www.kidney.niddk.nih.gov/kudiseases/pubs/uiwomen/index.htm
- National Library of Medicine
- National Statistics office. Globoscan: cancer incidence and prevalence worldwide. London: National Statistics Office; 2000.
- Nayan W, Schwarzern U, Klotz T, et al. Transcutaneous pelvic oxygen pressure during bicycling. BJU Int. 1999;83:623-5.
- Neal DE. The national prostatectomy audit. Br J Urol. 1997;79:69-75.
- Neumann P, Gill V. Pelvic floor and abdominal muscle interaction: EMG activity and intra-abdominal pressure. Int Urogynecol J. 2002;13:125-32.
- Newman DK. Behavioral treatment. In: Vasavada SP, Appell RA, Sand PK (Eds). Female urology. Urogynecology and voiding dysfunction. New York: Marcel Dekker. pp. 233-66.
- Newman DK. Clinical Manual for Pelvic Muscle Rehabilitation. Dover, NH. Prometheus, Inc; 2003. pp. 89-98.
- Newman DK. Managing and treating urinary incontinence. Baltimore: Health Professions Press; 2002:79-110.
- Newman DK. The Urinary Incontinence Sourcebook, 2nd edition. Los Angeles: Lowell House; 1999.
- Nicholson D. Teaching psychomotor skills. In: Shepard KF, Jensen GM (Eds). Handbook of Teaching for Physical therapists. Boston: Butterworth-Heinemann; 1997. p. 271.
- Noblett KL, Jeansen JK, Ostergard DR. The relationship of body mass index to intra-abdominal pressure as measured by multichannel cystometry. Int Urogynecol J Pelvic Floor Dysfunct. 1997;8:323-6.
- North American Menopause Society. www.menopause.org.
- Nygaard I, Bradley C, Brandt D; Women's Health Initiative. Pelvic organ prolapse in older women: Prevalence and risk factors. Obstet Gynecol. 2004;104:489-97.
- Nygaard I, Milburn A. Urinary incontinence during sexual activity: prevalence in a gynaecologic practice. J Women's Health. 1995;4(1):83-6.
- Nygaard IE. Nonoperative management of urinary incontinence. Curr Opin Obstet Gynecol. 1996;8:15.
- O'Connell HE, Sanjeevan KV, Hustson JM. Anatomy of the clitoris. J Urol. 2005;174(1):1189-95.
- O'Farrell TJ, Kleinke CL, Cutter HS. Sexual adjustment of male alcoholic: changes from before to after receiving alcoholism counseling with and without marital therapy. Addict Behav. 1998;23:419-25.
- Olsen AL, Smith VJ, Bergstrom JO, et al. Epidemiology of surgically managed pelvic organ prolapse and urinary incontinence. Obstet Gynecol. 1997;89:501-6.

- Oyama IA, Rejba A, Lukban JC, et al. Modified Thiele massage as therapeutic intervention for female patients with interstitial cystitis and high-tone pelvic floor dysfunction. Urol. 2004;64(5):862-5.
- Paddison K. Complying with pelvic floor exercises: A literature review. Nurs Stand. 2002;16(39):33-8.
- Park JM, Bloom DA, McGuire EJ. The Guarding reflex revisited. Br J Urol. 1997;80:940-5.
- Parks AG, Porter NM, Hardcastet JD. The syndrome of the descending perineum. Proc Royal Soc Med. 1966;59:477-82.
- Pastore AL, Palleschi G, Leto A, et al. A prospective randomized study to compare pelvic floor rehabilitation and dapoxetine for lifelong premature ejaculation. Int J Androl. 2012;35:528-33.
- Paterson J, Pinnock CB, Marshall VR. Pelvic floor exercises as a treatment for post-micturition dribble. Br J Urol. 1997;7:892-7.
- Pauker-Sharon Y, Arbel Y, Finkelstein A, et al. Cardiovascular risk factors in men with ischemic heart disease and erectile dysfunction (Editorial comment by Jacob Rajfer). Urology. 2013;82:377-81.
- Pauls RN, Berman JR. Impact of pelvic floor disorders and prolapsed on female sexual function and response. Urol Clin N Am. 2002;29:677-83.
- Peschers U, Gingelmaier A, Jundt K, et al. Evaluation of pelvic floor muscle strength using four different techniques. Int Urogynecol J Pelvic Floor Dysfunct. 2001;12:27-30.
- Peschers UM, DeLancey JOL. Anatomy. In: Laycock J, Haslam J (Eds). Therapeutic Management of Incontinence and Pelvic Pain. London: Springer Verlag; 2002. pp. 7-16.
- Phillips NA. Female sexual dysfunction: evaluation and treatment. Am Fam Physician. 2000;62(1):127-36.
- Pinnock CB, Stapleton AM, Marshall VR. Erectile dysfunction in the community: a prevalence study. Med J Aust. 1999;171:353-7.
- Planned Parenthood. "What is virginity and the hymen? | Losing your virginity." What is Virginity and the Hymen? N.p., 30 Nov. 2015. Web. 14 Feb. 2017.
- Plevnik S. New method for testing and strengthening of pelvic floor muscles. In: 15th Annual Meeting of the International Continence Society. London: ICS; 1988:95-1049.
- Pomfret I. Male incontinence. Community Outlook. 1993;45.
- Porru D, Campus GA, Madeddu G, et al. Impact of early pelvic floor rehabilitation after transurethral resection of the prostate. Neurourol Urodyn. 2001;20:53-9.
- Portman D, Gass M. Genitourinary syndrome of menopause: new terminology for vulvovaginal atrophy from the International Society for the Study of Women's Sexual Health and the North American Menopause Society. Menopause. 2014;21:1063-8.
- Pregnancy and Signs of Labor. WebMD, 28 Nov. 2016.
- Prota C, Gomes CM, Ribiero LHS, et al. Early postoperative pelvic-floor biofeedback improves erectile function in men undergoing radical prostatectomy: a prospective, randomized, controlled trial. Int J Impot Res. 2012;24:174-8.
- Rapp DE, Kobashi KC. Mid-urethral slings: Techniques and outcomes. Urology Times – Clinical Edition. 2008.
- References FOR FSFI
- Resnick MI. Carcinoma of the prostate. In: Resnick MI, Caldamone AA Spirnak JP (Eds). Decision making in urology, 2nd edition. Philadelphia: Decker; 1991. pp. 114-5.
- Ribiero LH, Prota C, Gomes CM, et al. Long-term effect of early postoperative pelvic floor biofeedback on continence in men undergoing radical prostatectomy: a prospective, randomized, controlled trial. J Urol. 2010;184:1034-9.

- Richardson A. The anatomic defects in rectocele and enterocele. J Pelvic Surg. 1995;4:214-21.
- Rittweger J, Beller G, Felsenberg D. Acute physiological effects of exhaustive whole-body vibration exercise in man. Clin Physiol. 2000;20:134-42.
- Rittweger J, Just K, et al. Treatment of chronic lower back pain with lumber extension and whole-body vibration exercise – a randomized controlled trial. Spine. 2002;27:1829-34.
- Rivalta M, Sighinolfi MC, De Stefani S, et al. Biofeedback, electrical stimulation, pelvic floor muscle exercises, and vaginal cones: A combined rehabilitative approach for sexual dysfunction associated with urinary incontinence. J Sex Med. 2009;6(6):1674-7.
- Rochera MB. Physiotherapy in treating sexual pain disorders in women: A systematic review. Sci Res. 2016;6(3):26-32.
- Roges J. Pass the cranberry juice. Nurs Times. 1994;87:36-7.
- Romanzi L, Polaneczky M, Glazer HI, et al. Simple test of Pelvic muscle contraction during pelvic examination: correlation to surface electromyography. Neurourol Urodyn. 1999;38(3):134-8.
- Rortveit G, Brown JS, Thom DH, et al. Symptomatic pelvic organ prolapse: Prevalence and risk factors in a population-based, racially diverse cohort. Obstet Gynecol. 2007;109:1396-403.
- Rosen R, Brown C, Heiman J, et al. The Female Sexual Function Index (FSFI): a multidimensional self-report instrument for the assessment of female sexual function. J Sex Marital Ther. 2000;26(2):191-208.
- Rosenbaum TY. Pelvic floor involvement in male and female sexual dysfunction and the role of pelvic floor rehabilitation in treatment: a literature review. J Sex Med. 2007;4:4-13.
- Rosenbaum TY. The role of physical therapy in female sexual dysfunction. Curr Sex Health Rep. 2008;5:97-101.
- Rubin C, Recket R, Cullen D, et al. Prevention of bone loss in a post-menopausal population by low level biomechanical intervention. Bone Min Res. 1998;23:1126.
- Rubin C, Turner AS, Bain S, et al. Anabolism. Low mechanical signals strengthen long bones. Nature. 2001;412:603-4.
- Salonia A, Munarriz RM, Naspro R, et al. Women's sexual dysfunction: a pathological review. BJU Int. 2004;93:1156-64.
- Salonia A, Zanni G, Nappi RE, et al. Sexual dysfunction is common in women with lower urinary tract symptoms and urinary incontinence: Results of a cross-sectional study. Europ Urol. 2004;45:642-8.
- Samples JT, Dougherty MC, Abrams RM, et al. The dynamic characteristics of the circumvaginal muscles. JOGNN. 1988;17(3):194-201.
- Sampselle CM, Brink CA, Wells TJ. Digital measurement of the pelvic muscles strength in childbearing women. Nursing Research. 1989;38(3):134-8.
- Samuelson EC, Victor FT, Tibblin G, et al. Signs of genital prolapse in a Swedish population of women 20 to 59 years of age and possible related factors. Am J Obset Gynecol. 1999;180:299-305.
- Sant GR, Long JP. Benign prostatic hyperplasia. In: Sant GR (Ed). Pathophysiologic principles of urology. Oxford: Blackwell Scientific; 1994. pp. 123-54.
- Sapsford R, Kelly S, Pilates CR. The pelvic floor. Abstract Physiotherapy Conference; 2004.
- Sapsford R. Pilates and the pelvic floor. Proceedings, 2nd Biennal Excellence Down-under. School of Physiotherapy, University of Melbourne, Australia; 2005.
- Sapsford R. The pelvic floor. A clinical model for function and rehabilitation. Physiotherapy. 2001;87:620-30.

- Schouman M, Lacroix P. Apport de la re-educationa pelvic-perineale au traitment des fuites veino-caverneuses. Ann Urol. 1991;25:92-3.
- Schussler B. Radiological evaluation of the pelvic floor and viscera. In: Schussler B, Laycock J, Norton P, Stanton S (Eds). Pelvic floor reduction: Principles and practices. London: Springer-Verlag; 1994:75-82.
- Segura JW, Opitz JL, Greene LF. Prostatosis, prostatitis or pelvic floor tension myalgia? J Urol. 1979;122:168-9.
- Sexuality Information and Education Council of the United States. www.siecus.org.
- Shafik A, El-Sibai O. Study of the pelvic floor muscles in vaginismus: a concept of pathogenesis. Eur J Obstet Gynecol Reprod Biol. 2002;10:105(1):67-70.
- Shafik A. The role of the levator ani muscle in evacuation, sexual performance, and pelvic floor disorders. Int Urogynecol J Pelvic Floor Dysfunction. 2000;11:361-76.
- Shaw C. A systematic review of the literature on the prevalence of sexual impairment in women with urinary incontinence and the prevalence of urinary leakage during sexual activity. Eur Urol. 2002;42:432-40.
- Shelly B, Knight S, King P, et al. Treatment of pelvic pain In: Laycock J (Eds). Therapeutic management of incontinence and pelvic pain. London: Springer-Verlag; 2002. pp. 177-89.
- Shepherd AM, Montgomery E, Anderson RS. Treatment of genuine stress incontinence with a new perineometer. Physiotherapy. 1983;69:13.
- Siegel AL. Pelvic floor training in males: practical applications. Urology. 2014;84:1-7.
- Simpson RJ, Fisher W, Lee AJ, et al. Benign prostatic hyperplasia in an unselected community-based population: a survey of urinary symptoms, bothersomeness and prostatic enlargement. Br J Urol. 1996;77:786-91.
- Singh NP, Sharp A, Ferro MA. Pulsed Short-wave therapy for chronic prostatitis [abstract]. Br J Urol. 1997;79(Suppl 4):69.
- Siroky MB. Electromyography of the perineal floor. Urol Clin North Am. 1996;23:299-307.
- Smith ARB, Hosker GL, Warrell DW. The role of partial denervation of the pelvic floor in the aetiology of genitourinary prolapsed and stress incontinence of urine. A neurophysiological study. Br J Obstet Gynaecol. 1989;96(1):24-8.
- Society for Sex Therapy and Research. www.sstarnet.org.
- Society for the Scientific Study of Sexuality. www.sexscience.org.
- Sotiropoulos A, Yeaw S, Lattmer JK. Management of urinary incontinence with electronic stimulation: observations and results. J Urol. 1976;116:747-50.
- Spence-Jones C, Kamm M, Henry M, et al. Bowel dysfunction: a pathogenic factor in uterovaginal prolapse and urinary stress in utero. Br J Obstet Gynaecol. 1994;101(2):147-52.
- Stewart WF, Van Rooyen JB, Cundiff GW, et al. Prevalence and burden of overactive bladder in the United States. World J Urol. 2003;20:327-36.
- Stief WE, Noack T, Djamilian MH, et al. Functional electromyostimulation of the penile corpus cavernosum (FEMCC): initial results of a new therapeutic option of erectile dysfunction. Urologe A. 1996;35:321-5.
- Stoddard H, Donvon J, Whitley E, et al. Urinary incontinence in older people in the community: A neglected problem? Br J Ger Pract. 2001;51:548-52.
- Subak LL, Brubaker L, Chai TC, et al. Urinary incontinence treatment network. High costs of urinary incontinence among women electing surgery to treat stress incontinence. Obstet Gynecol. 2008;1111(4):907.
- Subak LL, Van Den Eeden S, Thom D, et al. Reproductive Risks for Incontinence Study at Kaiser (RRISK) Research Group. Urinary incontinence in women: Direct costs of routine care. Am J Obstet Gynecol. 2007;197:1-9.

- Subak LL, Wing R, West DS, et al. Weight loss to treat urinary incontinence in overweight and obese women. N Engl J Med. 2009;360(5):481-90.
- Swift S, Woodman P, O'Boyle A, et al. Pelvic Organ Support Study (POSST): The distribution, clinical definition, and epidemiologic condition of pelvic organ support defects. Am J Gynecol. 2005;192:795-806.
- Tan RS, Philip PS. Perceptions of and risk factors for andropause. Arch Androl. 1999;43:227-33.
- Theofrastous JP, Wyman JF, Bump RC, et al. Effects of pelvic floor muscle training on strength and predictors of response in the treatment of urinary incontinence in women. Neurourol Urodyn. 2002;21:486-90.
- Thomas TM, Plymat KR, Blannin J, et al. The prevalence of urinary incontinence. Br Med J. 1980;281:1243-5.
- Thompson J, Briffa K, Court S. The comparison between transperineal and transabdominal ultrasound in the assessment of women performing pelvic floor exercises. In: Continence Foundation of Australia (CFA) 12th National Conference. Sydney: CFA; 2003:39.
- Tindall B, Torpy JM. Women's sexual concerns after menopause. JAMA. 2007;297(6):664.
- Tobani L, Fantl JA. Urinary incontinence in women and the use of bladder training for its management. Mature Medicine. 1999:90-3.
- Torvinen S, Kannu P, Sievanen H, et al. Effect of a vibration exposure on muscular performance and body balance. Randomized cross-over study. Clin Physiol Funct Imaging. 2002;81:449-54.
- Trinkaus M, Chin S, Wolfman W, et al. Should urogenital atrophy in breast cancer survivors be treated with topical estrogens? The Oncologist. 2018;13(3):222-31.
- Turner LA, Althof SE, Levine SB, et al. Twelve-month comparison of two treatments for erectile dysfunction: self-injection versus external vacuum devices. Urology. 1992;39:139-44.
- US News (2011). Brigham and Women's Hospital. 2011. Urinary Incontinence. [online]. Available from https://health.usnews.com/health-conditions/urology/urinary-incontinence/links [Accessed December 2018].
- Van Arsdalen, KA. In: Hanno, PM, Malkowicz SB, Wein AJ (Eds). Clinical Manual of Urology, 3rd edition. New York: McGraw Hill Co.; 2001. pp. 49-86.
- Van der Velde J, Everaerd W. Voluntary control over pelvic floor muscles in women with and without vaginismus. Int Urogynecol J. 1999;10:230-6.
- Van Kampen M, De Weerdt W, Claes H, et al. Treatment of erectile dysfunction by perineal exercise, electromyographic biofeedback, and electrical stimulation. Phys Ther. 2003;83(6):536-43.
- Van Kampen M. Male incontinence and importance [Ph.D dissertation]. Louvain; 1998.
- Viereck V, Peschers U, Singer M, et al. Metrische Quatifizierung des weiblichen Genitalprolapses: Eine Sinnvolle Neuerung in der Prolapsdiagnostik? GebusrtshFrauenheik. 1997;57:177-82.
- Wahl LM, Blandau RJ, Page RC. Effect of hormones in the public symphysis ligament of the guinea pig. Endocrinol. 1977;100:571-9.
- Walters MD, Taylor S, Schoentfeld LS. Psychosexual study of women with detrusor instability. Obstet Gynecol. 1990;75:22-6.
- Waterstone M, Wolfe C, Hooper R, et al. Postnatal morbidity after childbirth and severe obstetric morbidity. BJOG. 2003;110:128-33.
- Wein AL, Kavoussi LR, Nivick AC, Partin AW, Peters CA. Campbell-Walsh, Urology, 9th edition. US: Saunders; 2007.

- Wein AL, Kavoussi LR, Nivick AC, Partin AW, Peters CA. Campbell-Walsh, Urology, 10th edition. US: Saunders; 2012.
- Weiss JM. Pelvic floor myofascial trigger points: manual therapy for interstitial cystitis and the urgency-frequency syndrome. J Urol. 2001;166(6):2226-31.
- Weiss JP, Stember DS, Blaivas JG, et al. Nocturial in adults: classification and etiology. Neurourol Urodyn. 1998;17:467-72.
- Wells TJ. Additional treatments for urinary nocturia incontinence. Top Geriatr Rehabil. 1988;3:48-57.
- Wespes E, Nogueira MC, Herbaut AG, et al. Role of the bulbocavernosus muscles on the mechanism of human erection. Eur Urol. 1990;18:45-8.
- Wesselmann U, Burnnett AL, Heinberg LJ. The urogenital and rectal pain syndromes. Pain. 1997;73:269-94.
- Weston LC. (2008). Can't orgasm? Here's help for women. WebMD the Magazine (March–April). [online]. Available from www. webmd.com/sex-relationships/features/cant - orgasm - here - for – women [Accessed December 2018].
- Whitmore K, Kellog-Spradt S, Fletcher E. Comprehensive assessment of pelvic floor dysfunction. Issues in Incontinence. 1998:1-10.
- Willams G. Editorial comment. BJU Int. 2000;86:6.
- Willans A. The role of pelvic floor muscle exercise in the treatment of female sexual dysfunction. J Assoc Chart Physiother Women's Health, Autumn. 2014;115:22-9.
- Wise D, Anderson RU. A Headache in the Pelvis: A New Understanding and Treatment for Chronic Pelvic Pain Syndromes, 6th edition. National Center for Pelvic Pain Research; 2012.
- World Health Organization. (2003). World cancer report.
- Worth AM, Dougherty MC, McKey PL. Development and testing of the circumvaginal muscles rating scale. Nurs Res. 1986;35(3):166-8.
- Wurn LJ, Wurn BF, King CR, et al. Increasing orgasm and decreasing dyspareunia by manual physical therapy technique. MedGenMed. 2004;6:47.
- Wyman JF, Fantl JA, McClish DK, et al. Comparative efficacy of behavioral interventions in the management of female urinary incontinence. Am J Obstet Gynecol. 1998;179:999-1007.
- Wyman JF, Fantl JA. Bladder training in ambulatory care management of urinary incontinence. Urol Nurs. 1991;11:11-7.

Index

Page numbers followed by *b* refer to box, *f* refer to figure, and *t* refer to table.

A

Abdominal pain 93
Abdominal pressure 93
Abdominal surgeries 29
Accessory muscles 194
Adcirca 265
Adductor 30
    magnus 154
    stretch, integrated 279
Aginal flatulence 78
Alcock's canal 157
Alcohol abuse 164
Allergy 68
Alpha-blockers 293
American Academy of Family Physician 85
American Physical Therapy Association 23, 53, 149
American Psychiatric Association 176
    classification 108
American Urogynecologic Society 86
Anal canal 3, 10*f*
Anal sphincter 11, 15, 160, 168
Anal structures 10*f*
Anal wink test 151
Androgen therapy 274
Anismus 65, 289
Anorectal rehabilitation 295
Antibiotics 290
Antidepressants 29
Anus 11
    opening 14
    winks 51
Anxiety 82, 176
Arousal
    and lubrication 106
    and sensations, reduced 282
    disorders 108
Atrophic vaginitis 82
Auditory cues 224
Autoimmune disorders 68
Automatic defibrillator 201
Avanafil 265

B

Back pain prenatal 29
Bacterial infections 201
Bacterial prostatitis 159
Bariatric pelvic floor rehabilitation 302
Bartholin's gland 67, 100, 105, 106
Basson classification 108, 108b
Bed-wetting 178*f*, 301
Behavioral therapy 293
Biofeedback
    devices 196
    treatment 279
    types of 197, 198
Birth trauma 29
Birth weight 29
Bladder 3, 4*f*, 17, 125, 175, 229
    contractility, impaired 82
    diary 81
    drying agents 29
    emptying, incomplete 297
    fullness, sensation of 84
    function of 4
    functional capacity of 4
    health sample assessment 32
    incomplete emptying of 69
    neck 3
    pain 229
    reflex 5, 82
    suspensions 29
    syndrome, painful 68
    trauma 68
    wall
        chronic inflammation of 68
        severe inflammation of 68
Bloating 229
Blood supply 17, 136
BO intensive protocol 185
Body aches 157
Bony landmarks 30

Botulinum toxin 288
Bowel 229
   control
      pelvic floor muscles in 137
      reduced 163
   dysfunction 168
   impaction 84
Breast cancer 301
Bridge stretch, integrated full 241
Broad ligament 17
Bulbocavernosus
   contraction of 104
   muscle 15, 76, 114, 134, 150, 162
   reflex 104, 152
Bulbospongiosus 14, 15, 134
Bulbourethral glands 130
Burns 23, 201

C

Cancer 201
Cantienica 189, 190
Cardilology 302
Cardinal ligament 9
Cardiovascular diseases 201
Care, plan of 27
Ceftriaxone 289
Central nervous system 82
Central precocious puberty 24
Cervicopexy 293
Cervix 8, 100, 105
Cesarean section 66
   planed 22, 74, 77
Chemotherapy 116
Childbirth 22
Cialis 265
Clitoral
   details 104f
   glans 11, 102, 103
   hood 11, 102, 103
   shaft 102, 104
   structures of 102, 103f
Clitoris 14, 102
Coccydynia 65, 246, 288
Coccygeus 16, 30, 154
   muscle 16, 136
Coccygeus-levator spasm syndrome 67
Coccygodynia 232
Coccyx, transrectal traction of 233, 247, 279

Coital activity
   after 48, 221
   before 48, 221
Cold therapy 198
Colitis 108
Collagen diseases, active 201
Colorectal pelvic floor rehabilitation 302
Colpoperineorrhaphy 292
Colporrhaphy, anterior 292
Colposuspension 291
Combined dysfunction 141
Complete relaxation training 235
Condom cryotherapy 279
Connective tissue
   assessment 30
   manipulation 199, 230
Conservative therapy 291
Constipation 28, 69, 229, 290
   unspecified 297
Contracted muscles 59f
Core muscles, weakness of 108
Corporal veno-occlusive mechanism 165
Corpus cavernosa 102, 104
Corpus luteum 9
Corticosteroids 288
Cough
   allergies, sneezing 28
   reflex 5
Cowper's glands 130
Crescent stretch, integrated 239
Crohn's disease 69, 290
   surgery for 290
Crura 102, 104
Cryotherapy 230, 234
Cystitis 82, 108
Cystocele 24, 84, 89, 90f, 292
   lateral 297
Cysts 29

D

Daily living, activities of 28, 190
Danazol 289
Deep breathing exercise 190, 235
Deep frog stretch, integrated 238
Deep lean backstretch 237
Deep squat stretch 237
Deep tissue release 199, 230
Deep transverse perineal muscle 15, 135

Defecation
 difficulty in 94
 urgency of 94
Dehydrated vaginal tissues 67
Deliveries, type of 29
Depression 176
Detrusor muscles 82
 hypotonicity of 84
Detrusor overactivity 82
Detrusor sphincter dyssynergia 297
Diabetes 23, 301
 mellitus 84
Diagnostic tests 30
Diastasis recti 297
Digitation 94
Direct trauma 108
Disuse atrophy 23
Diuretics 29
Diurnal enuresis 177
Diurnal frequency 94
Doctors, benefits for 214
Dog stretch, integrated downward 239
Doxycycline 289
Ductus deferens 128, 130
Dysfunctional voiding 297
Dyspareunia 49, 64, 69, 89, 90, 91, 93, 94, 107, 108, 110, 229, 279, 281, 297
Dysuria 229

E

Eczema 201
Ejaculation
 delay 293
 female 105
Ejaculatory duct 130
Elastic vaginal tissues, less 67
Elasticity 5
Electrical stimulation 196, 230
 internal 230, 234
Electrodes placement 196f
Electromyography 30, 42, 196, 287
 assessment 59
 biofeedback 197, 234
 screen 234f
Electrotherapy modalities 196, 230
Elevator opening relaxation 235
Emergency cesarean section 22, 74, 77
Encopresis 178
 incidence of 178
 rehabilitation 301

Endometriosis 25, 66, 66f, 67f, 108, 289
Endometrium 7, 8
Endopelvic fascia 16
Endurance 59, 251
 protocol 209
 training 269
Enterocele 24, 89, 91, 91f, 292
Enuresis 176, 177, 301
 causes of 177
 continues 177
 incidence of 176
 types of 176, 177, 177b
Epididymis 128
Episiotomy 29, 51, 74, 76, 108
 painful 297
Erectile dysfunction 133, 136, 141, 144, 162, 163, 164, 201, 293, 295, 297, 301
 causes of 164
 classification of 166
 prevention of 261
 rehabilitation for 261
 treatment 265
Erectile functioning 145
Erectile tissue 130
Erection
 biomechanics of 165
 step by step mechanism of 165
Estrogen therapy 274
Excursion 51
Exercise 191, 229, 254, 256, 257
 training 235
External genitalia, female 101f

F

Fallopian tube 9, 9f, 17, 100
Fascial restrictions 30
Febrile condition 201
Fecal incontinence 28, 90
Feldenkrais method 189
Female organ, anatomy of 86f
Female pelvis, midsaggital section of 11f
Female sex health 113, 115-118
Female sexual
 desire 115
 dysfunction 99, 107, 108, 108b, 115, 116, 121, 212, 281, 282
 causes of 107
 rehabilitation 300

function 34, 37
    index 28, 113, 212
    health
        disorder 99
        dysfunction rehabilitation 275
Female sexuality 99
Fibroids 29
Fibrous tissue, abnormal bands of 67
Filling phase 6
Fimbriae 9
Finger test 42
First sensation 6
Fissures 69
Fistula 77
Fit pelvic floor 23*f*
Fitness 183
Flaccid-erect penis 165*f*
Flibanserin 274
Forceps 29
Fothergill operation 292
Friedreich's criteria 67

G

Garage door syndrome 82
Gastrointestinal-bowel dysfunctions 28
Genital hiatus 197
Genital organs
    anatomy of female external 100*f*
    female 100*f*
    thick male 23
Genital pain 157
Genitalia
    external 12*f*
    female 100
Genito-pelvic pain 108
Genitourinary organ 130
Genuine incontinence, grades of 81
Genuine stress incontinence 80, 291
Gestrinone 289
Glazer's pelvic floor rehabilitation protocol 278
Glazer's protocol 118, 209, 229, 230, 282
Gluteals 154
Gluteus maximus 14, 15
Gonadotropin-releasing hormone 289
Grafenberg spot 105
G-spo*t*, location of 106*f*
Gynecologic and breast cancers 115
Gynecological cancer 116
Gynecological history 29
Gynecological surgeries 29, 299

H

Hemorrhoids 28
Hamstring 30
    muscle stretch, integrated 279
Happy baby pose 236
Health Care Policy and Research 206
Healthcare providers, benefits for 214
Healthy sexual function 273
Heat therapy 198, 230
Hemorrhoids 69
    muscle 65, 94, 288
Het's BC protocol for male 269
Het's classification 24
Het's exercise protocol 243, 243*b*, 253
Het's female sexual function scale 34, 37
    interpretation of 40
Het's functional grade 46
Het's goal setting scale 251
Het's male sexual function scale, interpretation of 148
Het's manual muscle testing 30, 31, 42, 43
    grade 43, 45
    scale 45
Het's pelvic floor muscle 245*f*
    goals scale 244, 250
Het's protocol 229, 253, 254, 256, 257
Het's provider protection guidelines 296
Het's reflexive result scale 60, 177*t*, 252*t*
Het's rehabilitation protocol 244*b*
Het's relaxation protocol 229, 242
Het's ring
    clock assessment 55
    side section of 57*f*, 153*f*
Het's scale 268
Het's self test 42
Het's SERF assessment scale 59
Het's ultimate goal 59
High voltage galvanic stimulation 288
Hip adductors, integrated stretching of 236
Hold back gas 193
Hold time trainer 209

Holding technique 281
Holmium laser ablation of prostate 294
Home exercise plan 199
Home Exercise Program 191
Hormonal status 29
Hormone replacement therapy 29
Hot bath 230
Human papillomavirus 29
Hymen 11, 102, 105
Hyperactivity disorder, attention deficit 178
Hypermobile urethra 83
Hyper-reflexia 82
Hypertonic pelvic floor muscles 110
Hypertonous pelvic floor dysfunction 24
Hypertonus 24, 140, 141, 194, 201, 296
   conditions 200, 245, 268
   dysfunction 23, 141
Hypertonus muscle 121
   rehabilitation of 228
Hypertonus pelvic floor
   dysfunction 23f, 64, 156, 243b, 244b
   muscle 69, 121, 228, 229t, 277
      rehabilitation 243
Hypertrophy 192
   protocol 209
Hypotonus 140, 201, 296
   conditions 200
   dysfunction 23, 141, 163
   muscle 121, 242
Hypotonus pelvic floor
   dysfunction 23f, 24f, 72, 162
   muscle 73, 109, 118, 121
      causes of 73
      vagina-fit 47t
Hysterectomy 29, 108

I

Iliac spine
   level of anterior superior 30
   posterior superior 30
Iliococcygeus muscle 15, 16, 136, 243
Iliopsoas 236
   integrated 279
Incontinence during sex 94
Incontinence rehabilitation 298
Incoordination dysfunction 24, 141
Infections 48, 221
Infertility 279
Inflammation, acute 201
Inflammatory bowel disease 69, 290
Inflammatory conditions, chronic 108
Institute of Pelvic Floor Research Rehab and Education 214
Integrated stretching exercise 235, 236, 279
Intercourse 48, 221
   painful 87
Interferential therapy 198, 230, 233
International Continence Society 80, 196
Interstitial cystitis 25, 68, 290, 297
Intra-abdominal pressure 51
Intrauterine device 48, 201, 221
Intravaginal electrical stimulation 234
Intravaginal myofascial release 279
Introitus 102
Irritable bowel 28
   syndrome 25, 70, 108, 290
Ischemic compression technique 230, 231
Ischiocavernosus 134
   create penile erection 166
   muscle 14, 15, 114, 135, 150, 162

J

Joint mobilization 199, 230
JV Maigne's technique 279, 233, 247

K

Kegel's exercise 143, 185, 292
Kegel's training and protocols 185
Kelly's cystourethroplasty 292
Kidney 3, 201
Knack technique 267

L

Labia
   majora 11, 101
   minora 11, 101, 102, 105
Labor 22
   duration of 29
Laparoscopic surgery 29
Laparoscopic uterosacral nerve ablation 289
Laparoscopy 108
Laser therapy 294

Laxity-hypotonus 37
Laycock protocol 185
Laycock quantitative assessment scale 61, 154
Lefort's colpocleisis 293
Levator ani 16, 68, 243
   muscle 15
   stretch to 247
   syndrome 65, 288, 297
Levator prostate 136
Lifestyle modifications 274, 279
Lift penis 193
Lift testicles 193
Ligaments 17, 297
Liver failure 201
Local anesthetic injections 288
Lordosis kyphosis 42, 149
Love muscle 112
Low back pain 229, 297
Low self-confidence 176
Low self-esteem 176
Lower abdominal wall pain 229
Lower back pain 157
Lower estrogen level 116
Lower urinary tract 125
   infection 48, 221
Lumbar lordosis, increased 42, 149
Lumbar spine 30
Lumbopelvic junction 28
Lumbopelvic mobility 30
Lumbopelvic stretch, integrated 240
Lunge stretch
   deep side 237, 239
   half side 237

M

Mackenrodt's ligaments 292
Male pelvic floor
   hypertonus dysfunction 153
   rehabilitation focus 259
Manometric visual biofeedback 197
Manual muscle testing 151
   grading 43, 252
Mayo clinic protocol 185, 186
Medical and surgical management 285
Mediolateral incision 76
Menopausal
   changes 116
   issues 29
   vaginal rehabilitation 298

Menopause 23
Menstrual cycle, during 48, 221
Menstruation 201
Metal implants 201
Metronidazole 289
Micturition 6, 6f, 7
Modified oxford grading system 151
Monosymptomatic enuresis 177
Mons pubis 11, 101
Mons veneris 101
Motor learning 197
Move clitoris 193
Movement awareness 188
Movement training 242
Muscle 136, 154
   activation 188
   and tissue atrophy 297
   facilitation 242
   guarding reflexes 5
   identification 188, 242
   incoordination 297
   inner layer 16f
   memory, improves 205
   middle layer 15f
   spasm of 297
   test 150
Myofascial
   release 199, 230
   restrictions 160
Myomectomy 29
Myometrium 7, 8

N

National Institute of Health 85, 164, 179, 185, 186
Nerve
   stimulation 287
   supply 17, 131, 136
Neurogenic inflammation, primary 68
Neuromuscular re-education 270
   indirect 263
Nocturia 82, 157
Nocturnal enuresis 177, 297
Nocturnal frequency 94
Nonablative cosmetic intervention 201
Nonfunctional dysfunction 25, 142
Nonsteroidal anti-inflammatory drugs 288

O

Objective progressions system 208
Obstetric fistula 74, 77
Obstructive pulmonary disease, chronic 164
Obturator internus 16, 17, 30, 68, 136
Oncology 125
Operational design 207
Optional transrectal examination 153
Orchialgia 156
Organ
    bulging of 95
    dysfunction pain intensity 29
    falling out, sense of 87
Orgasm 12f, 36, 38, 146, 281
    disorders 108
    ejaculations 146
    reduced intensity of 166
Orgasmic disorder, female 108, 112
Orgasmic dysfunctions 282
Orgasmic platform 106
Orifices 8
Ovary 8
Overactive bladder 82, 168, 267, 291
    symptoms 69, 297
Ovum 8

P

Pacemaker 201
Pad test 81
Pain 65, 229
    and discomfort 145
    chronic 297
    medications 29
    nature and location of 29
    relief 233
    tightness and discomfort 35
    to perineum 153
    while intercourse 49
Painful stages 111
Pain-hypertonus 34
Pale vulvar tissues 67
Palpable bladder 84
Palpation periurethral muscles 57
Palpation, external 150
Paradoxic puborectalis contractions 229
Paradoxical relaxation 229, 230
    techniques, movement to movement 279
Paraphimosis 156
Paraurethral gland 105
Paraurethral implants 291
Partial bridge stretch, integrated 241
Pediatric pelvic floor 173
    dysfunction 178
    rehabilitation principles 179
Pelvic alignment 30
Pelvic cancer 300
Pelvic diaphragm 14, 15, 133, 135
Pelvic floor 3, 14, 19, 45, 67, 121, 133, 141, 204f, 199, 200, 214
    application of 202
    clinical research of 212
    desire enhancement by 121
    devices 274
    evaluation 28
    exercise, wakened 192f
    exerciser 45, 229
    facilitation 301
    hypertonus dysfunction, rehabilitation for male 243
    laxity 141f
    medical mechanics of 204
    repair 292
    sample protocol of 210
    spasms 112
    strengthening 219
    weakness 86f
Pelvic floor dysfunction 1, 22, 27, 42, 52, 99, 108, 123, 133, 139, 140, 144, 253, 295
    causes of 139
    classification of 24, 141
    combined 24
    common 297
    incoordination 24
    nonfunctional 24
    rehabilitation
        for hypertonus 228
        for hypotonus 250
        for male hypotonus 258
    relation of components to 40
    treatment of 293
        hypertonus 287, 291
        plan for 191f
    types of 23, 140, 140f
Pelvic floor muscle 3, 14, 17f, 14f, 22, 44, 46, 54, 64, 70, 74, 80, 85, 94, 99, 106, 120, 130, 136, 139, 143, 156, 162, 176, 185, 250, 228, 252, 270, 274, 298

and clitoris 104
and orgasm 106
assessment of 27, 57, 143
during coughing, observation of 51
dysfunction 22, 25, 68
   causes of 22
   management of 287
   types of 22, 23
examination, ultrasonic 58*f*
exercise 191, 192, 195*f*
facilitation 262
function of 14, 17, 18*f*, 22, 133, 136, 188
Het's assessment level for 60, 176
hypotonic 110
incoordinated 118, 121
instructions 259
laxity 88
layers 14, 133, 134*f*
location of 73*f*
prevent 137
rehabilitation 213, 259, 269
relaxation ability, testing 50
significance of 113
sphincteric function of 19*f*
strength, testing 46
strengthening 215
tight 229
training protocols 185, 185*b*
transrectal examination of 152
weakness, constipation 65
Pelvic floor rehabilitation 112, 185, 214, 234, 273, 274, 279
   foundation for 188
Pelvic girdle 30
Pelvic inflammatory disease 65, 108, 289
Pelvic joints, damage to 297
Pelvic muscle
   exercises 137, 168
   support 168
Pelvic organ 3, 11*f*, 22
   pathology 23, 108, 139
   prolapse 24, 28, 34, 48, 52, 86, 87*f*, 93, 95, 100, 143, 221, 269, 292
   types of 89
Pelvic pain 28, 52, 92, 133, 143, 156, 229
   chronic 246, 295
   female 297

posture
   chronic 42, 149
   typical 149
prevents 136, 137
rehabilitation 299
severe 52
syndrome 29
   chronic 160
unrelated to intercourse 229
Pelvic plexus 131*f*
Pelvic til*t*, anterior 42, 149
Pelvic trauma 23, 139
Pelvic viscera 135
Pelvis
   female 3
   male 125
   sprain of 297
   strain of 297
Penetration disorders 108
Penile discharge 157
Penile implant 266
Penile pump 266
Penis 130
   base of 153
   captivus 114
   erectile mechanism of 166
   medical anatomy of 129*f*
Perimetrium 7, 8
Perineal body 14, 134
   draws up 51
Perineal membrane 134
Perineal muscle 114*f*
   superficial transverse 14, 134, 150
Perineal pain 156, 160
Perineal tear 74, 76
Perineal trauma 23, 139
Perineum 94, 106
   elevation of 197
   observation 42, 50, 149
Peripheral arterial diseases 201
Peripheral nerve injury 297
Persistent genital arousal disorder 114
Peyronie's disease 156
Phasic enuresis 177
Photoselective vaporization of prostate 294
Physical activities 274
Physical Rehabilitation Programs 85
Physical therapists, benefits for 214
Pigeon stretch, integrated half 238

Piles 65
Piriformis 16, 17, 30, 136, 236
    stretch, integrated 279
Plyometric and coordination training 256
Poor body mechanics 108
Poor posture 23, 108
    health 133, 163, 168
Popping out sensations 87
Portability 207
Positive Thomas test 149
Postdefecation rectal prolapse 94
Posthysterectomy vaginal
    rehabilitation 299
Postpartum
    and postsurgery, six week 52
    period 201
    problems 29
Postpregnancy strengthening 48, 221
Postprostatectomy
    incontinence 170
    protocol 261
    rehabilitation 259
Postural assessment 30
Postural corrections 279
Postural reeducation 192, 229
Posture, assessment of 42
Postvaginal rejuvenation rehabilitation 299
Postvoidal dribbling 84, 141, 163, 267, 293
Prayers stretch, integrated 240
Pregnancy 22, 52, 74
    and deliveries, number of 29
    and labor 75
    and postpartum 48, 221
Premature ejaculation 141, 163, 166, 266, 293, 295
    rehabilitation 301
    treat 137
Prenatal rehabilitation 298
Prepregnancy strengthening 48, 221
Pressure release technique 231
Presurgical patients 48, 221
Priapism 156
Procidentia 92, 93
Proctalgia fugax 65, 156, 160, 288
Progressive resistance training system 206

Prolapse
    causes of 88
    organs, repair of 29
    rehabilitation 299
Proprioceptive neuromuscular
    facilitation 194, 192, 229, 298
Prostate 126
    benign hypertrophy of 168
    cancer 169, 169f, 294
        stages of 170f
    gland 125, 126, 127f, 259
    health, improve 137
    nonbacterial inflammation of 160
    pain 156
    rehabilitation 301
    surgery 163
    transurethral
        incision of 294
        resection of 168, 293
Prostatectomy 139, 170
Prostatic hyperplasia
    benign 159f, 168, 293
    stages of 168
Prostatitis 108, 139, 157, 157f, 158f
    acute 157
    chronic 160, 297
Prostatodynia 156, 160
Psoas 30
Psychological factors 148
Pubic bone 14, 17, 101, 193
Pubocervical ligament 9
Pubococcygeal muscles 243
Pubococcygeus 15, 16, 55
    muscle 16, 77, 135, 150, 153
        normal 234
Puborectalis muscle 16, 69f, 114, 136
Pubovaginal sling operations 292
Pubovaginalis 16
Pubovesical ligament 17
Pudendal arteries 17, 136
Pudendal canal syndrome 156, 157
Pudendal nerve 17, 64, 131, 136, 260, 297
    neuralgia 157
Pudendal neuralgia 64, 287
Pull penis 193
Pulse 211, 280
    trainer 209
Purandare's sling operation 293

Q

Quadratus lumborum 30

R

R Maigne's technique 233, 247, 279
Radical prostatectomy 169
Radiotherapy 116, 169
Rectocele 24, 89, 90, 91f, 292, 297
Rectum 3, 10
   and anus 65
   golf ball in 154, 243
Rectus femoris 236
   stretch 279
Referred pain 108
Reflex incontinence 82
Rehabilitation 183
   external 258
   postnatal 298
   techniques 229
Relax pelvic floor 236f
Relaxation techniques 279
Relaxation time 210
Relaxed healthy muscles 59f
Relaxed muscles 58f
Reproductive system
   female 7f, 11
   male 125f
Retropubic cystourethropexy 291
Retropubic midurethral sling 291
Retropubic prostatectomy 168
Round ligament 17

S

Sacral alignment pubic symphysis 30
Sacroiliac joint 30, 230
   mobilization, external 247
Sacrospinous colpopexy 293
Sacrospinous ligament 9
Sacrotuberous ligament 15
Sample treatment plan 247
Scar 30, 51
   painful 297
School of thoughts 61
Scleroderma 201
Scrotum 127, 128f
Sedentary lifestyle 23
Self test 150
Self vaginal examination 44
Self-care 287
Semen 130
Seminal vesicles 130
Sensation, lack of 94
Sensory deficit 88
Sensory information 197
Sensory urinary incontinence 83
Severe vaginitis 48, 49, 52, 221
   infection 52
Severe vestibulitis 48, 221
   infections 49
Sexual abuse 52, 111
   history of 29, 108
Sexual arousal 35, 38, 99, 145
   disorder 108-110
Sexual aversion disorder 108, 109
Sexual desire 35, 37, 145
   disorder 108, 109
      hypoactive 108, 109
Sexual dysfunction 107, 115
   guidelines for female 281
   history of 52
   rehabilitation
      for female 273
      for hypertonus 276
Sexual fitness, improves 136
Sexual function 229
   male 144
Sexual health 28
   dysfunction rehabilitation, stages of
      female 275t
   rehabilitation guidelines for
      hypotonus 279
Sexual intercourse 159
Sexual interest 108
Sexual overactivity 23
Sexual pain disorder 108, 110
Sexual problems 108
   postsurgical 117
Sexual sensation 24
Sexually transmitted infection 201
Sildenafil 265
Skeletal muscle ring 57f, 153f
Skene's glands 100, 105
Skin condition 51
Smoking 28
   stop 274
Soft tissue
   mobilization 199, 230
   release 233, 244

Sonography
   specialized 42
   visual biofeedback 197
Spasm 64
Spasmodic muscles 111
Spasmodic pelvic floor muscles 141
Spermatic cords 128
Spermatogenesis 127
Sphincter 6
   external 6
   internal 6
   urethera 15
Spinal cord
   injury 84
   trauma 68
Spinal range of motion, reduced 42, 149
Steroid use 23
Stimulate clitoris 120
Stimulates nerve endings 205
Stress 82, 176
   control 274
   female 297
   incontinence 48, 94, 220
   male 297
   test 81
   urinary incontinence 25, 80, 117, 167, 167f, 194, 267, 270
Stretching 192, 229
Suprapubic tenderness 84
Sweet-spot 231
   principle 230

T

Tactile biofeedback 207
Tadalafil 265
Teach pelvic floor muscle
   control 190
   exercise 193
Tear
   first-degree 76
   fourth-degree 76
   second-degree 76
   third-degree 76
Teflon 291
Temperature sensor safety 211
Tension myalgia 64, 160, 288
Tensor fascia lata 236
   stretch, integrated 279

Testicles 128
Testimonials 217
Thiele's massage 247
Thiele's release 279
Thiele's technique 230, 232
Thomas test positive 42
Thoracic spine 30
Thrombophlebitis 201
Thrombosis 201
Tobacco, use of 23
Tonic vibrathine reflex 262
Tonic vibration reflex 205, 206f, 254
Total knee replacement 259
Train intimate muscles 45
Training protocols 209
Transcutaneous electrical nerve stimulation 198, 230, 233
Transrectal assessment 233, 246, 247
Transrectal examination 153f
Transrectal manual therapy 246
Transrectal pelvic floor examination 57
Transurethral microwave thermotherapy 294
Transurethral needle ablation 294
Transvaginal examination 52
Transvaginal pelvic floor
   examination 42, 44
   muscle 54f
   exam 52, 54
Transverse cervical ligament 17
Trauma 163
Trigger point release 199, 279
   techniques 243
Trigger point symptoms 153
Tuberculosis 201
Tumor 82
   necrosis factor-alpha 290

U

Ulcerative colitis 69
   surgery for 290
Ultrasound, treatment 279
Upper urinary tract 3
Ureter 3, 125
Urethra 3, 5, 5f, 14, 125, 126
   compressor 15, 169f
   kinking of 80f
   nonbacterial inflammation of 160
   obstructed 158f

Urethral diverticulum 83
Urethral meatus 11
Urethral opening 102
Urethral pain 153
Urethral sphincter
   external 15, 135
   internal 170
Urethral stricture 84
Urethral syndrome 68, 290
Urethritis 82
Urethrovesical junction 57
Urge incontinence 48, 81, 94, 220, 229, 291
Urge urinary incontinence 82
Urgency-frequency syndrome 68
Urinary bladder, female 5f
Urinary continence 175
Urinary frequency 157, 297
Urinary health 22
   improve 137
Urinary incontinence 78, 79, 79f, 81, 82, 100, 117, 133, 143, 144, 163, 291
   mixed 83
   pathophysiology of 79
   rehabilitation principles for 267
   statistics for 84
   types of 79, 82
Urinary leakage 27
Urinary prolapse 297
Urinary symptoms 28
Urinary system 4f, 125, 126f
Urinary tract 3
   infection 82, 108, 177
Urination
   frequent 64, 89
   painful 157
Urine
   flow
      interrupted 84
      stop 193
   leakage 84
   stopping flow of 193
   stream
      difficulty starting 69
      reduced 84
Urogenital anatomy, male 129f
Urogenital and anal triangle 14, 133, 134
Urogenital diaphragm 14, 15, 133, 135
Urogenital system 101f
Uterine cavity 9f
Uterine ligaments 9
Uterine prolapse 89, 92, 92f, 292
   stages of 92, 93f
Uterosacral ligament 9, 17, 92
Uterus 3, 7, 17, 100, 102
   ligaments of 10f
   to sacrum posteriorly 17

V

Vagina 14, 45, 100, 105
   and bladder 77
   and rectum 77
   dilate 230
      device 49f
   fit 221
      device 46f
      use of 222
   gapping in 78
   looseness of 78
   splinting of 94
Vaginal bulge 87
Vaginal canal 3, 105
Vaginal delivery 74, 75
Vaginal dilators 198, 234
Vaginal estrogen 116
Vaginal heaviness 93
Vaginal hysterectomy 292
Vaginal introitus 105
Vaginal laxity 34, 48, 52, 72, 73, 77, 78, 84, 116, 143, 221, 269, 291
   consequences of 78
   dysfunction 24
Vaginal looseness 84, 95, 214
Vaginal lubrication 115, 116, 300
Vaginal muscles 45, 214
Vaginal opening 102, 105
   lump at 93
   system 234
Vaginal orifice 11, 102
Vaginal pain 89, 90, 92
Vaginal pelvic floor muscle
   examination 53
Vaginal penetration of penis 89
Vaginal pressure 91
   increased 87
Vaginal recovery 200

Vaginal spasm 64, 115
    dysfunction 24
Vaginal tightening rehabilitation 298
Vaginal vault prolapse 89, 93, 94f, 293
Vaginal vulva 12f
Vaginismus 49, 108, 111, 221, 229, 281, 297
Valsalva maneuver 54, 190, 197, 213
Vardenafil 265
Vas deferens 128
Vascular disease 201
Vascular surgery 266
Vestibular bulbs 105
Vestibule 11, 102
Vestibulitis 297
Viagra 265
Vicious cycle 70
Viral infections 201
Visceral dysfunction 24, 25, 142
Visceral manipulation 199, 230
Visceral pelvic floor dysfunction 24
Visual biofeedback 197
Visual cues 224
Visual input 207
Voice guided 207
Voiding 125
Vomiting 28
Vulva 11
    inspection of 51f
Vulvar ultrasound 198, 230, 233
Vulvar vestibulitis 67, 289
Vulvodynia 67, 289, 297

W

Warm compression 233
Warrier stretch, integrated 239, 240
Warts 29
Weak muscles bands 55
Weak pelvic floor 250
    muscles 87f
Weak prostate health 163
Weight gain 23
Wise-Anderson and Thiele technique 199, 230
Wise-Anderson pressure principle 231
Wise-Anderson protocol 230
Wise-Anderson sweet-spot release 279
Wise-Anderson technique 231
Woman's sex health 273
World Health Organization 107
WOW vagina-dilate 48, 235f, 279
    treatment 222
WOW vagina-fit 45, 218
WOW woman 214, 215, 217, 279
    placement of 216f

Y

Yoga, integrated 279

EU GSPR Authorised Reprsentative
Logos Europe, 9 rue Nicolas Poussin
1700, La Rochelle, France
Phone: +33 (0) 6 67 93 73 78
E-mail: contact@logoseurope.eu

www.ingramcontent.com/pod-product-compliance
Ingram Content Group UK Ltd.
Pitfield, Milton Keynes, MK11 3LW, UK
UKHW050428150426
5217IPUK00019B/1283